Coronary Heart Disease Prevention

FUNDAMENTAL AND CLINICAL CARDIOLOGY

Editor-in-Chief

Samuel Z. Goldhaber, M.D.

*Harvard Medical School
and Brigham and Women's Hospital
Boston, Massachusetts*

Associate Editor, Europe

Henri Bounameaux, M.D.

*University Hospital of Geneva
Geneva, Switzerland*

Additional Volumes in Preparation

Coronary Heart Disease Prevention

edited by

Frank G. Yanowitz

The Fitness Institute, LDS Hospital
and University of Utah School of Medicine
Salt Lake City, Utah

Marcel Dekker, Inc.   **New York • Basel • Hong Kong**

Library of Congress Cataloging-in-Publication Data

Coronary heart disease prevention / edited by Frank G. Yanowitz.
      p.   cm.
    Includes bibliographical references and index.
    ISBN 0-8247-8713-7 (alk. paper)
    1. Coronary heart disease--Prevention.   I. Yanowitz, Frank G.
    [DNLM: 1. Coronary Disease--prevention & control.   W1 FU538TD v.9
/ WG 300 P94542]
    RC685.C6P666   1992
    616.1'2305--dc20
    DNLM/DLC
    for Library of Congress   92-22168
                                           CIP

This book is printed on acid-free paper.

Marcel Dekker, Inc.
270 Madison Avenue, New York, New York 10016

Current printing (lst digit):
10 9 8 7 6 5 4 3 2 1

PRINTED IN THE UNITED STATES OF AMERICA

Series Introduction

Marcel Dekker, Inc. has focused on the development of various series of beautifully produced books in different branches of medicine. These series have
facilitated the integration of rapidly advancing information for both the clinical
specialist and the researcher.

My goal as editor of the Fundamental and Clinical Cardiology series is to
assemble the talents of world-renowned authorities to discuss virtually every area
of cardiovascular medicine. In the current monograph, Coronary Heart Disease
Prevention, Dr. Yanowitz has edited a much needed and timely book. Future
contributions to this series will include books on molecular biology, interventional
cardiology, and clinical management of such problems as coronary artery disease
and ventricular arrhythmias.

SAMUEL Z. GOLDHABER

Preface

I often tell this shaggy-dog story to medical students and house officers taking an elective in preventive cardiology:

It was graduation day at Harvard Medical School. Michael, the top student in his graduating class, was walking along the Charles River with a wise old professor of medicine. They were reminiscing about medical education and about Michael's many scholarly achievements during his 4 years at Harvard. In addition to gaining valuable experience in a research laboratory investigating mechanisms of atherosclerosis, Michael had encountered many patients on the medical wards with interesting and complex disease problems. His enthusiasm for an academic career in internal medicine had never been greater as he eagerly awaited his upcoming residency.

Suddenly, a loud cry was heard from the river: a man appeared to be drowning. Michael, an excellent swimmer, kicked off his shoes and dove into the river. Swimming fast, he arrived just as the the man disappeared under water. Michael dove, grabbed onto his shirt collar, and was able to swim back to shore with the victim's head held above water. On shore, the man was unconscious and not breathing. Michael immediately began closed-chest cardiac massage and mouth-to-mouth resuscitation, and within several minutes the victim regained consciousness. As an ambulance arrived, Michael was congratulated by the professor for a job well done. He was overwhelmed by a deep sense of personal satisfaction. He had saved a life! Wasn't this the epitome of his 4 years of medical school education?

They continued to walk. Although wet and somewhat fatigued, Michael was proud of himself for having the necessary skills and medical expertise to help others in need. He looked forward to his emerging career in medicine where he would have many opportunities to help the sick and injured. He also hoped to continue his research investigations into the basic mechanisms of disease.

Only several minutes later another cry for help came from the river. Unbelievable! Someone else appeared to be drowning. Without wasting a second, Michael dove into the river and once again rescued the drowning victim. Cardio-pulmonary resuscitation was successfully carried out on shore, and the second victim was transported to the hospital by ambulance. Michael was exhausted, but obviously thrilled by these two acts of emergency rescue and treatment.

More walking, more talking and, believe it or not, more people drowning in the river. Finally, after the sixth or seventh successful rescue, now thoroughly exhausted and very frustrated, Michael looked up at the professor. "What am I to do?" he pleaded, "I can't keep this up any more!" The professor thought for a moment before answering: "Why don't you walk upstream and stop whoever is pushing those unfortunate people off the bridge?"

As a physician, most of my medical education, like Michael's, focused on the diagnosis and treatment of disease. The emphasis was on saving or improving the lives of patients suffering from complex diseases or serious injuries. Today, we are awed by the technological advances of the late 20th century that enable hospitals and clinics to offer our patients an increasing array of sophisticated diagnostic and therapeutic services. The downside of these modern technologies, however, is the unrelenting upward spiraling of medical costs. Nevertheless, the continued influx of the sick and injured into the medical care system seems to justify giving most of our attention to those who are suffering, just as Michael gave all of his attention to the drowning victims.

A careful analysis of today's major causes of death and disability reveals that cardiovascular disease, cancer, and accidents head the list. Of necessity, our medical attention is primarily directed toward studying the *processes* of these serious problems in order to establish accurate diagnoses and determine the best treatments. But what about their *origins*? Wouldn't it be better if we could determine the origins of today's leading causes of death and disability before they become established and serious medical problems? This is not just wishful thinking. The scientific evidence is now overwhelming in support of the concept that these leading causes are largely due to self-destructive behaviors and adverse environmental influences that are potentially reversible and under our control.

It is not very surprising that the general public and many of our patients seem more interested in preventive health behaviors than the medical community does.

This is partly because we, as physicians, are too busy putting out fires to worry about the origins of these fires. It is time to face the reality of a growing crisis in 20th century medicine. Costs are astronomical, and large segments of our population are receiving inadequate or no medical care. The general public is demanding a greater role in their own health care, and they are asking for more information about disease prevention. Today's primary-care physicians are in an excellent position to promote accurate and effective programs designed to prevent the onset or slow the progression of today's chronic diseases.

This book presents practical strategies and guidelines for the prevention of coronary heart disease (CHD), our country's leading cause of death and disability. Although the focus is on heart disease prevention, many of the recommendations are also applicable to preventing several forms of cancer, respiratory disease, and other afflictions of civilization. This book is written for physicians and health care providers who are on the front lines of our medical care system, and who therefore have the greatest opportunity to serve the public in their health care needs. The chapters are organized to provide the reader with the scientific rationale for the various therapeutic strategies known to be effective in CHD prevention, as well as the nuts and bolts of delivering those preventive services.

The reader is also encouraged to consider seriously the limitations of modern medicine's successful biomedical model, which focuses primarily on mechanistic aspects of diseases such as CHD. An alternative and more encompassing medical model is offered that defines the patient, the disease, and the range of therapeutic interventions in a broader framework; the model includes societal, environmental, and psychological aspects of health and disease in addition to the more traditional biological factors. It is argued that bringing preventive medicine services into the mainstream of the medical care system will require us to expand our notions of scientific medicine to incorporate these nonbiological systems into our patient care and research activities. Let us all stop whoever is pushing those unfortunate people off the bridge.

FRANK G. YANOWITZ

Contents

Contributors

Ted D. Adams, Ph.D. The Fitness Institute, Division of Cardiology, LDS Hospital, and Department of Physical Education, University of Utah, Salt Lake City, Utah

Nemat O. Borhani, M.D., M.P.H., F.A.C.C. Department of Community and Family Medicine, University of Nevada School of Medicine, Reno, Nevada, Professor Emeritus, University of California School of Medicine, Davis, California, and Adjunct Professor, University of Tennessee, Memphis, Tennessee

Timothy G. Butler, M.S. Office of Health Promotion and Preventive Medicine Services, Intermountain Health Care Health Plans, Inc., Salt Lake City, Utah

Gerald A. Charlton, M.D. Department of Medicine, LDS Hospital, Salt Lake City, Utah

Chad E. Edgington, M.A. The Fitness Institute, Division of Cardiology, LDS Hospital, Salt Lake City, Utah

Paul S. Fardy, Ph.D. Department of Health and Physical Education, Queens College, Flushing, New York

Frances M. Gough, M.D.   Department of Medicine, University of Utah School of Medicine, Salt Lake City, Utah

Terryl Hartman, M.S., R.D.   Department of Human Development and Nutrition, School of Public Health, University of Minnesota, Minneapolis, Minnesota

John H. Holbrook, M.D.   Department of Internal Medicine, University of Utah School of Medicine, Salt Lake City, Utah

Paul N. Hopkins, M.D., MS.Ph.   Cardiology Division, Department of Internal Medicine, University of Utah School of Medicine, Salt Lake City, Utah

Arthur S. Leon, M.D., M.S.   Division of Kinesiology and Leisure Studies, College of Education and Division of Epidemiology, School of Public Health, University of Minnesota, Minneapolis, Minnesota

Herbert D. Ruttenberg, M.D.   Department of Pediatrics (Cardiology), University of Utah School of Medicine, Salt Lake City, Utah

Timothy W. Smith, Ph.D.   Department of Psychology, University of Utah, Salt Lake City, Utah

Paula G. Williams, M.S.   Department of Psychology, University of Utah, Salt Lake City, Utah

Roger R. Williams, M.D.   Department of Internal Medicine, Cardiovascular Genetics Research Clinic, University of Utah School of Medicine, Salt Lake City, Utah

Frank G. Yanowitz, M.D.   The Fitness Institute, Division of Cardiology, LDS Hospital, and Department of Internal Medicine, University of Utah School of Medicine, Salt Lake City, Utah

Coronary Heart Disease Prevention

1

Prologue: The First Medical Revolution and the Crisis in 20th Century Medicine

FRANK G. YANOWITZ
The Fitness Institute
LDS Hospital
and University of Utah School of Medicine
Salt Lake City, Utah

I. INTRODUCTION

As the 20th century draws to a close, a number of major strategies for the prevention of coronary heart disease (CHD) and its complications have been identified. Numerous clinical guidelines and recommendations have been published to assist practicing physicians in their efforts to prevent CHD. Much of this book discusses the implementation of these strategies including diet, weight control, exercise, smoking cessation, stress management, and the treatment of hypertension and hyperlipidemia. In spite of these widely published recommendations, however, there is reason to believe that a large majority of practicing physicians are not providing comprehensive services for the prevention of CHD (1–3).

Many reasons might be offered for the reluctance of physicians to provide preventive cardiology services (3–6). The primary emphasis of medical education has been the diagnosis and treatment of disease; disease prevention and health promotion, unfortunately, have always been given a lower priority among the subjects studied during physicians' medical training and in subsequent professional activities. Accordingly, many physicians feel that disease prevention lies outside of their usual professional activities and, as a result, they have very little commitment to preventive medicine. The promotion of preventive health behaviors is also very time-consuming and generally without adequate remuneration.

1

Finally, physicians frequently lack confidence in their ability to change patients' habits, and many patients appear to ignore their advice when time is taken to teach preventive strategies.

Beneath the surface of these obvious obstacles lies a more basic and perhaps more significant problem. The eventual restructuring of physician practices to include comprehensive preventive services may require a reconsideration of the fundamental scientific model or paradigm from which the clinical practice of medicine is derived. There is now considerable opinion that this model, the biomedical model, which views the patient, the disease, and its treatment in purely mechanistic terms, is no longer adequate for solving today's chronic disease burden (6–10). This model is extraordinarily successful in elucidating the biological mechanisms of the body in health and disease as well as providing the scientific rationale for many of today's complex diagnostic methods and therapies. However, the biomedical model may be unduly restrictive by failing to consider extrasomatic variables (psychological, social, cultural, and ecological) as important factors influencing the origins, progression, and treatment of disease.

As important as scientific models are for providing a solid foundation from which to structure our clinical activities, they are rarely the focus of our attention. Any discussion, therefore, of the relevance of one or another paradigm to clinical practice is likely to be met with some confusion by the general reader. There is a tendency for those practicing a particular scientific discipline such as medicine to take for granted or rarely consider the underlying presuppositions that form the basis for a world view (i.e., an understanding of reality) to which the scientist or practitioner is philosophically committed. Yet, throughout the history of science major and minor scientific revolutions have drastically changed our concepts of reality and, in turn, our subsequent scientific practices. According to Thomas Kuhn, in his seminal work, *The Structure of Scientific Revolutions* (11), these so-called "paradigm shifts" occur when the accumulated scientific evidence in a particular discipline is no longer consistent with the prevailing world view, and new theories must be conceptualized or invoked to explain the apparent anomalies. Acceptance of these new theories requires that scientists view the domain of their research engagement, and sometimes even the world they live in, differently.

In the field of medicine, especially as it applies to today's chronic diseases (cancer, cardiovascular disease, and other "afflictions of civilization") a substantial body of evidence suggests that the prevailing medical paradigm, the biomedical model, is outdated and that a new and more encompassing scientific model is needed to provide the theoretical and conceptual framework for solving today's medical problems (6–10). One such successor medical model founded on the 20th century "postmodern" sciences has recently been proposed by Foss and Rothenberg in their book, *The Second Medical Revolution: From Biomedicine to Infomedicine* (8). The proposed scientific model for medicine, while incorporating all of the previous successes of biomedicine, reconceptualizes our notions of disease, patient, health, and therapy with profound implications for primary care and preventive medicine. Because of the importance of these ideas to the implementation of preventive cardiology services, this introductory chapter will explore the basis of this proposed paradigm shift in medicine. To appreciate the revolutionary impact of any successor medical model, however, a brief review of the origins of medicine's first revolution, the biomedical model, is instructive.

II. A BRIEF HISTORY LESSON

Hundreds of years before the Scientific Revolution in the 17th century, Hippocrates, the father of western medicine, described health as "a state of equilibrium among the various internal factors which govern the operations of the body and the mind; the equilibrium in turn is reached only when man lives in harmony with his external environment" (12). This very holistic concept that equates health as a function of mind–body/nature equilibrium and, by implication, disease as a function of mind–body/nature disequilibrium, was shattered by the intellectual upheaval of the 17th century, leading to the birth of the Scientific Revolution and the subsequent Age of Enlightenment that lasted over 300 years. Although many contributed to the revolutionary ideas influencing scientific thought up to the 20th century, two stand out as having a profound impact on the subsequent emergence in the 19th century of scientific medicine and the biomedical model: René Descartes and Isaac Newton (8,13).

Descartes, regarded by some as the founder of modern philosophy, was troubled by the scientist's need to remain unbiased and free of prejudice when studying nature. His concept of scientific objectivity coupled with his mechanistic view of the "outside" world demanded that the rational behavior of the scientist (i.e., thoughts and ideas) be excluded from the natural phenomena being studied. Accordingly, he proposed two separate and independent divisions of reality; mind and matter (or body). He suggested that science be concerned only with issues relating to the material universe; issues relating to the mind were relegated to theologians and philosophers and later became the basis for the humanities. The resulting major implication for medicine of this mind–body dualism was the separation of the sick body, the primary focus of our medical attention, from mental phenomena and all other nonbiological influences (8).

Descartes' great hope was to be able to reduce all of nature to exact mathematical relationships. His most important contribution to scientific thought was the analytic method of reasoning, now called the Cartesian method or reductionism. This idea, that all complex physical phenomena can only be understood by reducing them to their component parts, has guided scientific endeavors and theories of natural phenomena until the 20th century, and continues to be the dominant medical paradigm today. The human body was viewed in Descartes' time as a machine, a complex clockwork described entirely in mechanistic terms.

William Harvey, a contemporary of Descartes, used this mechanistic approach in his detailed description of the heart and circulation, an achievement enthusiastically praised by Descartes himself. In today's scientific medical environment this concept has as its ultimate goal the explanation of all living phenomena in the language of molecular biology: physics and chemistry (6). Although enormously successful in explaining the biological mechanisms of health and disease, the Cartesian method fails to consider the one aspect that separates us from all other biological organisms: our humanness.

Although Descartes provided the conceptual framework for the mechanistic world view, Isaac Newton completed the Scientific Revolution in the 17th century by formulating a detailed mathematical description of nature in his "laws of motion" (8,13). Newton's widely acclaimed experimental method included elements of both the empirical, inductive method of investigation and the rational, deductive method of mathematical analysis; it became the dominant methodology upon which all the natural sciences since then have been based. In Newton's conceptualization of reality, all physical phenomena could be reduced, in principle, to the motion of elementary particles or atoms under the influence of gravity and governed by the mathematical laws of motion. Furthermore, these laws were independent of time and completely deterministic. That is, given the initial state of a physical system and the forces acting on it, one could not only predict (in theory) what would happen in the future but also could go back in time and explain whatever happened in the past. In medicine the idea that biological events have determinate, physicochemical explanations is a direct consequence of the Newtonian world view and a fundamental characteristic of the biomedical model.

A consequence of Newtonian mechanics and the Cartesian division between mind and matter was the belief that all of nature, including the human body, could be described objectively and understood by an independent scientific observer (8). This meant that scientists could remain separate from the subjects of their investigations. The objective description of reality became the ideal standard for all the physical sciences and strongly influenced medicine's first revolution, which occurred in the latter half of the 19th century.

The shift from the subjective doctor–patient dialogue to the study of objective patient data was a direct result of advances being made in the basic medical sciences: pathology, physiology, pharmacology, microbiology, and others. These scientific discoveries were the driving force behind the technologic developments that enabled medical scientists in the 20th century to probe more objectively into the workings of biological organisms, including the human body.

Newer technologic innovations led to an impressive array of diagnostic tools to provide the physician with more quantifiable measures of pathophysiological events (8). In particular, the physician's task evolved from a reliance solely on bedside observations (history and physical examination) to the use of increasingly more accurate instruments to study the sick patient and translate various pathophysiological processes into machine language. An unfortunate side effect of these technological advances, however, was an increase in both the physical and emotional distance between physician and patient, with a corresponding loss of the humanistic skills so characteristic of physicians in the past. The advances in biotechnology encouraged the medical scientist to adopt a particular strategy that viewed the patient, the disease, the diagnostic methods, and the treatment in purely mechanistic terms. So successful was this strategy in furthering our knowledge of disease and its treatment that it became the dominant modus operandi of Western medicine. Before discussing the limitations of this approach, however, a more formal description of the biomedical model is presented.

III. THE BIOMEDICAL MODEL

As discussed previously, advances in the physical sciences during the 17th to 19th centuries were primarily responsible for the adoption of a mechanistic approach to the science of medicine. The first notable achievement of scientific medicine was the elaboration of the "germ theory of disease" (the recognition that certain organic entities such as the tubercle bacillus caused specific diseases such as tuberculosis, and that these diseases could be prevented or treated with specific vaccines or drugs). The enormous success of these early advances in medical science set the precedent for a mechanistic medical paradigm that formed the basis for the biomedical model and defined the boundaries within which Western physicians have practiced ever since (8).

In the biomedical paradigm the practice of medicine is firmly founded on a double-tiered body of knowledge. At the lower level are the basic sciences (physics, chemistry, mathematics, and molecular biology), which are among the premedical courses of study during our undergraduate years. These "hard" sciences serve to underwrite the principles of the applied medical sciences (anatomy, pathophysiology, pharmacology, and others), which are concerned primarily with the structure and function of the body, and disease processes. Together these two tiers of knowledge define the legitimate problems of biomedicine and shape the diagnostic and therapeutic strategies that characterize the clinical practice of medicine (8). All physicians should recognize the role played by the basic and applied medical sciences in their medical education.

Underlying these sciences, however, lies still another tier: one that is rarely considered by medical researchers and practitioners but is nevertheless a necessary conceptual component of a legitimate scientific model. At this most fundamental level, called "tier 1" by Foss and Rothenberg (8), are the philosophical ideas and commitments that define how medical scientists and clinicians approach their world or subjects of inquiry. In the biomedical model, as previously discussed, these methodologic directives (reductionism, dualism, determinism, linear cause and effect, and objectivity) originated during the 17th century scientific revolution with the mechanistic world view of Descartes, Newton, and their successors. They were the guiding principles that powerfully influenced the direction of scientific research over the next 300 years. Successes in the physical sciences and the growth of scientific knowledge served to reinforce confidence in these directives, which have now become so ingrained in our standardized system that they are taken for granted and risk becoming dogma.

Figure 1 illustrates the three-tiered scientific model for medicine that defines the biomedical paradigm (8). Tier 1 includes the conceptual strategies used by scientists to understand better the real world and to conduct scientific investigations. These natural science directives, largely derived from classic physics, involve several assumptions previously discussed. The first is that all natural systems (physical, biological, psychological) can be understood by reducing them to their constituent elements. Implied in this assumption is the concept that all biological phenomena (i.e., all aspects of living organisms) can be explained by the principles of molecular biology. The second assumption is that events occurring in the physical world that are subject to scientific investigation have determinate explanations that obey natural laws and can be expressed in a unified physicalist language. Finally these directives presuppose an external permanency of the physical world that is separate from the scientist's thoughts and ideas. In particular, dualism implies that the sick body, the focus of biomedicine, is

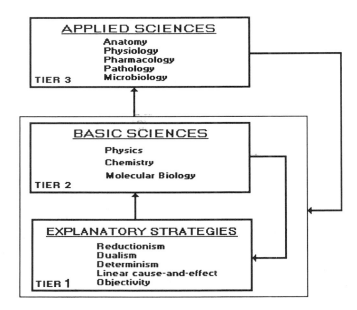

Figure 1   The biomedical model. (Adapted from Ref. 8.)

unaffected by any mental, social or cultural influences; that is, the thoughts of the patient, the physician, and significant others have no material impact on the course of physical events that determine states of health and disease (8).

Tier 2 consists of the basic physical and biophysical sciences that rely entirely on the assumptions and directives expressed at the tier 1 level. The remarkable discoveries in the physical sciences over the past 300 years have reinforced the validity of these directives, which in turn serve to define the scope of legitimate scientific problems. They also defined the permissible kinds of data obtained from research investigations, and what constitutes scientifically valid solutions to these problems.

The applied medical sciences represented in tier 3 have evolved directly from the scientific achievements in tier 2 and also depend upon the explanatory strategies and assumptions in tier 1. In turn, successes in the medical sciences reinforce the logic of method in tier 1 and the basic sciences from which they are derived. These three levels, therefore, provide the medical scientist with an integrated framework from which to approach questions of scientific interest. It is important to emphasize here that the range of legitimate scientific questions is dependent on the model used. This implies, for example, that questions relating to the possible health or disease implications of mind (thought)–body interactions would first have to be "rephrased" in the language of neurochemical processes and translated into the concomitant brain (physical)–body event, which could then be analyzed and explained in mechanistic terms (8).

On the basis of this three-tiered biomedical model, four important concepts that have characterized the practice of medicine for almost 200 years can be defined: the patient, the disease, the diagnostic process, and the treatment (8).

The patient is a complex biological machine best analyzed in terms of its parts: organ systems, tissues, cells, and subcellular components. These component parts are, in turn, described in the language of anatomy, physiology, biochemistry, and ultimately, molecular biology.

Disease is considered to represent a breakdown or malfunction in one or more of the body's component parts, usually resulting from an excess or deficiency of critical substances or from an intrinsically harmful physical agent.

The biomedical approach to detecting disease is analytic: a disease is diagnosed by studying organ systems, tissues, cells, and subcellular components, in a search for abnormalities in measurable biological parameters.

The therapeutic process is conceptualized as a physical intervention to correct the breakdown or malfunction of biological mechanisms using chemical, electrical, or mechanical treatments.

The mutual interrelationships of these four concepts are illustrated in Figure 2 (8). Diagnostic and therapeutic strategies are directly influenced by the mechanistic view of the patient as a biological organism and disease as a phenomenon confined to the body. It is no wonder that the outstanding scientific and technologic

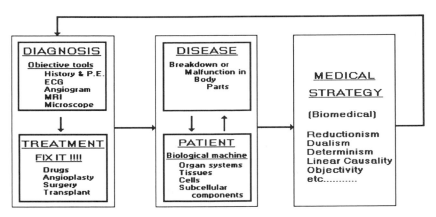

Figure 2 The loop-structured interaction between tier 1 strategies and the biomedical model's concepts of patient disease, diagnosis, and treatment. (Adapted from Ref. 8.)

achievements of 20th century biomedicine continue to reinforce the biomedical model as the only legitimate scientific model for medicine. As stated by Foss and Rothenberg (8, p. 43) and analogous to a self-fulfilling prophesy (Fig. 2):

> . . . we come full circle to the mutuality of philosophy, methodology, and clinical practice. Espousal of a philosophical framework shapes the direction of medical research and comes to define norms of success. Success in practice reinforces belief in the framework, assuring further application of the techniques used for carrying out the practice.

IV. THE CRISIS IN 20TH CENTURY MEDICINE

In spite of the impressive technologic successes of biomedicine, all is not well as the 20th century draws to a close. The costs of medical care in the United States are staggering and each year consume an increasing percentage of the gross national product. Because cardiovascular disease, and in particular coronary heart disease, continues to be the leading cause of death and disability in the Western world, the largest portion of medical expenditures goes towards the management of this major health problem. In 1991, for example, as reported by the American Heart Association, the estimated cost for treating cardiovascular diseases was over $100 billion (14).

Although many factors contribute to the total expenditures for heart disease in this country, there is no doubt that "high-tech" management of advanced, end-stage CHD is very expensive. This is exemplified by the recent emergence of "interventional cardiologists" with expertise in the mechanical alteration or removal of atherosclerotic plaque in the coronary and other arteries. A leading article in the *Journal of the American College of Cardiology* (April 1989) illustrates this trend by its title: "Crackers, Breakers, Stretchers, Drillers, Scrapers, Shavers, Burners, Welders and Melters—The Future Treatment of Atherosclerotic Coronary Artery Disease?" (15). There is no question that these new technologies, along with coronary artery bypass surgery, cardiac transplantation, and perhaps even use of the artificial heart, will have an important place in the treatment of advanced CHD. These high-cost procedures, however, represent the natural consequences of a mechanistic biomedical world view. Clearly this is not a very cost-effective approach to conquering our country's leading cause of death and disability. Also, it is unlikely that the trend in interventional cardiology can continue unabated, due to the increasing fiscal restraints being placed on the medical profession by government, industry, and insurance providers.

In addition to medicine's growing economic crisis, there is evidence of increasing public dissatisfaction with the medical profession's engineering approach to health and disease. Doctor–patient relationships are being eroded by technologic innovations that, although able to translate anatomical and pathophysiological findings into machine language, increasingly remove the physician from the bedside of the sick patient (7). As a result, physicians often perceive less need to deal with patients as people or to become personally involved in their illnesses. The growing reliance on objective, machine-language data has shifted physician attention from the patient as a sick person to the patient as a biological organism with a disease defined in purely somatic terms. This is also reflected by the career choices of today's medical students. Many are moving away from primary care practices toward more technically oriented specialties, reinforced by the biomedical emphasis of their educational experiences as well as by financial and lifestyle considerations (6,16).

At the same time that physicians are giving more of their attention to new technologies, an educated public is demanding a greater role in matters relating to their health and medical care (17). The biomedical model is perceived by many patients as too narrowly focused on biological information and inadequate to deal with many legitimate nonbiological aspects of health and disease. Dissatisfaction with the medical profession's commitment to high-cost technologies at the expense of more humanistic doctor–patient interactions has become a major factor in the current avalanche of malpractice litigations.

From this perspective it can be argued that medicine's current crisis is partly the result of a philosophical commitment to an unduly restrictive scientific model that views the sick patient, the disease, the diagnostic process, and the treatment in purely somatic or biological terms. No one doubts the importance of extrasomatic influences (psychological, social, ecologic, etc.) on the course of health and disease but, because these factors lie outside the boundaries defined by the biomedical model, they are rarely given the same careful attention as the more accepted biologic components. In fact, these nonbiological factors are generally relegated to the category of the "art of medicine" and investigating these factors often plays only a secondary role in the overall responsibilities of physicians.

Faced with the problems of today's chronic disease burden there is growing dissatisfaction from both inside and outside the medical community regarding biomedicine's limited focus. It is not surprising, therefore, that a number of countermovements have become established within the medical profession to focus attention on the extrasomatic (i.e., psychosocial) variables influencing health and disease (8). Of particular relevance to the prevention of CHD has been the holistic medicine movement, which emphasizes preventive health behaviors and encourages self-responsibility for the maintenance of good health (18). In addition, holistic health practitioners are convinced that mental processes such as attitudes and emotions can have a significant impact on the course of health and disease.

The emphasis of holistic medicine on preventive strategies (diet, exercise, stress management, and environmental safeguards) seems, at first glance, to complement the more traditional biomedical strategies already in place in today's medical establishment. The holistic approach fills a much needed gap by including those aspects of medical practice that are traditionally excluded by biomedicine. Most primary care physicians seem to accept these additional holistic strategies as legitimate and important adjuncts to their more traditional clinical activities, although, because of time and financial constraints, they rarely have more than a limited impact on patient care. Of greater concern, however, is the realization that the combined biomedical–holistic approach has serious conceptual problems that may potentially impede research and the delivery of comprehensive preventive services (8).

The problem with combining biomedical (curative) with holistic (preventive) strategies is that only the former are compatible with the prevailing biomedical paradigm and, therefore, "scientifically" based (8). The idea that social, psychological, or behavioral factors might serve as important determinants of diseases such as CHD violates fundamental tier 1 presuppositions of the biomedical model (reductionism, dualism, etc.). These extrasomatic factors have no physical basis and, although they may have physical consequences, they cannot themselves be reduced to physicochemical terms. They also cannot be placed within the biomedical model's definition of patient, disease process, or treatment. As a result, any application of holistic strategies to medical practice must be justified entirely on empirical observations that these strategies do, in fact, work. Moreover, since these strategies fall outside of biomedicine's scientific boundaries, it is unlikely that they will ever become fully integrated into the mainstream of medical education or clinical practice.

This presents an interesting dilemma to advocates of preventive medicine education (6). As will be seen in later chapters, an abundance of empirical data already supports various preventive strategies for lowering the risk of chronic diseases such as CHD, cancer, respiratory diseases, and other "afflictions of civilization." To a large extent these strategies fall outside the narrow confines of biomedicine since they involve interactions between the patient and the environment that are predominantly behavioral. At the same time, however, biomedicine, and especially cardiology, is becoming increasingly focused on molecular biology as its basic scientific discipline, essentially excluding the wealth of data from the social and behavioral sciences that emphasize prevention (19). Furthermore, the predominant biomedical orientation of medical education is attracting students interested primarily in mechanistic issues: molecular genetics, magnetic resonance imaging, cardiac transplantation, and others. It is no wonder that there is so much pessimism about incorporating prevention into the mainstream of medicine practice (6).

There may, however, be a way out of this dilemma. What is needed is a revised theory or medical model that puts the existing data on disease prevention into a legitimate scientific context. This would permit the discovery of new and unexpected findings, which, although incompatible with the present biomedical model, would be logically consistent with the premises of the revised theory. In fact, the articulation of such a revision based on the 20th century "postmodern" sciences is already underway and is seriously challenging the dominant paradigm in medicine, the biomedical model (7,8,13). To challenge the biomedical model effectively, however, any successor theory must offer an alternative, but internally consistent three-tiered structure, analogous to the three-tiered biomedical model. In the following section the initial contours of such a structure are described.

V. THE 20TH CENTURY SCIENTIFIC PARADIGM

While medicine continues to operate under the restricted biomedical framework, scientific advances during the 20th century have resulted in the emergence of new disciplines (relativity theory, quantum mechanics, irreversible thermodynamics, information theory, ecology, complexity, chaos theory, and others) that question concepts of reality in place since the 17th century (8,13,20,21). Beginning with the "new" physics in the early 20th century, scientists began to change profoundly their understanding of nature as new findings were discovered that were incompatible with a purely mechanistic model of the world. These "postmodern" sciences have seriously challenged the old tier 1 philosophical commitments to reductionism, dualism, determinism, and linear causality. Instead, a "systems" strategy based on nonreductionism, indeterminism, and interacting levels of organization is suggested. Furthermore, postmodern scientists have come to view the physical world as no longer separate from themselves but one in which their own thoughts or ideas might influence the outcome of their experiments and, in turn, have an impact on the nature of external reality (8,13). An obvious example in medicine is the placebo response: positive thoughts about the effectiveness of an intervention are documented as affecting the outcome.

A postmodern scientific model, if it is to succeed logically its predecessor, must not only explain all the scientific achievements of the past but also, at the same time, provide a conceptual framework for findings (i.e., anomalies) incompatible with the older theory. This has clearly been shown to be the case for sciences such as quantum mechanics and irreversible (far from equilibrium) thermodynamics (13,20). It is not possible in this brief discussion to present in detail all the components of a successor scientific model based on the postmodern sciences. It is clear, however, that the postmodern sciences (new tier 2) and their underlying assumptions (new tier 1) can serve as a foundation for a more comprehensive successor medical model (new tier 3). The interested reader will find a stimulating account of this revolutionary thesis in Foss and Rothenberg's book (8).

One very significant feature of the new model that has far-reaching implications for medicine is the concept of self-organizing systems, a term taken from general systems theory and thermodynamics but applicable to all complex systems, including the human patient. According to Foss and Rothenberg (8, p. 157), self-organizing systems differ qualitatively from simple mechanistic systems by exhibiting the properties of

> (1) *self-renewal*—the ability to continuously renew and recycle their components while maintaining the integrity of the overall structures, and (2) *self-transcendence*—the ability to reach out spontaneously beyond physical and mental boundaries in the process of learning, developing, and evolving (italics added).

It does not take a great deal of insight to realize that the human body, unlike a simple mechanical system, exhibits these properties of self-organization.

Self-organizing systems, therefore, are "open" systems capable of interacting with the environment to maintain stability or evolve (self-organize) to a higher level. Unlike in simple systems, which are "closed" to the environment, the behavior of self-organizing systems cannot be understood entirely by analyzing the component parts and their internal interactions. Instead, these complex systems exhibit properties of "wholeness" that are best described in terms of cybernetics or information theory. The behavior of a complex system (e.g., a person's blood pressure) at any one time is the result of rule-governed processes (negative and positive feedback loops) that control the exchange of information between the system's internal and external environments.

From a self-organizing systems perspective (Fig. 3), the human patient can be conceptualized as "a biopsychosocial entity in an open systems information exchange with the environment or, for short, an information processing system" (8, p. 156). In a cybernetic model various positive and negative feedback loops

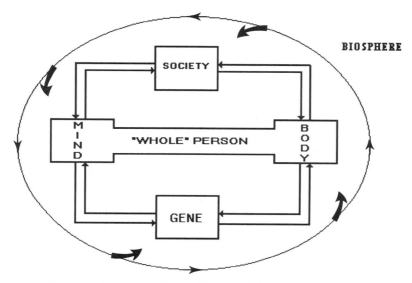

Figure 3 A proposed new scientific model for medicine—the "infomedical model"— based on self-organizing systems concepts. (Adapted from Ref. 8.)

mutually interconnect the patient, who is a complex hierarchy of systems, with other significant levels of organization (biological, psychological, social, etc.); the future state of the patient (e.g., health or disease) is more a function of the total exchange of information than a simple (linear) cause-and-effect mechanism.

This revolutionary concept has profound implications for modern medicine, because it redefines our notions of patient, disease, diagnosis, and therapy. No longer is the sick patient to be considered just a biological organism (i.e., a closed mechanical system reducible to cellular and molecular components). Instead, the patient, a human being, is now conceptualized as a mind–body unity, a complex system capable of interacting with the physical and social environment to evolve from a state of health to disease and then back to health again.

From this perspective a disease such as coronary atherosclerosis is more than just a breakdown or malfunction of the cardiovascular system. With mind and more complex social systems being given weight in this model, the disease equation must be enlarged to include nonbiological variables (e.g., behavioral and lifestyle factors). In a self-organizing systems paradigm, these nonbiological factors are now scientifically valid parameters for study; they fit within the new boundaries of the successor model. As a final point, given this expanded disease equation, the implications for prevention and treatment are equally profound, since it implies that not only must the traditional physical interventions be considered, but also behavioral, social, and environmental interventions must be emphasized.

VI. CONCLUSIONS

As is discussed in later chapters of this book, the prevention and treatment of coronary heart disease are tasks that require considerable attention to both biological and nonbiological disease variables. If the nonbiological variables cannot legitimately be included within the scientific framework for medicine, it is unlikely that they will ever receive the serious attention they deserve. Given the traditions of biomedicine with its emphasis on biological parameters, the incorporation of comprehensive preventive cardiology services into the practice of medicine seems far in the future. Yet the scientific rationale for preventing the onset and progression of atherosclerosis is known, and the data, largely accumulated in the 1980s, strongly suggest that prevention of CHD is within our grasp.

While the extraordinary successes of modern medicine are without question, a serious medical crisis nevertheless exists as the 20th century draws to a close. The costs of providing complex biomedical strategies for patients with far-advanced chronic diseases are prohibitive and continue to spiral upwards. Many in our society are becoming increasingly dissatisfied with the mechanical emphasis of medical care and are seeking alternative, and at times questionable, medical services. Yet students of medicine in increasing numbers are choosing to go into more technically oriented specialties at the expense of primary care careers, in part because of the biomedical emphasis of their education. As a result, interest in the study of prevention is on the decline.

An expanded medical model based on the postmodern sciences offers an attractive new strategy for incorporating preventive services into the mainstream of medical care. To be successful, however, it will require radical changes in our system of medical education, with the inclusion of courses in the social and behavioral sciences, epidemiology, information theory, ecology, and population biology. These curricular innovations will not be easy to implement, given the enormous influence of the biomedical model on institutionalized medicine: medical schools, academicians, professional organizations, hospital associations, insurance companies, the pharmaceutical industry, federal agencies, and other organizations that maintain and legitimize the current biomedical approach (8).

Nevertheless, there is reason for cautious optimism. The postmodern sciences are now recognized as legitimate academic disciplines, and they are having a profound effect on our understanding of reality and our approach to solving scientific problems. They also provide a solid foundation of basic sciences that can underwrite a new medical model based on a self-organizing systems perspective. Social, political, and economic forces are also beginning to exert their influence on medicine's infrastructure to increase the number of primary care physicians being trained and entering practice.

The chapters that follow provide the reader with the scientific basis for the practice of preventive cardiology. The authors focus primarily on the detection and management of the conventional coronary risk factors. A major emphasis will be given to changing patients' behaviors and modifying adverse lifestyles. Although we are still largely the product of a biomedically oriented medical education, the information presented in this chapter should at least bring attention to the need for a new perspective. In reference to today's chronic disease burden, Foss and Rothenberg conclude that there is "no overriding conceptual (as distinct from infrastructural) reason to wage today's war with weapons fashioned for yesterday's battle" (8, p. 311).

REFERENCES

1. Wechsler H, Levine S, Idelson RK, et al. The physician's role in health promotion—a survey of primary-care practitioners. N Engl J Med 1983; 308:97–100.
2. Rosen MA, Logsdon DN, Demak MM. Prevention and health promotion in primary care: baseline results on physicians from the INSURE project on lifestyle preventive health services. Prev Med 1984; 13:535–48.
3. Dismuke SE, Miller ST. Why not share the secrets of good health? The physician's role in health promotion. JAMA 1983; 249:3181–83.
4. Becker MH, Janz NK. Practicing health promotion: the doctor's dilemma. Ann Intern Med 1990; 113:419–22.
5. Kottke TE, Blackburn H, Brekke ML, et al. The systematic practice of preventive cardiology. Am J Cardiol 1987; 59:690–94.
6. Fried RA. Prevention in medical education: an uncertain future. J Gen Intern Med 1990; 5 (suppl):S108–S111.
7. Engel GL. The need for a new medical model: a challenge for biomedicine. Science 1977; 196:129–36.
8. Foss L, Rothenberg K. The second medical revolution—from biomedicine to info-medicine. Boston: New Science Library–Shambhala, 1987.
9. Freymann JG. The public's health care paradigm is shifting: medicine must swing with it. J Gen Intern Med 1989; 4:313–19.
10. Feinstein AR. The intellectual crisis in clinical science: medaled models and muddled mettle. Perspect Biol Med 1987; 30:215–30.
11. Kuhn TS. The structure of scientific revolutions, 2nd Ed. Chicago: University of Chicago Press, 1970.
12. Dubos R. Hippocrates in modern dress. Proc Inst Med Chicago 1965; 25:242–51.
13. Capra F. The turning point. Science, society and the rising culture. New York, Simon & Schuster, 1982.
14. 1991 Heart and Stroke Facts, 1991. Dallas: American Heart Association (AHA publication no. (COM) 55–0379).
15. Waller BF. "Crackers, breakers, stretchers, drillers, scrapers, shavers, burners,

welders, and melters"—the future treatment of atherosclerotic coronary artery disease? A clinical-morphologic assessment. J Am Coll Cardiol 1989; 13:969–87.

16. Lipkin M, Levinson W, Barker R, et al. Primary care internal medicine: a challenging career choice for the 1990s. Ann Intern Med 1990; 112:371–78.

17. Brody DS. The patient's role in clinical decision-making. Ann Intern Med 1980; 93: 718–22.

18. Pelletier K. Holistic medicine. San Francisco: Delacorte Press, 1979.

19. Conti CR. Clinical cardiology and molecular biology. Clin Cardiol 1990; 13:755–56.

20. Prigogine I, Stengers I. Order out of chaos. Man's new dialogue with nature. New York: Bantam Books, 1984.

21. Gleick J. Chaos: making a new science. New York: Penguin Books, 1987.

2

Atherosclerosis: Processes vs. Origins

FRANK G. YANOWITZ

The Fitness Institute
LDS Hospital
and University of Utah School of Medicine
Salt Lake City, Utah

The main error of the biomedical approach is the confusion between disease processes and disease origins. Instead of asking why an illness occurs, and trying to remove the conditions that lead to it, medical researchers try to understand the biological mechanisms through which the disease operates, so that they can then interfere with them.

Fritjof Capra, The turning point (1)

I. INTRODUCTION

"Processes" of disease refer to the underlying mechanisms responsible for the development of pathologic lesions and their subsequent evolution into the various clinical expressions of the disease. The biomedical approach to understanding atherosclerosis has primarily focused on the fundamental lesion, the atherosclerotic plaque, and the mechanisms by which these lesions lead to the clinical manifestations of disease. In particular, studies of the progression of coronary atherosclerosis have provided a very detailed description of the pathophysiological mechanisms responsible for the clinical syndromes of angina pectoris, unstable angina, myocardial infarction, sudden death, and congestive heart failure. There is no question that such studies have revolutionized the treatment of advanced coronary heart disease, with an impressive reduction in the morbidity and mortality resulting from these syndromes.

It is unfortunate, however, that this analytical and mechanistic approach to the study of atherosclerosis has done little to enhance our understanding of the "origins" or underlying causes of this disease. As a result, issues relevant to the prevention of coronary heart disease have not received adequate attention from many practicing physicians. While it is true that there is a large body of research into the causes of atherosclerosis, much of this research deals with disciplines that are less familiar to primary care physicians: cardiovascular genetics, clinical epidemiology, and the psychosocial sciences.

This chapter will contrast the two very important bodies of knowledge necessary for a comprehensive understanding of atherosclerosis: processes (mechanisms) and origins (causes). An appreciation of the distinction between these two knowledge bases is an important prerequisite to understanding the particular strategies needed for the prevention of coronary heart disease. Furthermore, as discussed in Chapter 1, the contrast between the biological mechanisms of atherosclerosis and the origins of this disease will reinforce the arguments for a more encompassing medical model, which goes beyond the purely reductionist biomedical approach so prevalent in today's medical environment.

II. ATHEROGENESIS: THE PROCESSES OF ATHEROSCLEROSIS

The mechanisms responsible for the development and subsequent progression of the atherosclerotic plaque are complex, fascinating, and only partially understood. Research into these processes has played a large part in establishing the careers of many scientists worldwide in their search for the fundamental mechanisms of atherosclerosis. It is not the purpose of this section to review in depth the current status of this research, but to summarize briefly our present understanding of these processes to set the stage for the preventive strategies discussed in later chapters. Much of what follows comes form several recent and excellent reviews on various aspects of atherogenesis (2–7). Readers interested in more detailed information on this subject will find informative references in these papers.

The human drama known as atherosclerosis, sometimes called "the Black Death of the 20th century," has an impressive cast of characters (Table 1). These factors interact over many years to produce the clinical syndromes of atherosclerotic cardiovascular disease, including coronary heart disease. The pathogenic mechanisms that lead to these syndromes have been reasonably well worked out by investigators using animal models of atherosclerosis as well as studying atherosclerotic plaques in humans. Our most recent understanding of the pathogenesis of atherosclerosis is based on the concept of chronic inflammation within the arterial wall, characterized by repetitive cycles of injury and healing occurring in an environment of hyperlipidemia or dyslipoproteinemia and involving myriad chemical mediators, genetic factors, and hemodynamic mechanisms (2).

In summarizing our current knowledge of atherogenesis, it is useful to organize

Table 1 Leading Roles in Atherosclerosis

Principal cell types
  Endothelial cells
  Monocyte/macrophages
  Smooth muscle cells
  Platelets
Lipoproteins
  Low-density lipoproteins (atherogenic)
  Very-low-density lipoproteins (atherogenic)
  Intermediate-density lipoproteins (atherogenic)
  High-density lipoproteins (antiatherogenic)
Chemical mediators
  Mitogens (growth factors)
  Chemoattractants
  Inflammatory cytokines
  Thrombogenic factors

the processes of atherosclerosis into three distinct phases: 1. fatty streaks, 2. fibrous plaques, and 3. advanced lesions. Although the clinical syndromes of coronary heart disease only occur in the setting of advanced or complicated coronary arterial lesions, success in preventing coronary heart disease requires aggressive intervention at earlier stages in the evolution of the atherosclerotic plaque.

A. Act 1: The Fatty Streak

Although ubiquitous in childhood, the fatty streak is widely believed to be the precursor of advanced atherosclerotic lesions in adults. These yellowish, flat intimal lesions appear in the aorta shortly after birth and accumulate in increasing numbers throughout the arteries of children, adolescents, and young adults. The fatty streak consists of macrophages and smooth muscle cells filled with cholesterol and cholesterol esters. These lipid-ladened cells are appropriately called "foam cells."

The mechanisms leading to the development of fatty streaks in humans is unknown. Nevertheless, from animal models of atherosclerosis, investigators have carefully described a sequence of events that is likely to be similar to that occurring in humans. In particular, studies by Faggiotto et al. (8) using hypercholesterolemic monkeys have shown that the first observable finding within days of initiating a high-fat, high-cholesterol diet is the attachment of circulating monocytes to the surface of arterial endothelium. These monocytes appear to migrate through the junctional areas between endothelial cells and establish residency as macrophages in the subendothelial space where they accumulate lipid and become foam cells. The beginning fatty streak enlarges by the addition of more macrophages from the circulation and the migration of smooth muscle cells from the media, which also accumulate lipid to become foam cells.

Just why circulating monocytes are recruited to set up housekeeping in the subendothelial tissues under conditions of hypercholesterolemia is the subject of intense investigation. A major hypothesis of atherosclerosis, discussed in depth by Ross and Glomset (5) and recently updated by Ross (6), focuses on the endothelial cells as key players in atherogenesis. In lesion-prone areas of endothelium, cells appear to become "injured" or, at the very least, activated in response to a variety of noxious stimuli including elevated blood levels of low-density (LDL) and very-low-density (VLDL) lipoproteins. The "response-to-injury" hypothesis states that certain presumably adverse conditions in the arterial blood or blood flow lead to morphologic and/or functional alterations in the endothelial cells. As a result potent vasoactive agents (growth factors, chemoattractants, and other endothelial cell products) are released that have profound effects on nearby blood constituents as well as in the subendothelial tissues. In particular, growth factors resembling platelet-derived growth factor (PDGF) attract circulating monocytes to areas of altered endothelium and also stimulate the migration of smooth muscle cells into the subendothelial tissues, where they proliferate, take up lipid, and form the fatty streak.

New findings on the metabolism of lipoproteins have led to an additional and intriguing hypothesis involving the oxidative modification of circulating LDL by endothelial cells (2–4). It has been found that elevated plasma LDL levels result in the oxidative modification of the LDL molecules by arterial endothelial cells. The oxidized forms of LDL are more rapidly taken up by subendothelial macrophages and smooth muscle cells than native LDL. Furthermore, it has been shown that macrophages and smooth muscle cells themselves are also able to oxidize LDL in the subendothelial tissues.

Oxidized forms of LDL are very toxic to the subendothelial tissues. Steinberg et al. (3) have proposed several mechanisms for the pathogenicity of oxidized LDL: 1. chemotactic attraction of circulating monocytes to the endothelial surfaces, 2. prevention of subendothelial macrophages form escaping back into the circulation, 3. increased uptake of modified LDL particles by macrophages and smooth muscle cells to form foam cells, 4. cytotoxicity to endothelial cells further accelerating the entry of circulating LDL and monocytes into the subendothelial space and eventually leading to endothelial disruption and denudation, 5. autoantibody response to modified LDL particles leading to the formation of immune complexes that are rapidly taken up by macrophages. Which of these mechanisms, if any, predominate in the evolution of the fatty streak remains open to question. However, considerable evidence already exists to support the atherogenecity of cell-induced oxidized LDL. It is even likely that other lipid particles including intermediate-density lipoprotein (IDL) and VLDL also contribute to foam cell formation in the fatty streaks.

B. Act 2: The Fibrous Plaque

The fundamental lesion of atherosclerosis, the atheroma or fibrous plaque, is believed to evolve directly from the fatty streaks, although not all fatty streaks progress to plaque lesions (Fig. 1). It is thought that in the presence of increased circulating LDL, the continued influx of oxidatively modified LDL particles into the subendothelial space exceeds the capacity of macrophages to remove them (2). The cytotoxic effects of these particles in the interstitium lead to the destruction of foam cells and other cellular components, with the subsequent accumulation of lipid and necrotic debris within the intima. The release of lipid into the interstitium also results in inflammation resembling a foreign body granulomatous reaction involving macrophages, lymphocytes, and multinucleate giant cells (2).

As described by Ross et al. (5), the fibrous plaque consists of a raised lesion

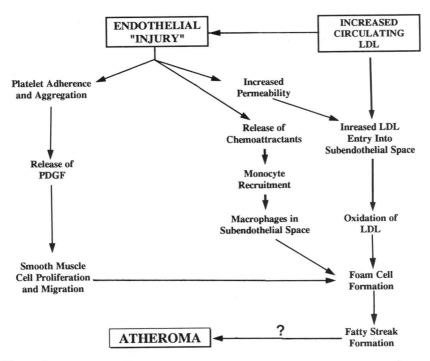

Figure 1 The process of atherosclerosis: interaction of circulating LDL with endothelial cells, monocyte/macrophages, and platelets in the evolution of the atherosclerotic plaque.

protruding into the lumen of the blood vessel and covered by a fibrous cap composed of alternating layers of modified smooth muscle and basement-membrane-like material. Beneath the fibrous cap is a highly cellular zone containing foam cells, leukocytes, and connective tissue, which, in turn, covers an area of necrotic debris, cholesterol crystals, and calcification. The development of fibrous plaques involves a continuation of those processes already at work in the formation of fatty streaks. Once mature, the fibrous plaque continues to exhibit dynamic changes that are the result of the complex interplay of factors influencing either growth or regression of atherosclerotic lesions.

Platelets are most likely to become involved in the process of atherosclerosis when endothelial injury permits a direct interaction between circulating blood components and subendothelial connective tissue. In their study of diet-induced atherosclerotic monkeys, Faggiotto et al. (9) observed the transition from fatty streaks to more advanced fibrous plaques at approximately 5 months after the onset of hypercholesterolemia. They described retraction of altered endothelial cells, particularly at branch points and bifurcations, resulting in exposure of the subendothelial collagen fibrils to circulating platelets. Platelet adherence, aggregation, and thrombus formation were observed at sites of endothelial injury.

A complex sequence of biochemical and mechanical events has been proposed to explain the platelet–subendothelial interactions that lead to fibrous plaque formation as well as the subsequent progression to acute coronary syndromes. For the moment, however, this discussion will focus on the initial role of platelets in the formation of atheroma.

There are many ways by which platelets may influence the process of atherogenesis. Perhaps the most obvious is the normal response of circulating platelets to endothelial injury: a reparative process to preserve hemostasis. Platelet adherence and aggregation result in the release of chemotactic and mitogenic growth factors as well as other constituents that induce smooth muscle cell migration and proliferation in the developing lesion (6). Furthermore, studies in both hypercholesterolemic animals and human subjects have shown an enhanced platelet sensitivity for these reactions over that in normolipidemic controls (10). This is one of the ways the hyperlipidemic state accelerates the atherosclerotic process.

It is unlikely that progressive atherosclerotic lesions would occur in the absence of continued exposure of the endothelium to injurious stimuli. This results in repeated disruption of endothelial cells at sites of injury or, at the very least, a loss of normal endothelial cell function at those sites (6). Under the appropriate atherogenic conditions, moreover, the injured endothelial cells facilitate the disease process by attracting additional platelets and monocytes to participate in the proliferative response. The progression of fibrous plaques to more advanced and complicated lesions is slow in humans, generally taking place over many years if the atherogenic milieu is maintained. Platelets continue to participate actively in the disease process and are especially important in the pathogenesis of the clinical syndromes of advanced coronary heart disease.

C. Act 3: The Advanced Lesion

The final phase in the drama of atherogenesis is in some ways the least predictable and in many ways the most dramatic. Up to this stage coronary artery disease is usually silent, since uncomplicated fibrous plaque lesions generally do not significantly interfere with myocardial blood flow. Although the transition from asymptomatic to symptomatic coronary heart disease may be insidious, it is often sudden and catastrophic. It is now widely accepted that rupture or fissuring of the fibrous plaque is the common underlying mechanism initiating the acute coronary syndromes: unstable angina, myocardial infarction, and sudden cardiac death.

Pathologic studies reported by Davies and Thomas (7) have beautifully demonstrated fissured plaques accompanied by new thrombus formation in patients dying of acute coronary syndromes. From these studies a reasonable sequence of events can be proposed. The fibrous plaque is covered on its luminal surface by a fibrous cap that is thinned at certain points along the crescent-shaped lesion. Rupture of the plaque at these sites may be the result of random, unpredictable stimuli possibly related to pulsatile blood flow, spasm, or other factors in the coronary circulation. In a sense, the events that follow are a "response to injury" phenomenon similar to what has been described previously for the developing fibrous plaque, but on a much grander scale. Exposure of the lipid-rich tissues to circulating blood results in acute formation of thrombi consisting of platelets, red blood cells, and fibrin. Fresh thrombus is often found within the lumen of the artery as well as inside the plaque itself as blood dissects into the lesion.

The fate of the fresh thrombus ultimately determines the clinical course following plaque rupture or fissuring (7). At least four possible outcomes can be envisioned: 1. incorporation of thrombus material into the plaque resulting in gradual growth of plaque without any acute clinical manifestations, 2. subtotal intraluminal occlusion causing varying degrees of obstruction and the syndrome of unstable angina pectoris, 3. total luminal occlusion that usually precipitates acute myocardial infarction, and 4. distal propagation of thrombus with embolization often leading to sudden ischemic death. These are clearly not independent outcomes, since each of these initial events may progress or regress into subsequent outcomes depending on many different factors including the body's own defense mechanisms, the natural history of the disease, and various medical interventions, if any.

D. Therapeutic Implications

An understanding of the processes of atherogenesis has resulted in major therapeutic advances during the last decade that have had a significant impact on the outcome of patients with coronary atherosclerosis. Several areas of clinical research stand out as therapeutic milestones in the war against CHD: 1. the demonstration that aggressive treatment of elevated blood LDL–cholesterol levels with diet and lipid-lowering drugs reduces the likelihood of new CHD events and potentiates regression of lesions (11,12), 2. the use of thrombolytic therapies in the early management of acute myocardial infarction to reduce both morbidity and mortality (13,14), and 3. the use of aspirin therapy in the prevention of acute coronary syndromes (15–18). These therapeutic advances have received much public and professional attention in recent years and have underscored the importance of basic research into the mechanisms of atherosclerosis.

A detailed discussion of hyperlipidemia and its management is presented in Chapter 8. The use of thrombolytic therapy in managing acute myocardial infarction is adequately covered in the medical literature (13,14) and not really pertinent to preventive cardiology. Aspirin therapy, however, deserves a brief discussion, since it is an intervention for preventing the manifestations of CHD and its mechanism of action is relevant to the preceding description of atherosclerotic processes.

Aspirin's antithrombotic effects are primarily the result of platelet inhibition (15). Aspirin inhibits the platelet's cyclo-oxygenase enzyme used in converting arachidonic acid into thromboxane A2, a potent vasoconstrictor and platelet-aggregating factor. The inhibition is permanent for the life of the platelet, which implies that a single small dose of aspirin will have an effect lasting several days. Larger doses, however, may have an adverse effect by inhibiting the formation in the blood vessel wall of prostacyclin, an important factor in vasodilation and the prevention of thrombosis.

There is conflicting evidence in the literature regarding aspirin's efficacy in the primary prevention of myocardial infarction. In a randomized, controlled study of 22,071 male U.S. physicians evaluated for 5 years, there was a 45% reduction of fatal and nonfatal myocardial infarctions in the aspirin-treated group (325 mg every other day); there was also a slight but significant increase in hemorrhagic stroke in those taking aspirin (16). Total cardiovascular deaths in the aspirin- and placebo-treated groups were identical. A 6 year British study of 5139 male physicians taking 500 mg aspirin daily did not show any significant cardioprotective benefits when compared to placebo, and again, there was a slight but significant increase in hemorrhagic stroke in the aspirin-treated group (17). In an observational study of 87,678 female U.S. nurses evaluated for 6 years, the use of one to six aspiring per week was associated with a 25% reduced risk of first myocardial infarction (18). This study, however, suffers from methodologic limitations (nonexperimental design), and further studies are needed to confirm these intriguing results.

Recommendations for prophylactic, low-dosage aspirin use in asymptomatic men and women have to be made with a great deal of caution because of the potential for undesirable side effects. At the present time it is reasonable to suggest the use of 325 mg aspirin every other day indefinitely for those patients at high risk for myocardial infarction (MI) who do not have significant hypertension or other risk factors for cerebral hemorrhage or gastrointestinal bleeding. The prophylactic use of aspirin therapy in patients with known coronary disease—unstable angina, non-Q-wave MI, and those who have undergone coronary revascularization—is less controversial and will not be considered further here.

Continued investigations into the mechanisms of atherosclerosis will no doubt lead to further therapeutic innovations aimed at controlling or reversing the atherosclerotic processes. New pharmacologic interventions are being sought that focus on inhibiting the oxidative modification of LDL particles to reduce their toxicity (3). Other areas of research are concerned with discovering ways to enhance HDL activity in order to augment removal of cholesterol from the arterial lesions (19). Pharmacologic agents are also being sought that interfere with monocyte recruitment and smooth muscle cell migration/proliferation in order to retard plaque formation (2). The search also continues for new genetic markers that may identify high-risk individuals as targets for early preventive strategies (2,20).

II. ORIGINS OF ATHEROSCLEROSIS

Throughout the history of medicine concepts of disease causation have been limited by the technologies available to study them and by the reigning scientific medical model (21). As our knowledge of the pathogenesis and epidemiology of today's chronic diseases evolved, so too did our understanding of their origins.

From the perspective of the biomedical model (Chap. 1) investigators have been probing deeper and deeper within the body (as a biological organism) to unravel the ultimate molecular and genetic defects responsible for atherosclerosis. Although these investigations provide most interesting insights into the complex biological mechanisms of atherosclerosis, they are simplistic in assuming that there must be a discrete, specific cause of the disease, one that will ultimately be explained in biological terms. This linear, deterministic view of disease causation is a modern expression of the 19th century "germ theory" of disease that assumed a single cause (e.g., tubercle bacillus) for each disease (e.g., tuberculosis). Such causative agents, when finally discovered, have certainly proven to be necessary but not sufficient causes of the diseases in question.

A complex interaction among physical agents, environmental factors, and host factors must be considered in the search for causal relationships in any disease (21). Host factors include a genetic predisposition, coexisting diseases, socioeconomic factors, behavioral and lifestyle factors, and hygienic practices, all of which have been shown to be important in determining the origins and progression of atherosclerotic diseases (22,23).

While the molecular aspects of cardiovascular genetics have proven to be fascinating avenues for research into the mechanisms of atherosclerosis, their importance must not be overestimated. Powles argues that hereditary factors might only become significant in disease causation when the host is exposed to stresses that are, in evolutionary terms, unusual (24). To illustrate this point he recalls Cleave and Campbell's analogy regarding the role of genetic factors in disease causation: "In populations that wear shoes the inherited variability of the build of the foot may well make some individuals more likely than others to develop bunions—but bunions only occur in populations that wear shoes" (25).

Studies of hereditary factors in CHD have likewise generally been carried out in industrialized populations, such as Framingham, Massachusetts, where the day-to-day stresses of modern living are naively assumed to be "normal." In fact, for most of the 50,000 generations in the last million years members of the genus *Homo* lived by hunting and gathering. Only 500 generations have passed since the agricultural revolution and a mere 15 since the industrial revolution (24). From an evolutionary perspective, therefore, our genetic make-up has been predominantly determined by the selection pressures associated with hunting and gathering. "Fight or flight" became the genetically programmed behavioral response to most stressful situations. The stresses and strains of modern industrialized life are, in evolutionary terms, very different from those of the hunter-gatherers, and fight or flight is no longer considered an appropriate response to stress. There are grounds to believe that today's chronic diseases, cardiovascular disease, cancer, pulmonary disease, and many others, occur, in part, because we are genetically unsuited for the stresses of modern industrial life (24). These diseases have therefore been characterized as "diseases of maladaptation" (24).

CHD is, in fact, the prototype of the afflictions of civilization, being the leading cause of death and disability in industrialized societies (26). It is now well recognized that external factors related to lifestyle, behaviors, and the environment are important contributors to atherosclerotic diseases especially as they relate to human patients. Since many of these extrasomatic factors fall outside the boundaries of biomedicine, they have been labeled "risk factors" rather than causative agents. Yet, from empiric and epidemiologic observations, many of these factors have been shown to satisfy the usually accepted criteria for disease causation (Table 2) (22).

Stamler uses the term "established major risk factors" to refer to those causative factors that are: 1. implicated in CHD causation, 2. widely prevalent in the population, and 3. amenable to prevention and control (22). According to these criteria diet-dependent hypercholesterolemia and hypertension, cigarette smoking, and non-insulin-dependent diabetes mellitus are the established major CHD risk factors and ones that are considered in subsequent chapters of this book (22). Other factors implicated as causes of CHD, including sedentary lifestyle, behavioral, psychosocial, and socioeconomic factors, are also of interest, although they may not be as fully "established" as the more traditional risk factors listed above. These too are discussed in subsequent chapters since they have important implications for those who wish to carry out comprehensive preventive cardiology programs.

Table 2 Criteria for Disease Causation

1. Strength of the association: incidence of disease is higher in those exposed than in those not exposed.
2. Graded nature of the association (dose–response): the relative risk of disease increases with greater exposure.
3. Time sequence of the association: exposure to suspected factor precedes the disease.
4. Consistency of the association: repeated demonstration of the association between suspected factor and disease in different populations and under varying circumstances.
5. Independence of the association: independent of other factors known or suspected to be involved in causing the disease.
6. Predictive capacity of the association: ability of the suspected factor to predict incidence rates in other population groups.
7. Coherence (plausibility) of the association: the epidemiologic findings are coherent with other types of biological investigations, and there are one or more plausible mechanisms by which the suspected factor causes the disease in question.

The evidence in support of Stamler's established major risk factors is substantial and well documented in the literature as well as in other chapters of this book (22,23). All seven criteria for causation listed in Table 2 have been fulfilled by careful epidemiologic and other types of scientific investigations. No one questions the validity of these studies because they fit very nicely into a biomedical framework, especially the requirement for coherence of the association (criterion 7 in Table 2). Coherence implies a plausible mechanism of action that can be understood in biomedical terms; that is, there is a biological explanation for the pathogenesis of these risk factors.

From a biomedical perspective it is more difficult to justify calling behavioral, psychosocial, or socioeconomic factors "causative agents" because there is no known mechanism of action or proven biological explanation for their causative role in atherosclerosis (i.e., they fail criterion 7 in Table 2). Yet there is considerable empiric evidence in favor of these factors in the causation of CHD (27–29). It is possible, moreover, to suggest plausible connections between the brain, the autonomic nervous system, and the neuroendocrine reactions to stress that might be involved in the pathogenesis of atherosclerosis (27). What is lacking are the specific links between the external behavioral factors and the biological pathways implicated in atherogenesis. If these links can be found, however, they could have a profound effect on our concepts of atherosclerosis as a disease, the patient, and the range of therapeutic options, including preventive strategies. These expanded concepts would lead us to abandon the simplistic biomedical notions of disease, patient, and therapy in favor of a more encompassing successor medical model discussed in Chapter 1.

IV. CONCLUSIONS

In summary, atherosclerosis has its origins in the complex interplay of causative factors occurring within the body, the mind, and the external physical and social environments. No longer is it possible to consider the disease a consequence of some initial set of conditions acting linearly to produce a final pathologic state. The causative model of atherosclerosis and many other chronic diseases is not characterized by determinism but by indeterminism. It is unlikely that we will ever be able to elucidate an exact "chain of events" linking the various causative factors from different hierarchic levels of organization (body, mind, external environment, etc.) to the specific expressions of CHD. In an indeterminancy model of disease the causes are multifactorial, and the occurrence of disease is probabilistic: dependent upon a particular mix of causative factors interacting at the proper time with a "host inhabiting a particular biopsychosocial space" (30). In addition, as stated by Evans (21), "different qualitative and quantitative mixes of agent, environment, and host may result in the same clinical and pathologic disease under different circumstances."

In a multifactorial model of atherosclerosis, both physical (e.g., hypercholesterolemia) and nonphysical (e.g., type A behavior) factors have been implicated in disease causation. Although preventive strategies, many of which are discussed in this book, have addressed both kinds of factors, only those therapies that deal with the physical causes are formally based on a sound biomedical framework and, therefore, lie within the domain of the traditionally trained medical practitioner. Accordingly, most of our current preventive efforts have been directed toward the management of hypercholesterolemia, hypertension, and smoking cessation, since these therapies are "scientifically" based.

Much less attention has been given by the medical profession to the detection and management of behavioral, psychosocial, and socioeconomic factors implicated in CHD causation. While there may be an empiric basis for these nonbiological factors in disease causation, they lie outside the boundaries of biomedicine and they do not have a mechanism of action explainable in biomedical terms (30). It is not surprising, therefore, that most physicians feel uncomfortable and unprepared when considering these kinds of factors. Yet these nonphysical factors lie within the scientific framework of the expanded, interactionist medical model of disease discussed in Chapter 1, and could play an important role in the design of effective preventive strategies in the future.

It is widely believed that the well-known CHD risk factors (hypercholesterolemia, hypertension, and cigarette smoking) explain only 50% of the premature CHD disease burden, leaving the other 50% caused by other yet-to-be-discovered factors (31). While it is still possible that some of these unknown factors will eventually be found within the physical domain, it is much more likely that a complete and satisfactory explanation for CHD causation will only occur when we

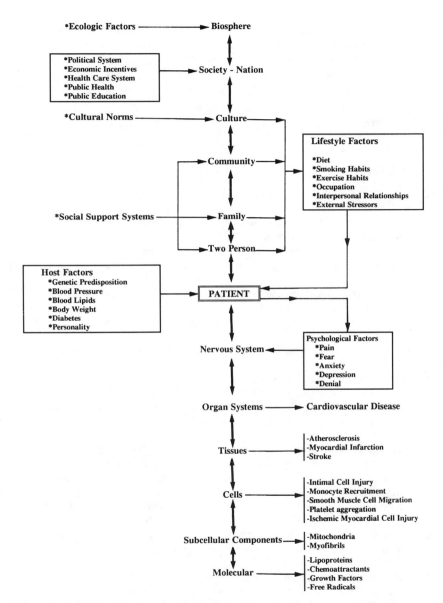

Figure 2 Hierarchy of systems—biological and nonbiological—that interact to determine the origins, progression, and clinical manifestations of coronary heart disease. (Adapted from Ref. 32.)

learn to integrate the extrabiological with the biological factors in a scientifically valid disease model. The challenge to primary care physicians interested in the prevention of CHD is to broaden their perspective to include in the domain of their clinical investigations the relevant data from all levels of organization (Fig. 2) (32). This will have important ramifications not only for CHD prevention but for most of the other 20th century "diseases of civilization" that make up today's chronic disease burden.

REFERENCES

1. Capra F. The turning point. Science, society and the rising culture. New York: Simon & Schuster, 1982.
2. Schwartz CJ, Valente AJ, Sprague EA, Kelly JL, Nerem RM. The pathogenesis of atherosclerosis: an overview. Clin Cardiol 1991; 14:I–1–16.
3. Steinberg D, Parthasarathy S, Carew TE, Khoo JC, Witztum JL. Beyond cholesterol. Modifications of low-density lipoprotein that increase its atherogenecity. N Engl J Med 1989; 320:915–24.
4. Steinberg D. Lipoproteins and the pathogenesis of atherosclerosis. Circulation 1987; 76:508–14.
5. Ross R, Glomset JA. The pathogenesis of atherosclerosis. N Engl J Med 1976; 295: 369–77.
6. Ross R. The pathogenesis of atherosclerosis—an update. N Engl J Med 1986; 314: 488–500.
7. Davies MJ, Thomas AC. Plaque fissuring—the cause of acute myocardial infarction, sudden ischemic death, and crescendo angina. Br Heart J 1985; 53:363–73.
8. Faggiotto A, Ross R, Harker L. Studies of hypercholesterolemia in the nonhuman primate. I. Changes that lead to fatty streak formation. Arteriosclerosis 1984; 4: 323–40.
9. Faggiotto A, Ross R. Studies of hypercholesterolemia in the nonhuman primate. II. Fatty streak conversion to fibrous plaques. Arteriosclerosis 1984; 4:341–56.
10. Aviram M, Brook JG. Platelet activation by plasma lipoproteins. Prog Cardiovasc Dis 1987; 30:61–72.
11. Blankenhorn DH. Prevention or reversal of atherosclerosis: review of current evidence. Am J Cardiol 1989; 63:38H–41H.
12. Lipid Research Clinics Program. The lipid research clinics coronary primary prevention trial results. I. Reduction in incidence of coronary heart disease. JAMA 1984; 251:351–62.
13. ISIS (Second International Study of Infarct Survival) Collaborative Group. Randomized trial of intravenous streptokinase, oral aspirin, both or neither among 17,187 cases of suspected acute myocardial infarction: ISIS–2. Lancet 1988; 2:349–60.
14. ASSET Study Group. Trial of tissue plasminogen activator for mortality reduction in acute myocardial infarction. Lancet 1988; 2:525–30.
15. Fuster V, Chesebro JH. Antithrombic therapy: role of platelet-inhibitor drugs. II. Pharmacologic effects of platelet-inhibitor drugs. Mayo Clin Proc 1981; 56:185–95.

16. The Steering Committee of the Physicians' Health Study Research Group. Preliminary report: findings from the aspiring component of the ongoing Physicians' Health Study. N Engl J Med 1988; 318:262–84.

17. Peto R, Gray R, Collins R, et al. Randomized trial of prophylactic daily aspirin in British male doctors. Br Med J Clin Res 1988; 296:313–16.

18. Manson JE, Stampfer MJ, Colditz GA, et al. A prospective study of aspirin use and primary prevention of cardiovascular disease in women. JAMA 1991; 266:521–27.

19. Gwynne JT. HDL and atherosclerosis: an update. Clin Cardiol 1991; 14:I-17–24.

20. Mahley RW, Weisgraber KH, Innerarity TL, Rall SC. Genetic defects in lipoprotein metabolism. Elevation of atherogenic lipoproteins caused by impaired catabolism. JAMA 1991; 265:78–83.

21. Evans AS. Causation and disease: a chronological journey. Am J Epidemiol 1978; 108:249–58.

22. Stamler J. Epidemiology, established major risk factors, and the primary prevention of coronary heart disease. In: Parmley WW, Chatterjee K, ed. Cardiology, vol. 2. Philadelphia: JB Lippincott, 1990.

23. Kannel WB, Schatzkin A. Risk factor analysis. Prog Cardiovasc Dis 1983; 26:309–32.

24. Powles J. On the limitations of modern medicine. Sci Med Man 1973; 1:1–30.

25. Cleave TL, Campbell GD. Diabetes, coronary thrombosis and the saccharine disease. Bristol, Wright: 1966.

26. American Heart Association. 1991 heart and stroke facts. AHA publication SS-0379(COM), 1991.

27. Manuck SB, Kaplan JR, Matthews KA. Behavioral antecedents of coronary heart disease and atherosclerosis. Arteriosclerosis 1986; 1:33–45.

28. Jenkins CD. Recent evidence supporting psychological and social risk factors for coronary disease. N Engl J Med 1976; 294:987–94.

29. The Review Panel. Coronary-prone behavior and coronary heart disease: a critical review. Circulation 1981; 63:1199–215.

30. Foss L, Rothenberg K. The second medical revolution—from biomedicine to info-medicine. Boston: New Science Library–Shambhala, 1987.

31. Newfield HN, Goldbourt U. Coronary heart disease: genetic aspects. Circulation 1983; 67:943–54.

32. Engel GL. The need for a new medical model: a challenge for biomedicine. Science 1977; 196:129–36.

3

Arguments for Prevention

FRANK G. YANOWITZ
The Fitness Institute
LDS Hospital
and University of Utah School of Medicine
Salt Lake City, Utah

GERALD A. CHARLTON
LDS Hospital
Salt Lake City, Utah

I. INTRODUCTION

In 1983 an editorial appeared in the *Journal of the American Medical Association* (1) entitled "Why not share the secrets of good health? The physician's role in health promotion." It pointed out that while physicians as a group were more likely than the general population to practice heart-healthy behaviors such as not smoking, exercising, and avoiding high-fat diets, they seemed reluctant or unable to communicate these behavioral skills to their patients.

A number of reasons were offered for this strange paradox. Much of the blame can be attributed to our medical education, which traditionally has not included courses on risk assessment, nutrition, exercise physiology, and the behavioral sciences. As discussed in Chapter 1, the focus of our medical education has always been on the mechanistic aspects of disease detection and treatment (the biomedical model) rather than on the origins and prevention of disease. Although there is a trend beginning in some medical schools to develop a curriculum for preventive and behavioral medicine, it will likely take years before the impact of these new approaches is seen.

Physicians may also be reluctant to promote preventive health behaviors because the evidence for these recommendations is still perceived as somewhat conflicting and controversial. Yet we are often willing to try new drugs and other therapeutic techniques on the basis of only preliminary evidence of efficacy, even

33

with the realization that these unproven therapies may be costly and associated with some risk to the patient. In contrast, the "evidence to date" for preventive health behaviors is substantial, and the recommended interventions are inexpensive and essentially without risk.

There are also many practical barriers to the implementation of preventive cardiology services (2). The primary care practice environment is generally not organized for the delivery of preventive services. If such services are offered they are usually provided without adequate reimbursement from insurance companies. Teaching preventive health behaviors to patients takes considerable physician time and may require additional staff to provide this service effectively. Many physicians lack confidence in their ability to change patients' behaviors or are pessimistic that their patients can actually change. This is especially true with smoking cessation. There is also an attitude among some physicians that the primary business of a medical practice is treating illness not keeping people healthy. In this view, prevention is seen more as a public health issue and not within the domain of primary practitioners of medicine (1).

This chapter presents the arguments for the prevention of coronary heart disease (CHD), focusing primarily on the role of practicing physicians. While there may be many barriers to the implementation of preventive cardiology services in clinical practice, we hope that the arguments are strong enough to convince the majority of physicians that such an approach is the only feasible method for conquering this most serious cause of death and disability in the Western world.

The arguments for prevention will center on five major issues: 1. health statistics indicating that while CHD is still our nation's number one cause of death and disability, there has been a significant decline in mortality in recent years, in part due to the adoption of healthier lifestyles by the general public; 2. the staggering costs of CHD to society; 3. evidence that lifestyle and risk factor interventions reduce first and subsequent CHD events; 4. the concept of reversal of atherosclerosis; and 5. the pivotal role of primary care physicians in the prevention of CHD.

II. STATISTICS: BAD NEWS AND GOOD NEWS

The bad news refers to the enormous burden cardiovascular disease has had on our society in recent years. This is illustrated in Figure 1, which shows the leading causes of death in the United States (3). In 1987 cardiovascular diseases accounted for more than twice the number of deaths due to cancer, the second leading cause of death, and 74 times the number of deaths from acquired immunodeficiency syndrome (AIDS), a syndrome that has captured a disproportionate amount of attention from the public and those in the medical professions. Figure 2 shows that more than half of these cardiovascular deaths resulted from myocardial infarction and its complications. The American Heart Association estimates that 1.5 million

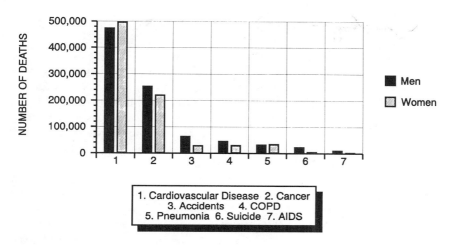

Figure 1 Leading causes of death in the United States. (Adapted form Ref. 3.)

Americans suffer acute myocardial infarction each year, of whom 300,000 will die before reaching a hospital (3). In fact, nearly half of all acute coronary events result in death, 25% of which are sudden, and 20% nonsudden. Survivors of such events are also five times more likely to die within the next 5 years.

This is not just a disease of the elderly either. Approximately 5% of all myocardial infarctions (75,000 Americans) occur in people under age 40, and

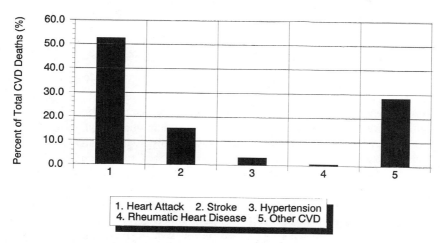

Figure 2 Estimated deaths from cardiovascular disease. (Adapted from Ref. 3.)

45% in those younger than age 65 (3). Myocardial infarction is the most common initial presentation of CHD in men, and those who survive often have catastrophic physical and emotional consequences. Cardiovascular disease accounts for 180,000 deaths per year in people under the age of 65. Many of these deaths could have been prevented by treating hypertension, smoking cessation, cholesterol lowering, and knowing the warning signs of myocardial infarction.

The good news is that deaths from CHD peaked in the 1960s and have been steadily declining by approximately 3% per year ever since (4). From the late 1960s through the mid-1980s CHD mortality fell more than 30%, resulting in over 800,000 lives saved (4). The reasons for the decline are complex but include healthier lifestyles, reductions in coronary risk factors, improved treatment of hypertension and hypercholesterolemia, earlier diagnosis and treatment of CHD, and improved interventional technologies. Although it is not possible to assess the specific contributions of each of these factors, considerable evidence suggests that preventive health strategies and risk factor modification have had a major impact on the decline in mortality.

In 1984 Goldman et al. (5) examined the decline in CHD mortality between 1968 and 1976 and concluded that more than 50% of the decline could be attributed to lifestyle changes, the most significant of which were reductions in serum cholesterol levels and cigarette smoking in the U.S. population. The remainder of the decline was attributed to improved medical and surgical interventions.

In support of these findings, Pell and Fayerweather analyzed long-term CHD incidence and mortality rates among Du Pont Company employees from 1957 through 1983 and concluded that the major cause for the fall in mortality was a reduction in the incidence of first acute myocardial infarctions rather than improved medical treatment (6). Primary care physicians have clearly played a role in these statistics by their more aggressive management of hypertension and counseling their patients to eat better, exercise more, and smoke less.

III. THE COST OF CARDIOVASCULAR DISEASES

As we enter the last decade of the 20th century there is growing concern about the increasing cost of health care in this country. Each year medical care costs consume a greater percentage of the gross national product. In 1987, for example, medical care in the United States cost $500.3 billion, approximately 11% of the gross national product (7). Because cardiovascular disease accounts for the largest share of our nation's mortality and morbidity, the cost to our economy is substantially greater than for any other diagnostic group. In 1990 the American Heart Association estimated that cardiovascular disease will cost $94.5 billion, of which $60.7 billion will pay for hospital and nursing home services, $13.6 billion for physician and nursing services, $4.7 billion for drugs, and $15.5 billion will be forfeited to the economy because of lost productivity (3). Almost 75% of these costs will be spent on coronary heart disease, stroke, and hypertension, diseases that can be prevented or reduced by risk factor modification and lifestyle changes.

IV. RISK FACTOR REDUCTION AND LIFESTYLE INTERVENTION

During the 1980s a substantial body of evidence accumulated to show that reduction of individual coronary risk factors can result in a significant lowering of CHD morbidity and mortality. The modifiable risk factors that have had the greatest impact on improving these disease endpoints are hypercholesterolemia, hypertension, and cigarette smoking. There is also increasing evidence to suggest that eliminating sedentary lifestyles in favor of more vigorous exercise programs and recreational activities may provide additional benefits in preventing CHD. Although subsequent chapters of this book review in some detail the implications of these many studies for clinical practice, several important highlights will be discussed briefly to strengthen the case for preventive cardiology.

A. Hypercholesterolemia

The relationship between high serum levels of low-density-lipoprotein (LDL)–cholesterol and CHD incidence has been well established and is generally accepted by the medical community. This relationship appears to be continuous and graded, not just confined to persons with serum levels above a certain threshold (8). An inverse relationship also exists between serum levels of high-density-lipoprotein (HDL)–cholesterol and CHD incidence, and the ratio of total cholesterol to HDL–cholesterol has become an important measure of CHD risk in asymptomatic individuals. Although there is still some skepticism in the lay press and medical literature regarding the "cholesterol myth" and the value of treating hypercholesterolemia, many studies have now shown unequivocally that lowering LDL–cholesterol with diet and drugs can significantly reduce the incidence of new CHD events in high-risk hyperlipidemic individuals (9–12).

In 1981 the results of the Oslo Study Group demonstrated a 47% decrease in the incidence of myocardial infarction and sudden death in high-risk, middle-aged men randomized to receive educational intervention aimed at lowering serum cholesterol levels through dietary means and smoking cessation (9). The mean cholesterol level in the intervention group was 13% lower than the controls who did not receive the educational intervention, and tobacco consumption per man decreased by 45%. This study was one of the first to demonstrate that a lifestyle intervention consisting only of patient education could lower CHD risk in an asymptomatic high-risk population.

The results of the well-known Lipid Research Clinics Coronary Primary Prevention Trial (LRC-CPPT) were published in 1984 and demonstrated conclusively that diet modification plus cholestyramine treatment could significantly lower serum cholesterol levels and CHD incidence in asymptomatic middle-aged men with primary hypercholesterolemia (10,11). In this randomized, multicenter study involving 3806 subjects, an 8% average reduction in cholesterol levels in the drug-treated group was associated with a 19% reduction in new CHD events compared to the controls who received only dietary intervention. For those patients able to tolerate the full dosage of cholestyramine (24 g/day) cholesterol levels dropped an average of 25% and the incidence of CHD events decreased by a remarkable 50%.

Three years after the LRC-CPPT results were published, the Helsinki Heart Study reported a 34% reduction in CHD incidence in hyperlipidemic middle-aged men randomized to receive the drug gemfibrozil (12). In this study involving over 4000 subjects, LDL–cholesterol levels fell approximately 9% in the drug-treated group, but, unlike the results of the LRC-CPPT, HDL–cholesterol levels increased by almost 10%. This is one of the few studies to associate a drug-induced increase in HDL–cholesterol with a reduction in CHD incidence.

The impressive results of these randomized studies coupled with the growing public and professional interest in CHD prevention led to the National Heart, Lung, and Blood Institute's (NHLBI) formation of an "expert panel" to develop new guidelines for the detection and management of hypercholesterolemia in adults (13). The expert panel's "Report of the National Cholesterol Education Program" was published in 1988 and had as its major goal "to establish criteria that define the candidates for medical intervention and to provide guidelines on how to detect, set goals for, treat, and monitor these patients over time." In addition to the published report the NHLBI mounted a national campaign to educate primary care physicians in the use of these guidelines and to encourage them to be more aggressive in the detection and treatment of hypercholesterol-emia. The specific recommendations of the expert panel's report are discussed in more detail in Chapter 8. Based on the recommendations of the panel, however, Sempos et al. (14) estimate that approximately 60 million Americans are candi-dates for medical advice and intervention for hypercholesterolemia.

B. Hypertension

In 1987 the American Heart Association estimated that 61 million Americans (approximately 40% of the U.S. population) had hypertension (defined as greater than 140/90 mmHg) (3). Without a doubt hypertension is one of the most common medical problems treated by physicians and continues to be a major risk factor for premature cardiovascular disease. The good news is that increasing numbers of hypertensive individuals are being detected and appropriately treated by the medical profession. The dramatic decline in death due to stroke and other cardiovascular diseases in recent years has reflected this more aggressive treat-ment approach.

In the 1970s the Multiple Risk Factor Intervention Trial (MRFIT) screened over 350,000 middle-aged men free of CHD and established the relationship of blood pressure to CHD risk with a degree of precision never before possible (8). The cardiovascular sequelae from high blood pressure were found to be directly proportional to levels of both systolic and diastolic blood pressures, with increasing morbidity and mortality observed from the lowest to highest pressures measured. For diastolic blood pressure the 6 year age-adjusted CHD mortality began to rise with levels above 75 mmHg and increased by 100% in the range usually considered to represent "mild" hypertension (90–104 mmHg). Of significance was that 25% of the total cohort (87,000 men) had blood pressures in this range, which included almost 90% of those with high blood pressure. For systolic blood pressure the relative risk began to rise at levels above 125 mmHg, with almost 25% of the excess CHD deaths occurring in those with blood pressure in the 130–139 mmHg range and another 25% in the group with blood pressure levels of 140–149 mmHg. These levels of systolic blood pressure usually are considered as only "borderline" elevated. These data clearly illustrate the enormous magnitude of the total blood pressure problem in the middle-aged U.S. population.

The benefits from treating hypertension in terms of reduced cardiovascular morbidity and mortality are well known in the medical community, although considerable controversy exists regarding the need for pharmacologic intervention in patients with diastolic blood pressures in the "mild" range (90–104 mmHg). The recently concluded Hypertension Detection and Followup Program (HDFP) clearly established the rationale for a "stepped care" antihypertensive drug regimen in this group of mildly hypertensive patients (15). There was a 20% lower mortality rate in patients vigorously treated by this approach compared to those randomized to a "referred care" group for whom treatment was guided by the then-prevailing care in the community. Treatment benefits included significant reductions in fatal and nonfatal stroke, myocardial infarction, angina pectoris, and left ventricular hypertrophy. Other studies have also confirmed the benefits of treating mild hypertension, although the major cardiovascular benefits are reductions in stroke morbidity and mortality (16). Only modest coronary disease prevention, if any, has been reported in the literature, although this is not surprising considering the relatively short duration of most studies compared to the much longer period of time required for coronary disease to progress.

C. Cigarette Smoking

The dramatic decrease in cigarette smoking among physicians in recent years underscores the importance of smoking cessation as the highest-priority preventive strategy in medicine. Smoking is particularly devastating to patients with atherosclerotic diseases, being responsible for an estimated 30% of deaths due to CHD annually (over 160,000 preventable deaths per year) (17). Although the exact mechanisms of tobacco toxicity in ischemic heart disease are not fully understood, nicotine's vasoconstrictive properties and carbon monoxide's ability to damage vascular endothelium are likely candidates in the progression of atherosclerosis.

Barry et al. (18) have recently shown with ambulatory monitoring that smokers with CHD had 3 times the number of ischemic episodes during daily activities and a 12-fold increase in the duration of ischemia compared to nonsmokers with CHD. Most disturbing, however, was that nearly all the ischemic episodes were silent. It is clear from studies such as this that smoking cessation should be given the highest priority among therapeutic interventions directed towards this population.

The good news is that successful smoking cessation has been associated with a reduction in morbidity and mortality from CHD. In 1988 the results of the CASS study showed an almost doubling of the 6 year mortality rate in CHD patients who continued to smoke compared to those who had quit smoking before the study began and had not smoked during the study (19). A number of studies have also shown that the risk of myocardial infarction in both men and women can be significantly reduced with 2 or 3 years of smoking cessation, essentially lowering the risk to that of a nonsmoker (20,21). A more detailed discussion of the cardiovascular hazards of cigarette smoking and strategies for smoking cessation is presented in Chapter 10.

V. REGRESSION OF ATHEROSCLEROSIS

From a preventive perspective, the most exciting evolving concept in athero-sclerosis research is that of regression of the pathologic lesions in the vasculature. Although hyperlipidemic animal models have been used for many years to document reversal of atherosclerosis with the administration of lipid-lowering agents, studies in humans with more advanced and complicated lesions have only recently appeared in the literature. The first studies to document regression of atherosclerosis in humans focused on peripheral vascular disease rather than coronary disease, because the quantitative angiographic techniques used were more easily applied to larger femoral arteries. Early studies from this country and abroad, although uncontrolled and involving small numbers of patients, demon-strated regression of atherosclerotic lesions in 10–30% of patients treated with hypolipidemic regimens (22). Randomized controlled studies reported in the 1980s clearly demonstrated the potential for regression of atherosclerosis in both coronary and peripheral arteries following treatment with lipid-lowering drugs (22).

The results of the Cholesterol Lowering Atherosclerosis Study (CLAS) provide the most compelling evidence to date that hypolipidemic therapy slows progres-sion, stops progression, or promotes regression of coronary atherosclerosis (23). This double-blind, placebo-controlled, randomized trial of 162 patients compared angiographically the effects of combined colestipol and niacin therapy on coronary artery and bypass graft atherosclerotic lesions. After 2 years of drug treatment there was a 26% reduction in total cholesterol, a 43% lowering of LDL–cholesterol, a 37% elevation of HDL–cholesterol, and improved coronary angiographic findings. Atherosclerosis regression was shown in 16% of the treatment group compared to 2.4% of the placebo-treated group. The treatment group also had fewer new lesions and lesions that progressed.

Ornish and his colleagues recently reported the findings of the Lifestyle Heart Trial, which was designed to test the hypothesis that comprehensive lifestyle changes including exercise, low-fat vegetarian diet, smoking cessation, and stress management can favorably alter the progression of coronary atherosclerosis (24). Although small numbers of patients were involved in this randomized clinical trial, there were significant angiographic changes toward regression in the experimental group at 1 year compared to the control group, whose angiograms showed progression of lesions.

The data from these and other studies suggest the potential for slowing, halting, or reversing the progression of existing atherosclerotic lesions and, it is hoped, preventing the development of new lesions. The challenge, therefore, is to identify individuals at high risk for coronary atherosclerosis in order to implement comprehensive preventive programs and reduce the risk of subsequent CHD morbidity and mortality. To meet this most important challenge primary care physicians must be motivated to provide these preventive services.

VI. THE ROLE OF PRACTICING PHYSICIANS

Regarding CHD, the traditional focus of physicians has always been the care of patients with clinically apparent disease: myocardial infarction, angina pectoris, arrhythmias, heart failure, and other symptoms. This disproportionate effort toward the treatment of symptomatic disease is often "too little, too late," since almost half of first coronary disease events result in death, and for those who survive there is often impaired cardiac function and a substantially greater risk of dying in the next 5 years (3). Also, as discussed previously, palliative therapy for advanced coronary disease is extremely expensive and likely to get even more costly as technologies for revascularization, heart replacement, and artificial hearts improve.

Practicing physicians today have an enormous potential for reducing the burden from CHD, since the American public is very receptive to receiving medical advice about preventive lifestyle changes (1). This is also a most opportune time for physicians to expand their systems of practice to incorporate preventive programs. The evidence that significant reductions in coronary events can be achieved by controlling the modifiable risk factors (cigarette smoking, hypertension, and hypercholesterolemia) is unequivocal. Strategies for risk factor intervention have been widely published and could easily be implemented by physicians in clinical practice, given the appropriate economic incentives. Major medical organizations including the American Heart Association, the American College of Cardiology, and the National Institutes of Health have mounted vigorous campaigns to convince physicians of the feasibility and effectiveness of preventive programs. It is time for physicians to take a more active role in the prevention of CHD.

Suggestions for implementing preventive cardiology services in clinical practice have been published in the report of the Bethesda Conference on Prevention of Coronary Heart Disease (25). Risk factor screening should become an integral part of all health care encounters and include information on smoking and exercise habits, blood pressure measurements, estimates of obesity, and lipid studies when appropriate. Physicians should also provide their patients with an estimate of their probability for developing acute coronary events based on age, sex, and risk factors and derived from the American Heart Association's updated "Coronary Risk Profile" (26). This information can also be used to motivate patients to change their lifestyles in order to lower their risk. Physicians who are unable to provide comprehensive preventive services in their offices should have a list of available community or hospital-based risk factor intervention clinics to refer their patients.

Dr. Henry McIntosh, a prominent advocate for preventive cardiology and an internationally renowned cardiologist, has suggested several general office strategies for reducing the risk of CHD (27). First, patients should be encouraged to change from being passive recipients of medical care to active participants by taking responsibility for their own health and well being. Second, physicians, regardless of their specialties, should focus on their patients' overall wellness by identifying modifiable risk factors and offering suggestions for change. Third, since patients generally respect their physician's advice, physicians should insist on positive lifestyle changes. Fourth, physicians should modify their office environments to include literature and other educational offerings dealing with disease prevention and healthy lifestyles. As a final step, patients should be rewarded by their physicians for successful modification of adverse lifestyles and risk factors.

The general public would become much more respectful of the medical profession if we would all follow McIntosh's (27) words of wisdom:

> . . . if a physician is to deserve the exalted stature, granted by society, he or she must have as a major concern, regardless of the degree of specialization or even subspecialization, the adoption by all of his or her patients of a life-style likely to minimize the development or progression or both, of degenerative diseases that will lead to premature morbidity or mortality.

REFERENCES

1. Dismuke SE, Miller ST. Why not share the secrets of good health? JAMA 1983; 249:3181–3.
2. Kottke TE, Blackburn H, Brekke ML, Solberg LI. The systematic practice of preventive cardiology. Am J Cardiol 1987; 59:690–4.
3. American Heart Association. 1991 Heart and Stroke Facts. AHA publication no. 55-0379 (COM).
4. Kannel WB. Meaning of the downward trend in cardiovascular mortality. JAMA 1982; 247:877–80.
5. Goldman L, Cook EF. The decline in ischemic heart disease mortality rates. Ann Intern Med 1984; 101:825–36.
6. Pell S, Fayerweather WE. Trends in the incidence of myocardial infarction and associated mortality and morbidity in a large employed population, 1957–1983. N Engl J Med 1985; 312:1005–11.
7. Letsch SW, Levit KR, Waldo DR. National health expenditures, 1987. Health Care Finance Rev 1989; 10:109–22.
8. Stamler J, Wentworth D, Neaton JD. Is relationship between serum cholesterol and risk of premature death from coronary heart disease continuous and graded? JAMA 1986; 256:2823–8.
9. Hjermann I, Holme I, Velve Byre K, Leven P. Effect of diet and smoking intervention on the incidence of coronary heart disease. Lancet 1981; 2:1303–10.
10. The Lipid Research Clinics Program. The Lipid Research Clinics Coronary Primary Prevention Trial results: I. Reduction in incidence of coronary heart disease. JAMA 1984; 251:351–64.
11. The Lipid Research Clinics Program. The Lipid Research Clinics Coronary Primary Prevention Trial results: II. The relationship of reduction in incidence of coronary heart disease to cholesterol lowering. JAMA 1984; 251:354–74.
12. Frick H, Elo O, Haapa K, et al. Helsinki Heart Study: primary prevention trial with gemfibrozil in middle-aged men with dyslipidemia. N Engl J Med 1987; 317:1237–45.
13. The Expert Panel. Report of the National Cholesterol Education Program Expert Panel on detection, evaluation, and treatment of high blood cholesterol in adults. Arch Intern Med 1988; 148:36–69.
14. Sempos C, Fulwood R, Haines C, et al. The prevalence of high blood cholesterol levels among adults in the United States. JAMA 1989; 262:45–52.
15. Hypertension Detection and Follow-Up Program Cooperative Group. The effect of treatment on mortality in "mild" hypertension. N Engl J Med 1982; 307:976–80.
16. Medical Research Council Working Party. MRC trial of treatment of mild hypertension: principal results. Br Med J 1986; 291:97–99.
17. Health Consequences of Smoking: Cardiovascular Disease: A Report of the Surgeon General. US Dept. of Health and Human Services, 1983, pp. 1–11.
18. Barry J, Mead K, Nabel EG, et al. Effect of smoking on the activity of ischemic heart disease. JAMA 1989; 261:398–402.
19. Hermanson B, Omenn GS, Kronmal RA, et al. Beneficial six-year outcome of

smoking cessation in older men and women with coronary artery disease: results form the CASS registry. N Engl J Med 1988; 319:1365–69.

20. Rosenberg L, Kaufmann DW, Helmvich SB, et al. The risk of myocardial infarction after quitting smoking in men under 55 years of age. N Engl J Med 1985; 313:1511–4.

21. Rosenberg L, Palmer JR, Shapiro S. Decline in the risk of myocardial infarction among women who stop smoking. N Engl J Med 1990; 322:213–7.

22. Blankenhorn DH. Prevention or reversal of atherosclerosis: review of current evidence. Am J Cardiol 1989; 63:38H–41H.

23. Blankenhorn DH, Nessim SA, Johnson RL, et al. Beneficial effects of combined colestipol–niacin therapy on coronary atherosclerosis and coronary venous bypass grafts. JAMA 1987; 257:3233–40.

24. Ornish D, Brown SE, Scherwitz LW, et al. Can lifestyle changes reverse coronary heart disease? The Lifestyle Heart Trial. Lancet 1990; 336:129–33.

25. Reeves TJ, Burnum JF, Farrand M, et al. Task Force 2: the physician in the office (adult medicine). Am J Cardiol 1981; 47:747–66.

26. Anderson KM, Wilson PWF, Odell PM, Kannel WB. An updated coronary risk profile. A statement for health professionals. Circulation 1991; 83:356–62.

27. McIntosh HD. Office strategies to reduce the risk of coronary heart disease. J Am Coll Cardiol 1988; 12:1095–7.

4

Genetics of Atherosclerosis: Can Early Familial Coronary Heart Disease Be Prevented?

ROGER R. WILLIAMS
Cardiovascular Genetics Research Clinic
University of Utah School of Medicine
Salt Lake City, Utah

I. GENETIC MECHANISMS IN ATHEROSCLEROSIS

Figure 1 illustrates multiple causes of coronary heart disease (CHD). They generally can be classified into three major categories: major gene traits that segregate in families and are candidates for specific genetic studies such as linkage and detection of mutations; polygenes, which blend to produce a continuous distribution of both high and low values for continuous traits such as blood pressure and cholesterol level; and environmental factors, which are both shared in families (thus contributing to familial aggregation) and unique to individuals.

As shown in Figure 1, there are overlapping contributions from each of these risk factors in given individuals. A person with high coronary risk from a major gene trait may have this risk either increased or decreased by the background of polygenic factors and by the modifiable environmental factors. Each of these factors will be discussed in greater detail.

A. Familial Aggregation of Early Coronary Heart Disease

Persons with manifestations of CHD such as myocardial infarction or coronary death often have siblings, parents, and even spouses who also have CHD. Since about one-third of all deaths in men and women are due to CHD, one would expect to see multiple cases among family members, especially in older people. However, among adults under age 55 myocardial infarction (MI) occurs in less than 2% of

45

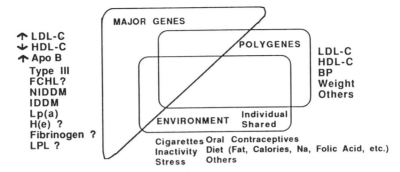

Figure 1 Multifactorial causes of coronary heart disease: major gene traits, polygenetic traits, and environment.

men and less than 0.3% of women (1). When CHD does occur at such an early age, other first-degree relatives will also have CHD in approximately two-thirds of the cases for both men and women (2,3). Families with two or more first-degree relatives with CHD at an early age represent only 2–6% of families in the general population (3,4) and yet they seem to account for approximately half of all cases of early CHD.

B. Genetic and Cultural Heritability of Coronary Risk Factors

Environmental factors such as smoking and dietary habits correlate significantly between spouses as well as blood relatives (5). Offspring often learn these habits from their parents. This sharing of environmental factors in families is sometimes referred to as "cultural heritability." For the major quantitative risk factors for coronary artery disease listed in Table 1, the proportion of the total variability attributable to genetic or cultural heritability has been estimated from the analysis of twins and pedigrees (5). As shown in Table 1, about half of the variability in quantitative coronary risk factors such as blood cholesterol level seems attributable to genetic effects, with measurable substantial cultural heritability also manifest for high-density lipoprotein (HDL)-cholesterol.

C. Polygenic Risk Factors

Both high and low levels of quantitative traits in the general population are usually thought to be due, in large part, to the blended effects of multiple genetic loci. For a trait such as low-density lipoprotein (LDL)-cholesterol, evidence of polygenic effects is clear when a woman with high values marries a man with low values. On average, all of their children will have values approximately half way between the two parents as a result of blending of polygenes. Superimposed upon this

Table 1 Genetic Heritability (H^2) and Cultural Heritability (C^2) of Coronary Risk Factors in Utah Families (%)

Risk factor	H^2 in twins	H^2 in pedigrees	C^2 in pedigrees
Total cholesterol	65	46	0
HDL-cholesterol	51	45	24
Triglycerides	75	13	0
Systolic BP	67	17	7
Diastolic BP	65	25	7
Body mass index	51	21	0

The proportion of total variance attributable to all genetic effects (H^2) or shared family culture (C^2) were estimated from 308 male twins (146 monozygous, 162 dizygous) and from 1102 adults (ages 18–83) in 182 sibships and 301 spouse pairs (5).

polygenic background, one can sometimes observe striking effects of certain major genes such as familial hypercholesterolemia. In general, the most common and pervasive genetic effect on coronary risk factors is due to polygenes in the general population. Whether a person is in the 95th percentile (high risk) or in the 10th percentile (low risk) for LDL-cholesterol, his or her baseline risk for this variable is determined mostly by polygenic effects. Dramatic changes in environment can have an additional effect superimposed upon this polygenic background. A person whose untreated LDL-cholesterol level is in the 90th percentile on a typical high-fat American diet can often drop his or her LDL-cholesterol level to the 75th percentile by strictly adhering to a diet that is very low in cholesterol and saturated fat. However, someone else with a more fortunate set of polygenes may enjoy eating a diet high in saturated fat and cholesterol and still maintain a low LDL-cholesterol level in the 10th percentile. Thus, genetic factors set the general "ballpark" of risk factor levels, but changes in lifestyle can change a person's position within that ballpark.

As indicated in Table 1, other common coronary risk factors such as HDL-cholesterol, blood pressure levels, and body mass index are also determined in large part by polygenic effects. In some persons, HDL-cholesterol, blood pressure, and weight can be significantly improved with lifestyle changes such as consistent aerobic exercise or dietary caloric restriction to encourage weight reduction.

D. Major Gene Coronary Risk Syndromes (Definite and Possible)

Specific major gene loci can dramatically increase risk for early CHD through such traits as high LDL-cholesterol levels in coronary-prone pedigrees. Such CHD risk loci have been inferred from segregation analysis and can be confirmed by genetic linkage analysis or DNA sequencing to detect specific point mutations for some coronary risk factors. This makes it possible to study contributions of individual genes and interacting risk factors for some persons with early familial coronary heart disease (EFCHD).

1. Familial Hypercholesterolemia

Familial hypercholesterolemia (FH) is the best understood genetic cause of EFCHD. FH is a dominantly inherited disorder causing almost twice normal LDL-cholesterol levels already manifest by age 2 and EFCHD at ages 30–60 in men and 50–80 in women (6). Drs. Goldstein and Brown received a Nobel Prize in 1985 for elucidating the LDL receptor defect responsible for this disorder. The gene responsible for LDL receptor defects has been mapped on human chromosome 19 (7).

The following observations support the clinical diagnosis of FH:

  1. Very high total cholesterol (generally above 350 mg/dl in adults over age 30) with normal triglyceride levels (generally below 200 mg/dl in adults).
  2. Children or grandchildren under age 20 who also have very high total cholesterol levels (generally above 250 mg/dl).
  3. Very high blood cholesterol in about half of first-degree relatives (parents, brothers and sisters, children) and normal cholesterol in the other half (i.e., bimodal distribution).

Figure 2 is a labeled diagram of a pedigree with FH. Six brothers in the second generation had early CHD (ages 34–45) and their father died of early CHD. Their strikingly high cholesterol levels (mid-300s) are almost double the 50th percentile for their age (200 mg/dl). About 50% of their offspring also have marked cholesterol elevations, while the other half are normal.

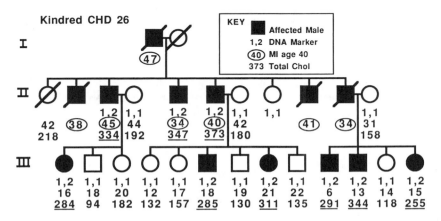

Figure 2 Diagram of a pedigree with familial hypercholesterolemia (FH). Affected men (squares) and women (circles) are shown in solid black. Other symbols are indicated in the key.

Figure 2 also illustrates the results of genetic linkage analysis using a DNA marker for the LDL receptor (7). Two polymorphisms for this locus were detected and tested using DNA extracted from white blood cells. As shown in Figure 2, persons with EFCHD and very high cholesterol levels consistently carry the number 2 allele at this locus. In a large number of relatives sampled by expanding this pedigree, cosegregation was consistently observed, establishing tight linkage without evidence of recombination. In other words, the gene that carries the coding sequence for the structural protein of the LDL receptor has been mapped to a specific location on human chromosome 19. A specific variation of this gene is consistently present in persons with FH in this pedigree. This indicates that the mutation responsible for very high LDL-cholesterol levels in this family is either in the LDL receptor gene or very close to this gene (i.e., genetically linked).

The gene frequency of heterozygotes with this condition has been estimated between 1:200 and 1:500. Although FH is often considered to be rare, the number of persons with FH in the United States is approximately the same as those infected with human immunovirus (8). Without treatment, the risk of early death is approximately the same in persons with FH as it is for acquired immunodeficiency syndrome (AIDS) and yet in contrast to AIDS, FH is currently very treatable. With a combination of diet and multiple prescription medications, most compliant patients with FH can achieve normal cholesterol levels (i.e., reductions from well above the 99th percentile to the 50th percentile). We need to increase public awareness and support for finding and helping persons with FH in parallel to efforts to control other health problems such as AIDS.

Because persons with FH (especially men) have a very high risk of early coronary death and because conscientious treatment can normalize cholesterol levels in these patients, it should be considered malpractice to ignore a patient with FH or to leave family members unscreened. It also ought to be considered poor medical practice to allow a person with FH to experience only partial success from treatment. Some patients on a single drug show a drop in cholesterol levels from 450 to 350 mg/dl. Although this is an improvement, to leave a patient at this level still leaves them at very high risk of early coronary disease. If a primary care physician tries to treat a person with FH for 6–12 months and fails to achieve normal cholesterol levels, the patient should be referred to a specialist who has experience treating many patients with FH.

2. Familial Type III Hyperlipidemia

Like FH, type III is a confirmed major gene abnormality leading to early coronary disease (9). Abnormalities in apolipoprotein E manifest as E2 phenotype result in the accumulation of beta very-low-density lipoprotein (VLDL), a lipoprotein that is highly atherogenic. Several laboratory tests can help identify persons with type III. In most persons, this is a recessive trait with two copies of the apo E2 phenotype detected by polyacrylamide gel electrophoresis. However, many per sons with the E2/E2 phenotype do not have lipid abnormalities or early coronary disease. It is thought that additional factors promoting dyslipidemia interact with this recessive genetic abnormality. Although beta VLDL can only be measured in a few specialized laboratories, the most common laboratory test to help infer this diagnosis is presence of both cholesterol and triglyceride levels above the 90th percentile and a VLDL to triglyceride ratio greater than 0.3 (using mg/dl units). This requires ultracentrifugation to measure actual VLDL levels (9a).

In several population studies, the frequency of the apo E2/E2 genotype varies from about 0.5 to 2.0% (10). The percentage of persons who have at least one E2 allele is estimated to vary from about 8 to 16% (10). Past studies suggest that only a small percentage of persons with E2/E2 phenotype develop serious lipid abnormalities and early atherosclerosis (10). In persons with FH, the E2 phenotype is more threatening. Unpublished findings in Utah FH families show that even one E2 allele (present in about 10% of the general population) can lead to type III hyperlipidemia in about 25% of persons with FH and may dramatically enhance the rate of progression of atherosclerosis, causing coronary disease to occur 10–20 years earlier than in other persons with FH without the apo E allele. Thus at present, the most practical setting in which evaluation of apo E phenotypes might be useful would be in persons who already have diagnosed FH. Also worth noting is the fact that the lipid abnormalities in familial type III hyperlipidemia are usually quite responsive to dietary modifications and medications such as nicotinic acid and gemfibrozil.

3. Familial Combined Hyperlipidemia

Familial combined hyperlipidemia (FCHL) is the most common syndrome of lipid abnormalities in persons with EFCHD. It was present in approximately one-third of population-based families with two or more first-degree relatives with coronary disease under age 55 (11). Unlike FH and type III, the specific genetic and biochemical mechanisms explaining the occurrence of FCHL have not yet been elucidated. It is currently thought that FCHL is probably a heterogeneous group of several different disorders with differing genetic and biochemical mechanisms. It is also possible that two genes may be required for its expression.

The clinical diagnosis is made by observing two or more first-degree relatives who among them have LDL and VLDL-cholesterol (VLDL-C) levels above the 90th percentile (e.g., a man with high LDL-C whose brother has high VLDL-C). As long as the triglyceride level is below 350, LDL-C and VLDL-C can be estimated from the measurements of cholesterol, triglyceride, and HDL. A person with FCHL may have isolated elevated LDL-cholesterol, isolated elevated VLDL-cholesterol, or elevations of both forms of cholesterol. How this may be logical is worth explaining.

VLDL-cholesterol is a precursor of LDL-cholesterol. It is thought that persons with FCHL have an overproduction or increased turnover rate for VLDL-cholesterol. Once they have a genetic tendency to have increased levels of VLDL-cholesterol, their final measured lipid profile would depend upon how quickly VLDL-cholesterol is converted to LDL-cholesterol. If this conversion takes place as an average rate, both LDL-C and VLDL-C will be elevated (i.e., high total cholesterol and triglycerides). If this conversion takes place very rapidly, VLDL-C (and triglycerides) could be normal whereas only LDL-C (and total cholesterol) would be elevated. If conversion takes place very slowly, only VLDL-C (and triglycerides) would be elevated and LDL-C may be normal. Even though the exact genetic and biochemical basis of FCHL has not been determined, some important clinical features described below suggest that it is clinically useful to understand, diagnose, and manage this disorder.

Many patients with FCHL also have low HDL-cholesterol levels, diabetes or glucose intolerance, obesity (especially "central obesity"), and hypertension (11–14). This would indicate that it is important to look for multiple risk factors for EFCHD in persons suspected of FCHL. This emphasizes the need to evaluate all common CHD risk factors in persons with a family history of EFCHD. Once a particular constellation of risk factors is detected in a given individual, practical opportunities for intervention are already well known. For example, two brothers with LDL-C and VLDL-C abnormalities compatible with FCHL may also have low HDL-C levels, moderate obesity, glucose intolerance, and hypertension. In addition to the standard pharmacologic approaches to the treatment of hypertension and lipid abnormalities, these brothers could probably also benefit greatly from regular exercise and dietary modifications. Studies suggest that aerobic exercise and achievable amounts of weight reduction may help resolve all of the abnormalities present in these individuals and may even reduce or eliminate the need for medication (15–17). It is thought that fatty acids and obesity can induce insulin insensitivity, which in turn leads to hyperinsulinemia and a host of subsequent outcomes including aggravation of dyslipidemia, hypertension, diabetes, and eventually early CHD.

4. Isolated Low HDL-Cholesterol

Approximately 15% of families with EFCHD have low HDL-cholesterol level with normal total cholesterol (11). Some of these individuals have elevated triglyceride levels and some of them have pure low HDL-cholesterol (HDL-C). While familial low HDL-C is defined as two or more first-degree relatives below the 10th percentile of standard population data for HDL-C, many of these families show levels well below the fifth percentile. In some cases, this has been shown to segregate as a major gene characteristic and to be associated with coronary heart disease at ages 40–60 (18). It would appear that LDL-cholesterol plays a very important role in persons who have these very low HDL-C levels. Even normal or "permissive" levels of LDL-C would seem to be sufficient to allow the very low HDL-C to promote early CHD. In one Utah family with segregating major gene effects for very low HDL-C (approximately 20 mg/dl), it would appear that they were able to avoid EFCHD because they also had LDL-C levels below the 10th percentile (18).

Persons with familial low HDL-C and a strong family history of EFCHD should be considered as candidates for weight reduction (if obese) and routine aerobic physical activity. In our experience, some will respond quite well and others may not respond at all. Thus it is very important to measure follow-up HDL-C levels to assess the success of these interventions. Since national guidelines are not yet available for the treatment of low HDL-C we are currently dealing with the "art" of medicine. In persons who have very low HDL-C and are not overweight, another dietary approach to consider is reduction of LDL-C using a diet low in cholesterol and saturated fat. It is quite possible for a person with a "permissive" LDL-cholesterol level in the 50th percentile to reduce that below the 10th percentile (i.e., "preventive" levels) to help reduce the risk of future EFCHD. If all nonpharmacologic approaches fail to improve significantly the risk profiles of persons in early CHD families with very low HDL-C, one could also consider the use of several medications such as nicotinic acid or gemfibrozil, which have been shown to raise HDL-C levels significantly. As with any other medications, one must weigh the risks and benefits of treatment and consider the advice of experts as it becomes available through programs such as the National Cholesterol Education Program (19).

5. Familial Dyslipidemic Hypertension

In a study of early familial hypertension, it was discovered that dyslipidemia was the most common concordant biochemical abnormality in two siblings with hypertension diagnosed before the age of 60 (13). The appearance of hypertension together with lipid abnormalities (LDL-C and/or triglyceride > 90th percentile and/or HDL-C below the 20th percentile) has been descriptively labeled familial dyslipidemic hypertension (FDH). Subsequent studies of persons with this disorder (14) have demonstrated high fasting insulin levels, increased frequency of central obesity, high levels of apolipoprotein B, and a strong family history of early coronary disease. FDH was found to be present in 21% of population-based families with EFCHD (11). Some of these persons meet classic criteria for FCHL and others meet criteria for isolated low HDL-C. Treatment of patients with FDH and one of these two lipid disorders can follow the same recommendations described above for FCHL or low HDL-C. When treating patients with FDH, remember that some antihypertensive medications (e.g., diuretics and some beta blockers) may make their lipid abnormalities worse. Thus, diagnosing FDH has practical merit for tailoring the treatment of both hypertension and lipid abnormalities to match the findings of blood tests.

6. Elevated Lipoprotein (a)

Elevations of lipoprotein (a) (Lp(a)) have been associated with a two- or threefold increased risk for CHD and stroke (20–22). While measurement of Lp(a) is currently a research test, it may soon become available from clinical laboratories on ordinary blood samples. About 15% of persons with EFCHD seem to have elevated Lp(a). The gene for the apolipoprotein for Lp(a) has been fully sequenced and shows remarkable homology to the plasminogen gene on chromosome 6, to which high levels of Lp(a) have been genetically linked (23). In a segregation analysis of Lp(a), the genetic heritability estimate was 95% (24). Lp(a) levels can be reduced by treatment with nicotinic acid. Another practical approach to help persons with high Lp(a) should be to modify other coronary risk factors (smoking, dyslipidemia, etc.) to prevent multiplicative interactions that magnify the risk for coronary disease, as discussed below.

7. Elevated Apolipoprotein

Apolipoprotein B (apo B) is the molecule that carries most of the LDL-cholesterol in the blood. Elevated levels of apo B have been observed to segregate as a major gene trait in some pedigrees with EFCHD (25,26). It would appear that the same treatments used for high LDL-cholesterol level would be appropriate for persons with high apo B. More studies need to be done to define exactly how much extra benefit could be gained from measuring and treating high apo B in addition to LDL-cholesterol, since many persons with high apo B have high LDL-C and vice versa.

8. Hyperhomocyst(e)inemia

It has been known for several years that homocystinuria, a rare recessive disorder, is associated with arterial thrombosis and occlusion throughout the body. New laboratory methods make it easier to detect moderately elevated blood levels of homocyst(e)ine, which have been found to be associated with EFCHD in two recent case control studies (27,28). Concordant high levels of homocyst(e)ine (H(e)) seem to be present in approximately 15% of families with EFCHD. The suggestion that high H(e) levels can usually be modified simply by supplementing the diet with folic acid (29) should increase the interest in this risk factor. Intervention and prevention of EFCHD in persons with this risk factor may be even easier than in persons with other more classic risk factors.

9. Diabetes Mellitus

Both insulin-dependent diabetes (IDDM) and non-insulin-dependent diabetes (NIDDM) are well-established risk factors for early coronary disease. Both are thought to occur in large part due to major gene susceptibility, although the exact genetic mechanisms and mode of inheritance have not yet been established for either type of diabetes.

Evidence for major gene susceptibility to IDDM is provided from studies of the human leukocyte antigen (HLA)DR locus. It has been found that the lifetime risk of IDDM is about 3% for persons with DR3/4 heterozygotes compared to only 0.04% for controls (30). Further evidence of the association of diabetes risk with specific HLA genotypes has been found from studies of sibships in which at least one person has IDDM. The risk of IDDM among the other siblings is only 1.1% if they share no HLA haplotypes. The risk increases to 4.4% for siblings sharing one haplotype with an IDDM index case and to 14% for siblings who are HLA identical with the IDDM proband (30).

Although no genetic markers have identified a major gene locus causing susceptibility to NIDDM, it appears to be highly genetic and even more penetrant than IDDM (31). Among identical twins selected for at least one having diabetes, concordance for NIDDM is usually very high (60–90%) whereas concordance for IDDM is usually less than 50% (32–33). Thus, whatever the genetic factors that predispose to NIDDM, they must be quite strong. Many investigators believe that they probably involve some major gene traits.

The exact mechanisms by which diabetes promotes atherosclerosis are not fully understood. Suggested hypotheses include immunologic injury of endothelium for IDDM, dyslipidemia secondary to poor glycemic control for both IDDM and NIDDM, or even the direct effects of insulin itself as a potential coronary risk factor (31). Recent studies show that the duration of NIDDM is not a risk factor for early CHD (31). Studies also show that hyperinsulinemia without diabetes is a prospective risk factor for coronary heart disease (31). The same pathophysiology being considered to explain familial dyslipidemic hypertension may also be in operation in patients with NIDDM. The initial abnormality may actually involve insensitivity to insulin with subsequent hyperinsulinemia and secondary effects of this metabolic imbalance on lipids, hypertension, and other aspects of atherogenesis involving platelets and endothelium. As mentioned above, NIDDM occurs more often than expected among persons with FCHL, and recent unpublished data indicate that FDH is just as common among normoglycemic relatives of diabetic persons as it is among persons with hypertension.

Despite many unanswered questions regarding the exact pathophysiological mechanisms relating diabetes to CHD, several important, practical approaches emerge from our current understanding. In persons with a positive family history of EFCHD, one should also carefully search for a family history of diabetes. When present one should also look carefully for hypertension and lipid abnormalities, which are common in families with NIDDM and even more common in families in which both diabetes and early coronary disease are found. In the near future it may also be common practice to obtain fasting or glucose-stimulated insulin levels to assess coronary risk and the need for intervention. Exercise and dietary modification to reduce weight or control hyperglycemia and hyperlipidemia are reasonable interventions for persons with hyperinsulinemia. The type of diet that helps reduce hyperinsulinemia may also help prevent dyslipidemia and hypertension associated with insulin resistance.

It is important to consider the interaction between diabetes and the commonly associated risk factors of hypertension and dyslipidemia. As with other coronary risk factors, it is suspected that a multiplicative interaction occurs. Two risk factors lead to greater CHD risk than one would expect by simply adding their independent contributions to risk. Especially in diabetic persons with a positive family history of early CHD, one should aggressively screen for and treat high LDL-C, high triglycerides, and low HDL. All are commonly seen in diabetic persons, especially those with poor glycemic control. Careful management to normalize blood glucose levels should be the first step in treatment and often produces significant improvements in all three of these lipid parameters. However, if normalization of glucose levels is not sufficient to produce normal lipid values, treatment with medication should be strongly considered just as hypertension should also be aggressively treated in diabetic subjects to prevent future complications of atherosclerosis, nephropathy, and retinopathy.

10. *Other Potential Genetic Mechanisms*

Other potential genetic mechanisms facilitating atherosclerosis are either very rare or not fully proven (9). Elevated fibrinogen levels are becoming well established as a risk factor for coronary disease (34). The genetic heritability of fibrinogen levels has been estimated at 51% (35) and a significant amount of the determination of plasma fibrinogen levels has been associated with restriction fragment length polymorphisms of the fibrinogen gene (36).

Mutations have been identified for the gene coding for the enzyme lipoprotein lipase (LPL) (37). Persons with one LPL mutation produce normal amounts of a defective enzyme that results in significantly reduced lipoprotein lipase activity. Homozygotes of this condition are very rare and have very high triglyceride levels (mostly in chylomicrons and therefore not atherogenic). However, heterozygotes are much more common and have recently been found to have high VLDL-cholesterol and low HDL-cholesterol levels first manifest after about age 30 (37). Since these lipid abnormalities are known to be associated with increased risk of coronary disease, this could be another major gene predisposition affecting coronary risk. The exact frequency of early coronary disease among persons carrying one copy of this LPL mutation remains to be determined.

Several other rare recessive lipoprotein disorders that have been associated with early CHD include Tangier disease, apolipoprotein E absence, beta-sitosterolemia, cerebrotendinous xanthomatosis, fish eye disease, and lecithin cholesterol acyl transferase deficiency (9). Studying these rare conditions has helped to improve our understanding of the metabolic mechanisms of atherogenesis.

11. *Genetic Syndromes Protecting Against Early CHD*

While discussing genetic mechanisms and early CHD, one should not gain the idea that all genes are bad. Many people in the general population have very high HDL levels and/or very low LDL levels that cannot be attributed to any special dietary maneuvers or other modifications of their environment. Genetic resistance to early CHD is certainly just as interesting and maybe just as common as genetic susceptibility. Some families have been found to have total cholesterol levels below 100 of which only a small fraction is found to be LDL-cholesterol. A study of such a family has identified genetically determined very low levels of apolipoprotein B linked to a DNA polymorphism for the structural gene for this protein (38). Individuals found to carry this gene were often living in their 90s. Many older relatives died from cancer rather than coronary disease. Such families can be identified through a strong family history for longevity.

E. Gene–Environment and Gene–Gene Interactions

Common diseases such as CHD rarely occur from a single risk factor. Even when one major risk factor is identified (e.g., FH), other well-known common coronary risk factors often play a significant role in either accelerating or delaying the progression of atherosclerosis and age at which coronary events occur. One major goal of current research into the causes of CHD is to identify specific gene–environment and gene–gene interactions to explain with greater precision and detail the exact reasons for EFCHD in specific individuals.

1. *Cigarette Smoking*

Cigarette smoking has always been one of the most prominent risk factors in persons with early CHD. In a study of women with CHD before age 55, 48% of them had a history of smoking compared to 16% of age-matched female controls (2). In a study of men dying of CHD by age 45, 84% had a history of cigarette smoking compared to 47% in age-matched male controls (3). In both of these studies, two-thirds of the men and women with early CHD had first-degree relatives with early CHD. Thus, both smoking and a positive family history were very common among these persons with early coronary events, indicating that both risk factors working together help to foster the occurrence of early coronary disease.

The multiplicative interaction of smoking with a positive family history of CHD is illustrated in Figure 3. The two dotted lines in the lower portion of the graph illustrate coronary rates for smokers and nonsmokers in ordinary families without a positive family history. As reported by many population studies, smokers have approximately a doubled risk of CHD compared to nonsmokers (3). This corresponds to approximately 2–3 years difference in longevity between smokers and nonsmokers in the general population. The two solid lines in the

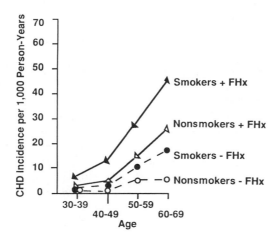

Figure 3 Coronary heart disease incidence rates related to cigarette smoking, family history, and age. Solid lines indicate positive family history (FHx); dotted lines indicate negative FHx; solid circles and triangles indicate smokers; open circles and triangles indicate nonsmokers.

upper portion of the graph illustrate coronary rates among smokers and non-smokers who are relatives of two or more persons with early CHD. Especially at younger ages (30s and 40s), the relative risk for smoking is increased approximately fourfold (rather than doubled), indicating a multiplicative interaction between a positive history and cigarette smoking. A practical example of this has been reported in families with FH in which two affected brothers had dramatically different longevity associated with their smoking status. A brother who smoked died at age 32 whereas a brother with FH who did not smoke died at age 45 (6).

2. *Dietary Fat Intake*
Even in persons with familial hypercholesterolemia, early myocardial infarction in men seems to be dependent upon an interaction with environmental factors. In a family with EFCHD due to FH, Utah pioneer ancestors traced to have this same gene from pedigree analysis were found to survive into their 60s and 80s while living in a frontier environment and consuming a diet devoid of saturated fat and cholesterol (6). Strict dietary fat reduction of current FH descendants following the "pioneer diet" shows that serum cholesterol levels can fall from the mid-300s to mid-200s (6). There are probably more instances of dietary interaction with factors such as folic acid levels influencing homocyst(e)ine in persons with genetic tendencies to high levels, or dietary calorie and fat intake affecting the expression of persons with genetic tendencies toward hyperinsulinemia.

3. *Type III Hyperlipidemia and FH*

Recent unpublished data show a dramatic example of gene–gene interaction leading to early coronary disease. In normal persons, one copy of the E2 allele does not produce elevated levels of beta-VLDL (type III hyperlipidemia) and early coronary disease. However, in persons with familial hypercholesterolemia, one copy of the E2 allele adds significant risk. We have found that one copy of the apo E2 allele results in type III hyperlipidemia and increased beta-VLDL levels in approximately 25% of these persons with both FH and apo E. Furthermore, we have observed an earlier age at onset of CHD manifestations in patients with FH who also have one or more apo E2 alleles. Among five sisters with FH who had one apo E2 allele, coronary disease occurred in the 40s and 50s (about 10–20 years earlier than usual in women with FH). In one young woman with FH and angina pectoris, percutaneous transluminal coronary angioplasty (PTCA) was required at age 28 during her third trimester of pregnancy to avoid myocardial infarction due to severe coronary atherosclerosis. This young woman had a DNA-confirmed LDL receptor defect leading to FH and had two copies of the E2 allele resulting in type III hyperlipidemia. As mentioned above, genetic and biochemical tests make it possible easily to diagnose both FH and type III hyperlipidemia and current medications make it possible to normalize lipid levels in both conditions. Thus, it seems possible that an understanding of gene–gene interactions may help us to detect persons likely to develop myocardial infarctions at very early ages that could be prevented or delayed with proper early diagnosis and focused treatment.

II. TECHNIQUES FOR ASSESSING FAMILY HISTORY AND FINDING HIGH-RISK FAMILIES

Family history assessment is considered to be a standard component of a physician's evaluation of any new patient. When we reviewed hundreds of hospital charts (24), we usually found some mention of family history in the physician's admission notes. However, details were usually very brief and further notes regarding the follow-up and management of patients with early coronary disease seldom reveal any practical application of this information. The goal of this section is to show how a properly collected family history can lead to specific approaches that will help prevent early coronary disease among patients and their close relatives.

A. How Strong a Risk Factor is a Positive Family History?

As shown in Table 2, a positive family history is a strong predictor of future CHD. A weakly positive family history (one parent or sibling with CHD at any age) is found in 38% of adults and predicts about a tripled risk for future CHD among men ages 20–39. In men the same age with a strongly positive family history (two or

Table 2 Relative Risk of Future Coronary Disease According to the Strength of a Positive Family History

Positive family history		Relative risk for CHD	
Definition	Frequency (%)	Men (20–39)	Women (40–49)
2 < age 55	2	12.7	12.9
2 + any age	8	5.9	4.8
1 < age 55	13	3.9	2.5
1 + any age	38	2.9	1.7

Data from 15,250 Utah families (38). "Definition" column indicates number of first-degree relatives experiencing coronary events.

more first-degree relatives with CHD before age 55), the risk of future coronary disease is now increased more than 12-fold (39). Only 2% of men and women in the general population would have such a strong family history, but these are the high-risk persons who should be identified using family history evaluation so that targeted preventive measures can be instituted to lower their familial risk for CHD.

B. Family History: Powerful and Practical for Prevention

Like other tests used to assess coronary risk and design intervention strategies, a medical family history will only lead to practical benefit if the physician collects the data properly and has a plan of what action will be taken depending upon the outcome of the test. When, why, and how to collect a family history and what can be learned from a detailed family history are summarized in Table 3 and discussed below.

1. When and Why Collect a Family History?

There are three clinical settings in which a family history has practical value. In the most important setting, a detailed family history should be collected from all patients with early CHD events occurring before age 55. Data would indicate that approximately two-thirds of these individuals will have other close relatives with early CHD (2,3). If the family history is positive, detailed information you collect will help identify which specific risk factor is responsible and also indicate which close relatives are likely to share the risk and should be screened and treated for this risk factor to help prevent early CHD. For example, a man with MI at age 42 is found to have a total cholesterol of 450 and reports that his older brother and father had coronary events at similar ages and similarly elevated total cholesterol levels. This strongly suggests the diagnosis of familial hypercholesterolemia. This patient's four teenage children and three nieces and nephews (offspring of his affected brother) should all be tested to find the approximately 50% who will also

Table 3 Medical Family History: Powerful and Practical Tool for Prevention

When?	*Why?*
1. Patient with early CHD. MI, CABG, PTCA before 55. Collect detailed family history.	1. In family history is positive find responsible risk factor(s). Help close relatives avoid early CHD.
2. Patient might have early CHD. Possible angina before age 45. Check brief family history.	2. Positive family history increases suspicion, justifying special tests (full blood lipid battery, treadmill ECG, etc.). Confirm diagnosis of coronary artery disease early and help prevent early MI.
3. Routine new patient hisotry. About 2–5% will have strong positive family history of early CHD.	3. Find persons with familial predisposition. Plan targeted screening and risk reduction.

How? (What data should be collected?)
1. Brief: Parents or siblings with MI, CABG, PTCA or death before age 55?
2. Detailed: For parents, siblings, spouse, children, grandparents, aunts, and uncles.
   Age, gender, living or dead, blood relative or not?
   Any evidence of CHD (MI, CABG, PTCA, angina)? Age at first diagnosis?
   Any known risk factors present (lipids, smoking, high blood pressure, diabetes, etc.)?
   Severity of risk factors? Years of exposure? Modification and outcome?

What can be learned from a detailed family history?

1. Does EFCHD run in this family?	5. Know gene or pathophysiology?
2. How strong is the tendency?	6. Which relatives need help?
3. Usual age at MI, death, CABG?	7. Age to start screening?
4. Which risk factors involved?	8. Best way to screen and reduce risk?

CABG = coronary artery bypass graft.

have familial hypercholesterolemia and who can benefit substantially from conscientious dietary and pharmacologic intervention to normalize their blood cholesterol levels.

In the second clinical setting, a family history can be used to help determine the likelihood of a diagnosis of early CHD in a person who has suggestive symptoms. For example, a 35-year-old man who complains of vague chest discomfort might have angina but his symptoms are not typical and diagnostic. His resting electrocardiogram (ECG) is normal and the physician still does not know whether his chest discomfort is due to common ailments such as indigestion or musculoskeletal pain or whether it is due to less likely but more serious coronary atherosclerosis. If a brief family history shows that this person has a brother and father who experienced MIs before age 55, the physician would have a much stronger suspicion of CHD. Because of this strong positive family history, the physician would be justified in ordering special tests such as a full blood lipid battery and treadmill ECG. This can help to diagnose coronary disease at an early stage and lead to measures to help prevent early MI.

The most commonly used setting for family history evaluation is the routine new patient work-up. Only 2–5% of persons in this setting will have a strong positive family history of EFCHD. However, persons who do have this strong family history can then be scheduled for targeted screening and risk reduction.

2. How To Collect a Useful Family History

As a routine screening tool or when evaluating a young man with vague chest discomfort, a brief family history is adequate. Even one simple question is useful as long as the patient fully understands: "Have your mother, father, brothers or sisters, grandparents, aunts or uncles died before age 55 or had any hospitalizations for heart disease before age 55?" (If the answer is yes, further details should be collected regarding myocardial infarction, coronary artery bypass graft surgery or percutaneous transluminal coronary angioplasty, etc.)

Once a family is found that has a serious treatable risk factor for EFCHD (such as familial hypercholesterolemia), a detailed family history is required to find close relatives who need screening and treatment. A detailed family history is also needed if CHD is known to run in a particular family but the exact risk factor mechanism has not yet been identified.

A detailed family history requires the collection of collecting specific information for all first- and second-degree relatives of the affected index case. First-degree relatives include parents, brothers, sisters, and children. While children may be too young to have coronary disease, they are old enough to have risk factors such as IDDM or familial hypercholesterolemia. Second-degree relatives include grandparents, aunts and uncles, and grandchildren.

A detailed family history for each of these persons should determine their age, vital status, and whether or not they are a blood relative (some of them may be adopted or have step relationships). Asking whether they are blood relatives or not is also useful when inquiring about aunts and uncles since social relationships are often equally close to the spouses of aunts and uncles as they are to blood relatives. For any of these persons who have evidence of CHD, it is important to document the age of first diagnosis. Even if CHD is not present, it is important to inquire regarding common risk factors. People usually know if their relatives have problems with obesity, smoking, and serious illnesses such as diabetes. For less prominent risk factors such as hypertension or lipid abnormalities, a positive report often leads to useful information but a negative report has to be considered possibly unreliable. Relatives either may not have been screened for these abnormalities or may not have mentioned routine treatment for these asymptomatic disorders. As we seek to learn more about the responsiveness of specific genetic syndromes to specific diets or medications, it will probably be useful to inquire about the success of specific treatments in close relatives sharing the same genetic predisposition.

3. *What Can Be Learned from a Detailed Family History?*

If you want to assess how successful you have been in collecting useful family history information, see how well it helps you answer the eight questions listed at the bottom of Table 3.

If two or more first-degree relatives experience CHD events before age 55, it clearly runs in the family. Multiple CHD events occurring in older ages may not be more than expected from population rates applied to the age distribution of relatives. For example, two second-degree relatives dying of CHD in their 70s is common and should not be considered a positive family history. The earlier the age of onset of CHD and the larger the number of relatives, the stronger the tendency to CHD. If multiple family members share a common genetic trait leading to early CHD, they will often have a fairly similar age at onset of coronary manifestations such as MI or CHD death. This is illustrated by six brothers with FH illustrated in Figure 1, all of whom had MI between the ages of 35 and 45. This is clinically useful information for cardiologists in deciding whether or not other members of this family with FH need to undergo special tests such as treadmill ECG or coronary angiogram.

Some persons with a positive family history will be able to report that well-known risk factors such as very high cholesterol levels have been found in relatives with early CHD. Often we must contact other family members and their physicians to obtain risk factor information to complete a detailed family history. Because informative blood tests and DNA markers are now becoming available, a complete family history can also include obtaining results of special blood tests from available relatives to define a specific biochemical or genetic syndrome such as FH, type III hyperlipidemia, low HDL-cholesterol, or hyperhomocyst(e)inemia. Just as a bacterial culture and indication of sensitivity will help determine the best antibiotic to use for a patient with a serious infection, making the proper genetic diagnosis through careful family history evaluation and blood tests will also enable a physician to provide the best possible treatment and prevention strategies for persons with specific genetic predispositions to EFCHD.

Treating only patients in your office and ignoring their relatives is not a responsible approach for familial problems such as FH or familial combined hyperlipidemia. A detailed family history should help physicians identify close relatives who need screening. Assessment of risk factors among relatives can also identify unaffected branches of the family that need to be reassured that they do not share the inherited risk found among their relatives.

If a detailed family history evaluation including blood test results in a specific genetic diagnosis, it can answer important questions such as what is the best age to start screening and the best tests to perform and treatments to give. For example, familial hypercholesterolemia is expressed in preschool children whereas most other lipid disorders are not manifest until adult years. For coronary risk associated with low HDL-cholesterol level or high homocyst(e)ine levels, the nonspecific approaches of testing total cholesterol and putting persons with a positive family history on a low-fat diet will not be effective. Specific blood tests are needed to allow physicians to choose screening tests and treatments properly tailored to the genetic syndrome in specific families.

This expanded concept of what constitutes a detailed family history may not sound feasible for the average physician. If it is not feasible for physicians to obtain this kind of information, they should refer their patients with strong positive family history to specialists who are willing to do the type of detailed family history evaluation described above. These physicians who specialize in high-risk families often work with the help of trained nurses, dietitians, and geneticists.

C. Tracing Medical Pedigrees to Find More Early Diagnoses and Prevent Early Deaths (MED PED)

MED PED is a pilot effort sponsored by the U.S. Centers for Disease Control to test the feasibility and cost-effectiveness of pedigree tracing as a public health tool to find and help all persons in Utah with familial hypercholesterolemia. If it works well in Utah, it will be tried in other states. Computerized genealogic methods already in use in Utah could be used to coordinate the tracing of FH pedigrees with members in many states. One seven-generation pedigree in Utah has already led to relatives with FH in 10 other states.

Procedures for project MED PED include the following steps:

1. Ascertain index cases with confirmed FH.
   a. Referrals from physicians treating patients with FH.
   b. Laboratory surveillance for very high LDL-cholesterol levels.
   c. CHD families found in a collaborative "high-risk" family program being carried out by the University of Utah, the Utah Department of Health, and Utah School Districts.
2. Contact index cases by mail and phone to find close relatives needing screening.
3. Use computers and genealogic library tools to extend pedigrees four to seven generations to find many distant relatives with the same FH gene.
4. Encourage all of these persons closely related to cases with FH in high-risk pedigrees to undergo cholesterol tests and receive treatment if they are found to have FH.
5. Assemble and train a network of physicians and dietitians willing to learn and apply state-of-the-art methods to treat FH.
6. Track patients and their treating physicians and dietitians over time to assess their success rate in normalizing cholesterol levels.
7. Assess the cost-effectiveness of this approach compared to conventional cholesterol screening and treatment.
8. Consider the feasibility of expanding this program to other states.

Some aspects of this program could already be implemented by physicians with special interest in FH. Whenever an index case is found it is easy to identify parents, aunts and uncles, brothers and sisters, nieces and nephews, and first cousins. Among these individuals, we often find 5–20 other relatives with FH. Many of them may live in the same community and could be evaluated by the same physician treating the index case.

III. IMPLICATIONS FOR PREVENTING CHD

In the past, some physicians and their patients have falsely assumed "since you can't change your genes, a genetically determined risk of early heart attacks cannot be modified." This false assumption ignores the possibility of using or understanding of gene–environment interaction and new medications essentially to normalize the risk for persons with well-defined genetic disorders such as familial hypercholesterolemia. The emphasis of the details reviewed above is to show how understanding and applying these principles can have a significant benefit to patients in high-risk families.

A. Current Usual Status of Persons in High-Risk Pedigrees

After 14 years' experience working with high-risk families in Utah, we find that most adults with FH have not received sufficient treatment to normalize their cholesterol levels. Many of their school-age children have never had their blood tested for this disorder, and few of them have had intensive counseling by a dietitian who has learned to lower cholesterol levels successfully in persons with inherited dyslipidemias. If the kind of knowledge reviewed above is conscientiously applied, all of this should change.

It is also important to consider more common (but less well defined) familial syndromes such as familial combined hyperlipidemia (FCHL). In our experience studying families with FCHL, we find that very few of these persons have ever received this diagnosis from practicing physicians. This is also true of sibships with strikingly low HDL-cholesterol levels and early CHD. If physicians gain an increased awareness of treatable familial syndromes, they should be more motivated to apply the family history assessment tools described above to find and help these persons.

B. How Preventable is Early Familial CHD?

With the help of proper blood tests, it is relatively easy to diagnose FH and type III hyperlipidemia. Twice-normal LDL-cholesterol levels observed in FH can usually be brought to the 50th percentile with conscientious compliance with diet and one or two medications. The high beta-VLDL and triglyceride levels of type III hyperlipidemia are very responsive to diet and medication. While the CHD risk is very severe without treatment, it seems reasonable to expect that early diagnosis and treatment of these conditions in young adults should lead to relatively normal life expectancy.

Familial combined hyperlipidemia and familial dyslipidemic hypertension are less well defined in terms of pathophysiology but much more common in the general population. Their association with early coronary risk is clear. The constellation of elevated LDL-C and VLDL-C as well as low HDL-C provides a logical explanation for the EFCHD found in these families. Although a consensus on the exact therapeutic approach to these problems (especially high triglyceride and low HDL-C levels) is still being formulated, well-accepted interventions such as weight reduction, aerobic exercise, and well-known prescription medications can normalize the lipid profiles in these patients. Clinical trials are necessary to prove clearly that such treatment will in fact reduce CHD risk; nevertheless, there is precedent for trying to treat and help these persons while waiting for results of such clinical trials. Medications were in common use for hypertension for more than a decade before clinical trials conclusively demonstrated a decreased rate of stroke events among treated hypertensives. Many of us still treat hypertension with the expectation that we are preventing coronary disease despite the fact that clinical trials are still trying to find conclusive proof that antihypertensive therapy could delay or prevent CHD.

Diabetes is well known for its high risk of cardiovascular disease. In the past, much attention has focused on normalizing blood glucose levels in the hopes of preventing early atherosclerosis. Although the debate continues on how effective that approach is, it seems prudent to treat aggressively dyslipidemia, hypertension, and obesity in persons with diabetes, especially in light of the expanding information on the pathophysiological mechanisms involving insulin resistance and hyperinsulinemia.

Regardless of the underlying genetic mechanism for EFCHD, programs to help members of high-risk families stop smoking or to help their children avoid taking up the habit have great practical merit. Data such as those shown in Figure 3 document a strong multiplicative interaction between environmental factors such as smoking and inherited risk. Even if nothing can be done for the primary risk factor, these data would suggest that helping a person with a strong family history of CHD to avoid smoking would probably increase their lifespan by 10–15 years (3,6). Similar interactions may be occurring for other environmental risk factors such as dietary fat intake and physical exercise levels.

New research efforts are opening on the horizon to other approaches for preventing familial CHD. Recent data suggest that homocyst(e)ine will probably be verified as a familial risk factor for early coronary disease. It might be easily treated by simple vitamin therapy with folic acid. Approaches already partially validated using aspirin and other approaches to the participation of platelets and clotting factors in atherogenesis may have even greater utility as fibrinogen and other risk factors in this area are better understood. Lp(a) is highly genetic and a strong risk factor for coronary disease. Niacin therapy helps, but more knowledge is needed regarding potential approaches for intervention. There is hope that a better understanding of the pathophysiology of this and other risk factors could open still other avenues for prevention.

C. High-Risk Families Require High-Intensity Risk Reduction

We often find members of high-risk families getting the same average attention promoted for a general population for coronary risk. This is often inadequate. The difference in normalizing a cholesterol of 265 vs. 450 is very different. A careful evaluation of family history and genetic risk factors can help identify the very-high-risk people who require intensive help. In many cases, this also requires the involvement of a person with special expertise and experience. We suggest that a family physician can try treating one of these persons for 6–12 months. If after that period of time they find they have not normalized risk levels such as cholesterol for a person with FH, they should refer this patient to a specialist who can provide more intensive treatment.

Since many factors such as cigarette smoking show a multiplicative interaction, there is also reason to provide even more intervention on these risk factors. This justifies greater expense and more aggressive encouragement from medical professionals when dealing with members of high-risk families.

D. Future Promise: Gene Markers and Tailored Therapy

In the past, all persons with hypertension were considered "essential hypertensives" and often given the same medications regardless of family history status. Persons with high cholesterol level were also considered in the same category regardless of family history status and treated with the same approach as for lipid intervention. In the future, we should be able to make specific diagnoses based on an exact genetic mechanism and tailor specific medications to a knowledge of the underlying pathophysiology. As a good example of beginning success in this direction, a knowledge of the exact biochemistry of LDL-cholesterol and the LDL receptors led to the development of HMG Co-A-reductase inhibitors, which have helped make normalization of cholesterol levels possible for the first time in history for persons with FH. Nicotinic acid seems to be specific in helping persons with type III hyperlipidemia. Again, the analogy of obtaining a culture and sensitivity for infections seems to be appropriate. Some of our current failures to improve significantly the risk of patients with very low HDL levels or high Lp(a) levels should be overcome in the future as we gain a better understanding of the pathophysiology and obtain focused approaches that utilize that information.

Studies of hypertension indicate that some patients may have specific mechanisms that will be more responsive to angiotensin converting enzyme inhibitors or calcium channel blockers, whereas other persons may have conditions that are responsive to the usual diuretic and beta blocker approaches.

IV. SUMMARY: MAJOR CONCEPTS WORTH REMEMBERING

About half of all coronary events can be accounted for by only 5% of families in the general population that have a strong familial predisposition to EFCHD. Affected persons in high-risk families often share a single concordant risk factor that points to a causal mechanism. Inherited major gene lipid disorders such as familial hypercholesterolemia and type III hyperlipidemia are two good examples and others are rapidly emerging. More common conditions such as familial combined hyperlipidemia and familial dyslipidemic hypertension occur in 2 or 3% of the general population and account for approximately half of EFCHD. While we wait for the exact genetic mechanisms to be determined for these disorders, we already know some practical approaches to help persons with these diagnoses. Cigarette smoking plays a very important role in EFCHD. In conjunction with other risk factors, smoking magnifies their liability and reduces their longevity by 10–15 years. Evidence has been presented for preventing or delaying EFCHD in high-risk families using four practical tools:

1. Precise family history assessment
2. Timely screening of targeted individuals
3. Tailored interventions matched to their risk profile
4. Persistent follow-up to ensure adequate response to prescribed interventions

It is also suggested that we expand our concern to include close relatives to make sure that persons with early coronary risk do not go undiagnosed and untreated until it is too late to prevent EFCHD. Current experience indicates that most patients in high-risk families are probably not getting adequate help. Physicians who learn to apply the principles described in this chapter should have exciting opportunities for finding and helping new patients. Detailed discussions on the management of hyperlipidemia are found in Chapters 7 and 8.

REFERENCES

1. Moriyama I, Krueger, DE, Stamler J. Cardiovascular diseases in the United States. Cambridge, MA: Harvard University Press, 1971.
2. Hunt SC, Blickenstaff K, Hopkins PH, Williams RR. Coronary disease and risk factors in close relatives of Utah women with early coronary death. West J Med 1986; 145:329–34.
3. Hopkins PN, Williams RR, Hunt SC. Magnified risks from cigarette smoking for coronary prone families in Utah. West J Med 1984; 141:196–202.

4. Williams RR, Hunt SC, Barlow GK, Chamberlain RM, Weinberg AD, Cooper HP, Carbonari JP, Gotto AM. Health family trees: a tool for finding and helping young family members of coronary and cancer prone pedigrees in Texas and Utah. Am J Public Health 1988; 78:1283–6.

5. Hunt SC, Hasstedt SJ, Kuida H, Stults BM, Hopkins PN, Williams RR. Genetic heritability and common environmental components of resting and stressed blood pressures, lipids, and body mass index in Utah pedigrees and twins. Am J Epidemiol 1989; 129:625–38.

6. Williams RR, Hasstedt SJ, Wilson DE, Ash KO, Yanowitz FG, Reiber GE, Kuida H. Evidence that men with familial hypercholesterolemia can avoid early coronary death: an analysis of 77 gene carriers in four Utah pedigrees. JAMA 1986; 255:219–24.

7. Leppert MF, Hasstedt SJ, Holm T, O'Connell P, Wu LL, Ash KO, Williams RR, White RL. A DNA probe for the LDL receptor gene is tightly linked to hypercholesterolemia in a pedigree with early coronary disease. Am J Hum Genet 1986; 39:300–6.

8. Heyward WL, Curran JW. The epidemiology of AIDS in the US. Sci Am 1988; 259:72–81.

9. Hopkins PN, Williams RR. Human genetics and coronary heart disease: a public health perspective. Ann Rev Nutr 1989; 9:303–45.

9a. Wu LL, Warnick GR, Wu JT, Williams RR, Lalouel JM. A rapid micro-scale procedure for determination of the total lipid profile. Clin Chem 1989; 35:1486–91.

10. Mahley RW, Rall SC. Type III hyperlipoproteinemia (dysbetalipoproteinemia): the role of apolipoprotein E in normal and abnormal lipoprotein metabolism. In: Scriver CR, Beaudet AL, Sly WS, Valle D, eds. The metabolic basis of inherited disease. 6th ed. New York: McGraw-Hill, 1989: 1195–1213.

11. Williams RR, Hopkins PN, Hunt SC, Wu LL, Hasstedt SJ, Lalouel JM, Ash KO, Stults BM, Kuida H. Population-based frequency of dyslipidemia syndromes in coronary-prone families in Utah. Arch Intern Med 1990; 150:582–8.

12. Iverius PH, Brunzell JD. Obesity and common genetic metabolic disorders. Ann Intern Med 1985; 103:1050–1.

13. Williams RR, Hunt SC, Hopkins PN, Stults BM, Wu LL, Hasstedt SJ, Barlow GK, Stephenson SH, Lalouel JM, Kuida H. Familial dyslipidemic hypertension: evidence from 58 Utah families for a syndrome present in approximately 12% of patients with essential hypertension. JAMA 1988; 259:3579–86.

14. Hunt SC, Wu LL, Hopkins PN, Stults BM, Kuida H, Ramirez ME, Lalouel JM, Williams RR. Apolipoprotein, low density lipoprotein subfraction, and insulin associates with familial combined hyperlipidemia: study of Utah patients with familial dyslipidemic hypertension. Arteriosclerosis 1989; 9:335–44.

15. Kaplan NM. The deadly quartet: upper-body obesity, glucose intolerance, hyper-triglyceridemia, and hypertension. Arch Intern Med 1989; 149:1514–20.

16. Krotkiewski M, Mandroukas K, Sjostrom L, Sullivan L, Wetterqvist H, Bjorntorp P. Effects of long-term physical training on body fat, metabolism, and blood pressure in obesity. Metabolism 1979; 28:650–8.

17. Rocchini AP, Key J, Bondie D, Chico R, Moorehead C, Katch V, Martin M. The effect of weight loss on the sensitivity of blood pressure to sodium in obese adolescents. N Engl J Med 1989; 321:580–5.

18. Hasstedt SJ, Ash KO, Williams RR. A re-examination of major locus hypotheses for high density lipoprotein cholesterol level using 2,170 persons screened in 55 Utah pedigrees. Am J Med Genet 1986; 24:57–67.
19. Grundy SM, Goodman DS, Rifkind BM, et al. The place of HDL in cholesterol management. A perspective from the National Cholesterol Education Program. Arch Intern Med 1989; 149:505–10.
20. Berg K, Dahlen G, Frick MH. Lp(a) lipoprotein and pre-beta$_1$-lipoprotein in patients with coronary heart disease. Clin Genet 1974; 6:230–5.
21. Dahlen G, Berg K, Gillnas T, Ericson C. Lp(a) lipoprotein/pre-beta$_1$-lipoprotein in Swedish middle-aged males and in patients with coronary heart disease. Clin Genet 1975; 7:334–41.
22. Murai A, Miyahara T, Fujimoto N, Matsuda M, Kameyama M. Lp(a) as a risk factor for coronary heart disease and cerebral infarction. Atherosclerosis 1986; 59:199–204.
23. Drayna DT, Hegele RA, Haas P, Emi M, Wu LL, Eaton DL, Lawn RM, Williams RR, White RL, Lalouel JM. Genetic linkage between lipoprotein (a) phenotype and a DNA polymorphism in the plasminogen gene. Genomics 1988; 3:230–6.
24. Hasstedt SJ, Wilson DE, Edwards CQ, Cannon WN, Carmelli D, Williams RR. The genetics of quantitative plasma Lp(a): analysis of a large pedigree. Am J Med Genet 1983; 16:179–88.
25. Kwiterovich PO Jr, Bachorik PS, Smith HH, McKusick VA, Connor WE, et al. Hyperapobetalipoproteinaemia in two families with xanthomas and phytosterolaemia. Lancet 1981; 1:466–9.
26. Hasstedt SJ, Wu LL, Williams RR. Major locus inheritance of apolipoprotein B in Utah pedigrees. Genet Epidemiol 1987; 4:67–76.
27. Williams RR, Malinow MR, Hunt SC, Upson B, Wu LL, Hopkins PN, Stults BM, Kuida H. Hyperhomocyst(e)inemia in Utah siblings with early coronary disease. Coronary Artery Dis 1990; 1:681–5.
28. Genest J (Jr), McNamera JR, Salem DN, Wilson PWF, Schaefer EJ, Malinow MR. Plasma homocyst(e)ine levels in men with premature coronary artery disease. J Am Coll Cardiol 1991;
29. Malinow MR. Hyperhomocyst(e)inemia: A common and easily reversible risk factor for occlusive atherosclerosis. Circulation 1990; 81:2004–6.
30. Ryder LP, Svejgaard A. The association between HLA and insulin-dependent diabetes mellitus (IDDM). In: J Nerup, T Mandrup-Poulsen, B Hokfelt, eds. Genes and gene products in the development of diabetes mellitus: basic and clinical aspects. Amsterdam/New York/Oxford: Excerpta Medica, 1989; 7–21.
31. Williams RR, Schumacher MC, Hunt SC, Wu LL, Hopkins PN, Kuida H. The genetics of hypertension, coronary atherosclerosis, and non insulin dependent diabetes mellitus (NIDDM): heterogeneity and covariation. In: J Nerup, T Mandrup-Poulsen, B Hokfelt, eds. Genes and gene products in the development of diabetes mellitus: basic and clinical aspects. Amsterdam/New York/Oxford: Excerpta Medica, 1989; 387–97.
32. Gottlieb MS, Root HF. Diabetes mellitus in twins. Diabetes 1968; 17:693.
33. Tattersall RB, Pyke DA. Diabetes in identical twins. Lancet 1972; 2:1120.
34. Wilhelmsen L, Svardsudd K, Korsan-Bengsten K, Larsson B, Welin L, et al.

Fibrinogen as a risk factor for stroke and myocardial infarction. N Engl J Med 1984; 311:501–5.

35. Hamsten A, Iselius L, deFaire U, Blomback M. Genetic and cultural inheritance of plasma-fibrinogen concentration. Lancet 1978; 2:988–91.

36. Humphries SE, Cook M, Dubowitz M, Stirling Y, Meade TW. Role of genetic variation at the fibrinogen locus in determination of plasma fibrinogen concentrations. Lancet 1987; 1:1452–5.

37. Wilson DE, Emi M, Iverius PH, Hata A, Wu LL, Hillas E, Williams RR, Lalouel JM. Phenotypic expression of heterozygous lipoprotein lipase deficiency in the extended pedigree of a proband homozygous for a missense mutation. J Clin Invest 1990; 86:735–50.

38. Leppert M, Breslow JL, Wu L, Hasstedt SJ, O'Connell P, Lathrop M, Williams RR, White R, Lalouel JM. Inference of a molecular defect of apolipoprotein B in hypobetalipoproteinemia by linkage analysis in a large kindred. J Clin Invest 1988; 82:847–51.

39. Hunt SC, Williams RR, Barlow GK. A comparison of positive family history definitions for defining risk of future disease. J Chron Dis 1986; 39:809–21.

5

Preventive Cardiology in Children

HERBERT D. RUTTENBERG
University of Utah School of Medicine
Salt Lake City, Utah

I. INTRODUCTION

It is widely believed that coronary atherosclerosis, the precursor to coronary heart disease (CHD), begins in childhood. Of considerable interest, therefore, are the questions: Will the reduction of risk factors during childhood significantly lower the incidence, morbidity, and mortality of CHD in later life? Does the risk/benefit ratio justify the tremendous expenditure of money and time that would be needed to reduce significantly risk factors in children? To answer these questions scientifically would require a prospective, randomized study of a large pediatric population, altering single or combinations of major risk factors in separate but comparable groups of children. Moreover, the experimental and control populations would have to be tracked for 50–60 years. It is very unlikely that this type of investigation will ever be done. Given the enormity of the problem of proving that modifications of risk factors in children will substantially reduce coronary heart disease in adults, we are limited to using circumstantial evidence, tracking studies, and data from adult studies to formulate guidelines for CHD prevention in children.

It is not uncommon in medical practice to begin using a given therapy based on preliminary clinical data. Advances in medicine occur not infrequently by the application of a seemingly logical principle, drug, or technique to a specific disease. In other words, a new therapy or procedure is tried and, if effective, it is implemented in clinical practice, even without the benefit of a prospective, randomized trial. A case in point was the introduction and subsequent use of coronary bypass surgery for the treatment of coronary arterial obstruction.

In the case of atherosclerosis, the vast majority of physicians in cardiovascular medicine have accepted the concept that lowering risk factors will lower CHD morbidity and mortality, even though the concept is not completely supported by hard scientific data (1,2). The application of prevention strategies to children does not have as much widespread support, with the exception of pediatric cardiologists (3). Nevertheless, it is appropriate to address the issue in this chapter. Evidence that atherosclerosis begins in childhood will be reviewed, risk factors in children will be identified, and methods of prevention will be discussed.

II. PEDIATRIC ORIGINS OF CHD

The pediatric age group extends at least through adolescence (18–21 years of age). For the most part, young adults are ignored in atherosclerosis research. Yet studies during the past 40 years have suggested that many young adults already have atherosclerosis, albeit asymptomatic. Moreover, it is very likely that this process started years before they reached adulthood (4).

A. Pathologic Studies

A landmark report was the necropsy study of young American soldiers killed during the Korean War (5). Coronary atherosclerosis was found in 77.3% of 202 soldiers whose ages ranged from 18 to 48 years with a mean age of 22 years. Additional evidence was reported in 1974 (6) from the necropsy study of 105 previously healthy American soldiers killed during the Vietnam War; coronary artery disease was found in 45% of men with an average age of 22.1 years. These studies strongly suggested that if men 22 years of age already had significant atherosclerosis, the disease process must have begun in early childhood. Strong and McGill (7) in 1961 proposed the pediatric origin of coronary artery disease when they found increasing prevalence of fatty streaks in coronary arteries from the first through the third decade of life. The same workers (8) in 1969 demonstrated in almost 5,000 necropsies the gradual progression from fatty streaks to fibrous plaques beginning in late childhood and up to 39 years of age.

Although there is still controversy over the significance of fatty streaks in predicting future CHD, most workers in the field are willing to accept these lesions as precursors to more advanced atherosclerotic plaques (see Chap. 2). Newman and co-workers (9) reported that fatty streaks found in adolescents and young adults correlated with levels of total serum cholesterol (TC, low-density lipoprotein (LDL) cholesterol (LDL-C), and very-low-density (VLDL) cholesterol (VLDL-C), as well as with blood pressure.

B. Tracking Studies

Tracking studies involving longitudinal observations over time have provided an enormous database with which to evaluate coronary risk factors in children. Data from large populations in Bogalusa, Louisiana (10), Muscatine, Iowa (11), Cincinnati (12), and Beaver County, Pennsylvania (13) indicate that CHD risk factors found in children are predictive of future adult levels. These risk factors include abnormal serum lipid and lipoprotein levels, obesity, high blood pressure, diet, use of contraceptive pills or androgenic–anabolic steroids, and cigarette smoking. Most authorities agree that these risk factors are likely to be causal mechanisms in the early stages of atherosclerosis and therefore strongly suggest that prevention of CHD should begin in childhood.

Although tracking cholesterol levels from childhood to adulthood has produced useful data, the most recent analysis from the Muscatine study suggests that many children with high cholesterol levels do not necessarily have high cholesterol levels as adults (14). Using criteria of the National Cholesterol Education Program, the investigators reported that of children with total cholesterol levels above the 75th percentile on two occasions, 75% of girls and 56% of boys would not qualify for hyperlipidemic intervention as adults. Of those with total cholesterol levels above the 90th percentile on 2 occasions, 57% of girls and 30% of boys would not qualify for intervention as adults. However, more sensitive markers of hyperlipidemia such as levels of apolipoproteins A and B are presently being evaluated that might permit investigators to identify higher percentages of children who would be at risk for CHD in adulthood.

C. Risk Factors

In the adult population, coronary risk factors are classified into unalterable risk factors (male sex, family history of premature CHD, and age) and alterable risk factors related to lifestyle (cigarette smoking, diet, sedentary living, use of contraceptive pills or androgenic–anabolic steroids, and stress). Diabetes and hypertension are also important risk factors that can be favorably altered but may not be completely eliminated.

As alluded to earlier, the identification of a coronary risk factor does not necessarily imply that modifying the factor will significantly reduce morbidity and mortality due to CHD. That requires carefully controlled, randomized prospective clinical trials. Although adult studies such as the Lipid Research Clinics Coronary Primary Prevention Trial (15) and the Helsinki Heart Study (16) provided convincing evidence that controlling hyperlipidemia reduces CHD events, no such studies have been performed, or even begun, in children.

III. PREVENTIVE CARDIOLOGY TECHNIQUES IN CHILDREN

If we accept the concept that preventive measures in children might significantly reduce premature CHD in adults, how is this best accomplished? How can the habits of American children be changed to produce healthier lifestyles? Primary health care providers, especially pediatricians and family practitioners, are in an excellent position to accomplish this. This section discusses various aspects of preventive cardiology, including cholesterol screening, smoking cessation, diet modification and weight control, hypertension detection and control, and recommendations for physical activity.

A. Cholesterol Screening in Children

1. *International Studies*

International epidemiologic studies have demonstrated that lipid profiles of American children are considerably more atherogenic than those in other countries. Knuiman and co-workers (17) compared serum lipid levels in boys from 16 countries and found that total serum levels were highest in American boys and boys from some European countries where coronary heart disease is highest. Total cholesterol levels were lowest in West African countries where prevalence of CHD is low. Intermediate levels of total cholesterol were found in the Philippines, Greece, Portugal, and Hungary (Table 1). Lower levels of serum cholesterol in Third World countries were primarily related to lower LDL levels, not to inadequate caloric intake. In populations where the prevalence of adult CHD is low, mean levels of total serum cholesterol in children are 100–150 mg/dl. In popula-

Table 1 Average Serum Total Cholesterol Concentrations in Boys 7 and 8 Years of Age from 16 Countries

Countries	Rural [No.] mmol/L (mg/dl)	Urban [No.] mmol/L (mg/dl)
Africa	3.01 [3] (115.8)	33.5 [3] (128.8)
United States	4.35 (167.3)	—
Asia	3.74 [2] (143.8)	3.93 [2] (151.1)
Europe	4.4 [6] (169.2)	4.4 [9] (169.2)
Finland	5.16 (198.5)	4.82 (185.3)
Greece	3.78 (145.4)	—
Portugal	3.76 (144.6)	3.94 (151.5)

Number in brackets is number of countries. Source: Ref. 17.

tions with a high incidence of adult CHD, total serum cholesterol levels in children are 150–200 mg/dl (18–20).

2. Cholesterol Screening in the Office

As part of the well-child visit, every primary care provider should identify the child who is at risk for CHD in adulthood. Parents should be asked to fill out questionnaires to identify risk factor profiles based on family history, cigarette smoking, diet, level of physical activity, and other diseases such as diabetes, hypertension, and peripheral vascular disease. The physician must follow up the questionnaire with a careful inquiry about family members with cardiovascular diseases, especially before age 55. It is important in taking the family history to ask about these diseases in immediate family members and in their first-degree relatives, including grandparents, uncles, and aunts (see Chap. 3). This should lead to identification of at least 50% of children at risk. There is no controversy regarding the need for cholesterol screening in this group of high-risk children. To evaluate serum lipid and lipoprotein levels in children, it is necessary to have the normal ranges for age, sex, and race available. "Normal" ranges will also vary depending on their ethnic group and where they live. Serum lipid and lipoprotein values for age, sex, and race are found in Tables 2 to 5 (21) and in Figures 1–8 (22).

3. Universal Screening vs. Screening Only High-Risk Children

There is no consensus about the need to screen all children or only "high-risk" children. Although some authorities advocate cholesterol testing only for those

Table 2 Plasma Total Cholesterol (mg/dl) in White and Black Males and Females

	Age (Years)	N	Overall (Mean ± S.E.)	Percentiles						
				5	10	25	50	75	90	95
Black males	0–9	351	165.6 ± 1.5	129	134	148	162	182	201	214
	10–19	1000	160.4 ± 0.8	120	129	142	158	177	195	205
White males	0–4	238	154.6 ± 1.8	114	125	137	151	171	186	203
	5–9	1253	159.9 ± 0.7	121	130	143	159	175	191	203
	10–14	2278	157.6 ± 0.5	119	127	140	155	173	190	202
	15–19	1980	149.9 ± 0.6	113	120	132	146	165	183	197
White females	0–4	186	156.0 ± 2.0	112	120	139	156	172	189	200
	5–9	1118	163.7 ± 0.7	126	134	146	163	179	195	205
	10–14	2087	159.6 ± 0.5	124	131	144	158	174	190	201
	15–19	2079	157.6 ± 0.6	120	127	140	155	172	191	203
Black females	0–9	362	171.3 ± 1.6	128	136	150	170	186	211	222
	10–19	991	165.0 ± 0.9	124	131	146	163	182	202	211

Source: Data from Ref. 21.

Table 3 Plasma LDL-Cholesterol (mg/dl) in White Males and Females

	Age (Years)	N	Overall (Mean ± S.E.)	Percentiles						
				5	10	25	50	75	90	95
White	5–9	131	92.5 ± 1.8	63	69	80	90	103	117	129
males	10–14	284	96.5 ± 1.4	64	72	81	94	109	122	132
	15–19	298	94.4 ± 1.3	62	68	80	93	109	123	130
White fe-	5–9	114	100.4 ± 2.1	68	73	88	98	115	125	140
males	10–14	244	97.3 ± 1.3	68	73	81	94	110	126	136
	15–19	294	95.8 ± 1.5	59	65	78	93	111	129	137

Source: Data from Ref. 21.

children with a family history of premature morbidity or mortality from CHD (23), persuasive arguments can be made in support of universal screening, even though the yield is low. Recent studies (24,25) have shown that screening only high-risk children will miss approximately 50% of children with elevated total cholesterol levels. If cholesterol screening in children is part of a comprehensive, office-based or community-based preventive cardiology program, it may be worthwhile (3).

Universal cholesterol testing in children has not yet been recommended by the American Academy of Pediatrics, the American Academy of Family Practice, or other professional medical societies. Moreover, the guidelines of the National Physicians Cholesterol Education Program do not recommend testing all children. However, many pediatricians have begun to include cholesterol testing in their preschool examinations and have purchased equipment to perform fingerstick total serum cholesterol determinations. This screening test may not be as accurate as a lipoprotein profile performed in a clinical laboratory, but it is reliable to within

Table 4 Plasma HDL-Cholesterol (mg/dl) in White Males and Females

	Age (Years)	N	Overall (Mean ± S.E.)	Percentiles						
				5	10	25	50	75	90	95
White	5–9	142	55.5 ± 1.0	38	42	49	54	63	70	74
males	10–14	296	54.9 ± 0.7	37	40	46	55	61	71	74
	15–19	299	46.1 ± 0.6	30	34	39	46	52	59	63
White fe-	5–9	124	53.2 ± 1.1	36	38	47	52	61	67	73
males	10–14	247	52.2 ± 0.7	37	40	45	52	58	64	70
	15–19	295	52.2 ± 0.7	35	38	43	51	61	68	74

Source: Data from Ref. 21.

Table 5 Plasma Triglycerides (mg/dl) in White and Black Males and Females

	Age (Years)	N	Overall (Mean ± S.E.)	Percentiles						
				5	10	25	50	75	90	95
White	0–4	238	54.6 ± 1.6	29	33	40	51	67	84	99
males	5–9	1253	55.7 ± 0.6	30	33	40	51	65	85	101
	10–14	2278	65.6 ± 0.6	32	37	45	59	78	102	125
	15–19	1980	78.0 ± 0.9	37	43	54	69	91	120	148
Black	0–9	351	52.3 ± 1.0	31	34	40	47	60	75	88
males	10–19	1000	58.6 ± 0.8	31	35	42	53	67	88	102
White	0–4	186	63.9 ± 1.8	34	38	45	59	77	96	112
females	5–9	1118	60.3 ± 0.8	32	36	44	55	71	90	105
	10–14	2087	75.4 ± 0.7	37	44	54	70	90	114	131
	15–19	2079	75.2 ± 0.7	39	44	53	68	87	114	132
Black	0–9	362	55.7 ± 1.2	33	35	41	50	63	83	94
females	10–19	991	64.6 ± 0.8	36	39	47	60	76	95	110

Source: Data from Ref. 21.

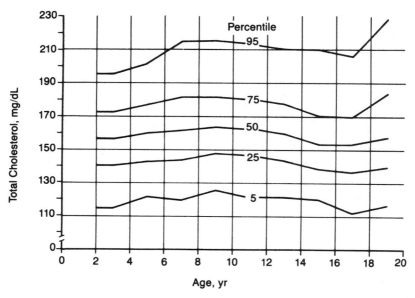

Figure 1 Selected percentiles of serum total cholesterol levels by age for 5,250 fasting children and young adults aged 2–19 years. Three patterns related to age are notable: 1. relatively stable levels from age 2 years until puberty; 2. a decline during adolescence; and 3. a sharp increase between ages 17 and 19 years. (Data from Ref. 22.)

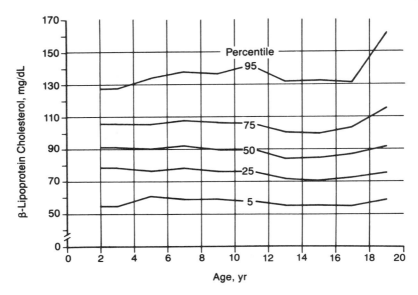

Figure 2   Selected percentiles of serum β-lipoprotein cholesterol (LDL-C) levels by age for 5,250 fasting children and young adults aged 2–19 years. Electrophoretic nomenclature is shown because of laboratory methods. (Data from Ref. 22.)

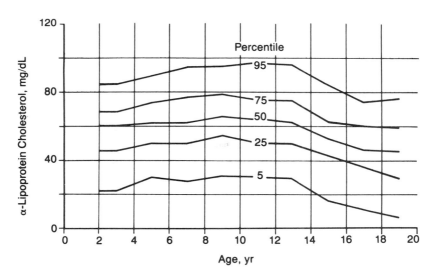

Figure 3   Selected percentiles of serum α-lipoprotein cholesterol (HDL-C) levels by age for 1,730 fasting white boys and young men aged 2–19 years. Electrophoretic nomenclature is shown here because of laboratory methods. A marked decline in levels occurred during adolescence. (Data from Ref. 22.)

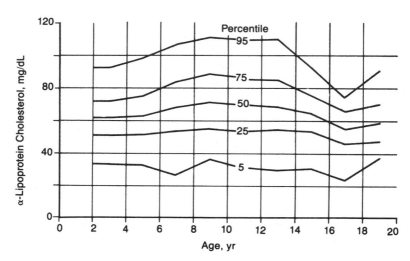

Figure 4 Selected percentiles of serum α-lipoprotein cholesterol (HDL-C) levels by age for 936 fasting black boys and young men aged 2–19 years. (Data from Ref. 22.)

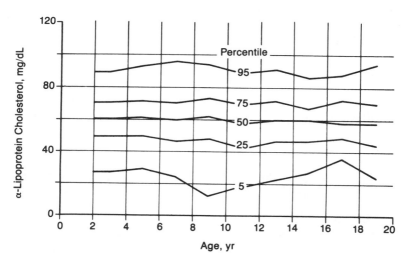

Figure 5 Selected percentiles of serum α-lipoprotein cholesterol (HDL-C) levels by age for 1,684 fasting white girls and young women aged 2–19 years. (Data from Ref. 22.)

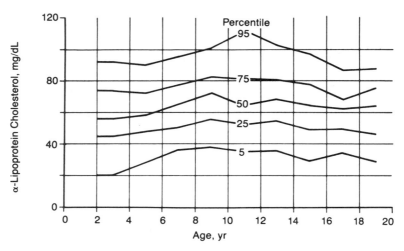

Figure 6   Selected percentiles of serum α-lipoprotein cholesterol (HDL-C) levels by age for 900 fasting black girls and young women aged 2–19 years. (Data from Ref. 22.)

±10%. If abnormally high values are obtained with the fingerstick method, confirmation by a reputable laboratory is recommended.

If routine cholesterol testing in children is used not only to identify high-risk patients but also as an educational opportunity, the cost–benefit ratio becomes more acceptable. Cholesterol testing in conjunction with a preschool examination gives the health care provider an excellent opportunity to teach parents about risk factors for CHD. Most parents are already familiar with the relationship between serum cholesterol and coronary heart disease. When a health care provider sits down with parents and discusses the implications of their child's cholesterol level, parents are likely to be motivated to develop a more healthy lifestyle for the whole family. Educational materials can also be provided at this time. If appropriate, referral to a dietitian may be very helpful in teaching the family how to prepare heart-healthy meals. Another argument in favor of universal cholesterol testing in children is the identification of adult relatives at risk for CHD. Recent studies (26,27) have shown a high prevalence of unrecognized and untreated hyperlipidemia in parents and first-degree relatives of hyperlipidemic children.

4. *Secondary Hyperlipoproteinemias*

Abnormally high serum cholesterol and lipoprotein levels are not uncommon in children and are occasionally secondary to other diseases rather than the result of unhealthy lifestyles or hereditary lipid disorders (Table 6). When these secondary hyperlipoproteinemias are ruled out by results of the usual laboratory and clinical

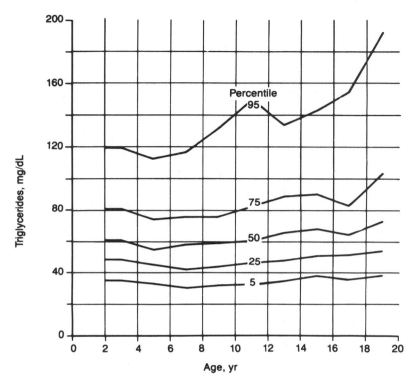

Figure 7   Selected percentiles of serum triglyceride levels by age for 3,414 fasting white children and young adults aged 2–19 years. Percentile levels are higher in white children than black children (Fig. 8) at every age shown. Adolescent increase in levels is most evident at 95th percentile. (Data from Ref. 22.)

investigations, a diagnosis of primary hyperlipoproteinemia is established and appropriate therapy instituted.

5. *Guidelines for Evaluating Serum Lipoproteins*

Guidelines for the management of children and youths aged 2–19 years with abnormal lipoprotein profiles are found in proceedings of the NIH Consensus Conference on Lowering Blood Cholesterol to Prevent Heart Disease (28). When total cholesterol levels are above the 75th percentile for age, sex, and race, a fasting lipoprotein analysis should be made to clarify further the type of hyper-lipidemia. Children with cholesterol levels between the 75th and 90th percentile should be counseled on diet and other risk factors and be rechecked in 1 year. Those above the 90th percentile need special dietary instructions and close supervision with evaluation of all risk factors (Fig. 9). It is important to emphasize

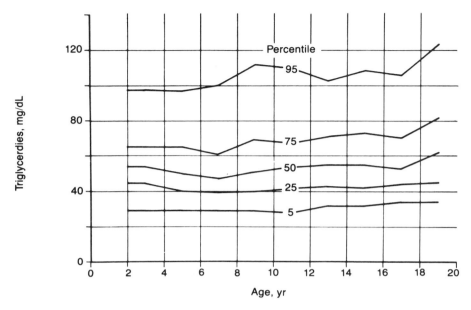

Figure 8   Selected percentiles of serum triglyceride levels by age for 1,836 fasting black children and young adults aged 2–19 years. Percentile levels were lower in black children than in white children (Fig. 7) at every age shown. (Data from Ref. 22.)

Table 6   Secondary Hyperlipoproteinemias: Diseases that Can Cause Dyslipoproteinemias

---

Juvenile-onset diabetes mellitus
Nephrosis and chronic renal failure
Hypothyroidism and Cushing's disease
Drugs and exogenous hormones
  Adrenal steroids
  Contraceptive hormones
  Androgenic–anabolic steroids
  Immunosuppressive drugs
Obstructive liver disease, pancreatitis
Dysgammaglobulinemia
Storage diseases
  Gaucher's disease
  Gierke's disease
  Nieman-Pick disease
Acute intermittent porphyria

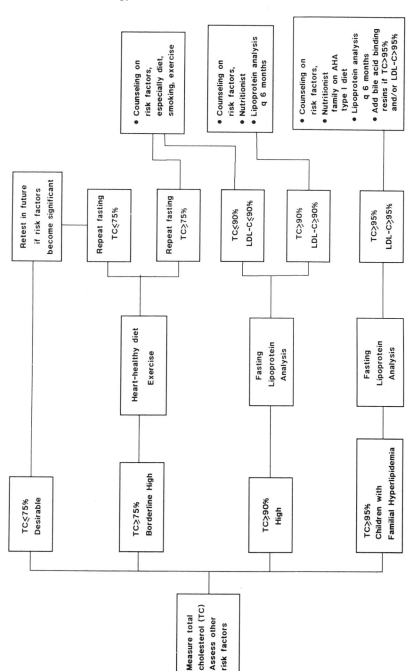

Figure 9 Algorithm for cholesterol screening of children and management of primary hyperlipidemia. %, percentile. See Tables 2–5 and Figures 1–8 for lipoprotein ranges and values.

that these guidelines are based on cumulative data, and there is considerable variation based on sex, race, and ethnic background. Physicians should be prudent in applying these data to their patients.

6. *Management of Children with Abnormal Serum Lipoproteins*

Children with hereditary hyperlipoproteinemias will, with few exceptions, have total cholesterol and LDL cholesterol levels far above the 95th percentile. These children should be referred to a specialized lipid clinic, if possible. Diet alone is rarely effective in reducing lipid levels to normal levels. These children will need drug therapy as well as strict dietary control. Only bile acid sequestrants (cholestyramine and colestipol) are currently approved for use in children. Even with the use of low-fat diets, bile acid sequestrants, weight control, and increased physical activity, many of these children will continue to have levels of total and LDL cholesterol above the 95th percentile. Compliance is also a major problem with these drugs because children do not easily tolerate the side effects of bile acid sequestrants or other drugs such as niacin. 3-hydroxy-3-methyl-glutaryl-coenzyme A (HMGCoA) reductase inhibitors (e.g., lovastatin) have been proven to be very effective in the treatment of hereditary hyperlipidemias in adults and have minimal side effects. Although lovastatin is not yet approved for children, a prospective study is underway and this drug may soon become available for use in patients of this age.

7. *Physician Education*

If preventive cardiology is to become an integral part of pediatric practice, physician education should be a prerequisite. Many primary care physicians are now poorly informed about cardiovascular risk factors. There is an urgent need to educate physicians not only about risk factors but also how to incorporate preventive cardiology into their practice (29). The Physician's Cholesterol Education Program, sponsored by the American Heart Association and the National Institutes of Health, is an excellent example of what is being done to enlighten physicians and prepare them better for this aspect of preventive medicine.

B. Diet and Weight Control

Diet is an important risk factor for several reasons. First, high-risk (atherogenic) diets are associated with high-risk lipoprotein profiles. Second, excessive caloric intake relative to energy expenditure results in obesity, which in itself is a significant risk factor for CHD and type II diabetes mellitus in adults. The high salt content of some diets may also predispose to hypertension.

There is no controversy concerning the effect of diet on blood lipids in children. Many studies have demonstrated the effects of altering dietary cholesterol, saturated, and polyunsaturated fats on blood lipids (30–33). The question remains as to whether a "heart-healthy" diet throughout childhood will alter the morbidity and mortality due to CHD in later life. It is now widely accepted that high serum cholesterol levels are directly related to the prevalence of CHD. Studies (15,16,34) have indicated that for each 1% reduction in blood cholesterol, there is about a 2% reduction in CHD. It is not surprising that leaders in cardiology recommend a "heart-healthy" diet for all Americans. The American Academy of Pediatrics and American Heart Association (35) have also recognized the importance of a low-fat diet and have recommended a "heart-healthy" diet for all children over 2 years of age (Table 7). The Academy, however, believes that a low-fat diet in the first 2 years of life may be deleterious to the rapid growth that occurs during this period. The average infant quadruples its birth weight by 2 years of age. During the early growth period, fat is needed in relatively large quantities for structural lipid as well as for high-energy requirements. There is still controversy concerning what type of fat should be included in the diet in the first years of life and whether "dietary lifestyle" tends to be imprinted on the baby's future behavior.

There is no strong evidence that obesity per se is an independent risk factor in childhood. Studies have demonstrated that childhood obesity is associated with increased serum cholesterol and triglyceride levels and that obesity tends to track from adolescence to young adult years (11,36,37). Also, reversing obesity in children results in reductions in serum cholesterol and triglyceride levels and increases in blood HDL (38). It is likely that obesity indirectly increases the risk of CHD because of its effect on blood lipoproteins and blood pressure and because it is often associated with other negative lifestyle factors such as sedentary living and high-fat diets.

C. Cigarette Smoking

There is no question that cigarette smoking increases morbidity and mortality not only by increasing the risks of CHD (39) but also by increasing the risk of cancer and chronic lung disease. It is unfortunate that while the prevalence of smoking in

Table 7 Step 1 American Heart Association Diet

Dietary components	% of daily calories
Total fat	30
Saturated	10 or *less*
Monounsaturated	10
Polyunsaturated	10
Cholesterol	100 mg/1000 calories, 300 mg maximum daily
Protein	15
Carbohydrate	55% primarily from *complex* carbohydrates

Dietary guidelines for children over 2 years of age who are at risk for CHD as adults.
Source: Ref. 36.

older adults is steadily decreasing, the highest prevalence of smoking is found in teenagers and young adults. A recent study on the effects of cigarette smoking on blood lipids in children 8–19 years of age (40) found increased levels of triglycerides, VLDL, and LDL cholesterol and decreased HDL cholesterol levels, similar to changes found in adults. Tracking studies have shown deleterious effects of cigarette smoking (as well as obesity and oral contraceptive use) in childhood on later adult cholesterol levels and lipoprotein fractions (11,37,41).

Parents should be told that environmental tobacco smoke (ETS) or passive smoking has been shown to be a risk factor for CHD, pulmonary cancer, bronchitis, and asthma. ETS-induced heart disease accounts for 10 times as many deaths as ETS-induced lung cancer, and ETS is the third leading preventable cause of death, after primary (or active) smoking and alcohol (42). A recent study (43) has demonstrated adverse alterations in systemic oxygen transport and lipoprotein profiles in preadolescent children exposed to long-term ETS. This suggests that children exposed to long-term ETS may be at increased risk for CHD.

There is virtually no disagreement that cessation or prevention of cigarette smoking is a very important goal in preventive cardiology, but changing the habits of adolescents and young adults is not easy (44). Primary care physicians have an important role in the promotion of smoking cessation or prevention. Perry and Silvis recommend the following behavioral prescriptions for pediatricians and other primary care providers (45). Their approach to reducing the effects of cigarette smoking is dependent on the age of the child (Table 8).

For *infants*, education of parents on the adverse effects of passive smoking is of primary importance. If parents have confidence in their child's physician, they will be strongly influenced by the advice offered. The infant chronically exposed to tobacco smoke is at high risk for sudden infant death syndrome (SIDS), pneumonia, bronchitis, asthma (46) and, later in life, increased morbidity and mortality from CHD (42). Parents who smoke around their children should be told that they provide unhealthy role models. This concept should increase their motivation to stop smoking.

Children will respond to direct education by the physician during the office visit. The goal in this age group is to prevent the onset of cigarette smoking.

Adolescents are the group at highest risk of beginning to smoke, and they are the most difficult group to influence since advice about the long-term adverse effects of smoking has very little effect. The greatest risk of starting to smoke occurs during the ages of 12–16 years. The most effective approach by the physician is to emphasize the immediate negative physiological and social consequences of smoking. The physiological effects of nicotine are increased heart rate and blood pressure and less steadiness of hand movements. The negative social effects to emphasize are bad breath, smelling of cigarette smoke, and staining of the fingers and teeth. The physician can use a digital ecolyzer, which measures carbon monoxide in the expired air. This will determine if the adolescent patient is

Table 8 Office-Based Strategies to Prevent Smoking and Motivate Children to Stop Smoking

	Objectives	Targets	Strategy
I.	To reduce passive smoking	Parents who smoke	Motivate those who pollute the child's environment to stop smoking by educating parents Discuss smoking habits of parents. Point out multiple risks to their children.
II.	To promote nonsmoking by children	Preadolescent school children	Direct teaching of children by physician. Harmful social and physiological effects. Addiction to nicotine. Misleading tobacco advertisements. Encourage children to oppose smoking by those in their environment.
III.	To influence adolescents to not start or to quit smoking	Adolescent children	Direct education of adolescent. Point out immediate social and physiological adverse consequences. Discuss ways to deal with peer pressure. Provide alternatives to smoking.

smoking, and it offers an opportunity for the physician to discuss the harmful effects of carbon monoxide as well as other negative aspects of smoking. On the positive side, the physician may suggest alternatives to improve lifestyle such as regular aerobic activities, selecting those most attractive to the individual adolescent.

D. Essential Hypertension

Essential hypertension is common in adults and is an important risk factor for CHD. Although high blood pressure is very uncommon in children, there is evidence that the onset of essential hypertension begins in childhood (47). Tracking studies in school children found that blood pressures (BP) did not track as well as height, weight, and serum lipids (9,48,49). Perhaps this was related to the difficulty in obtaining accurate BP in children and the lack of sophisticated tests to seek out hyperresponders and children with labile hypertension. Also, subtle cardiac changes can be detected with mild intermittent hypertension (50), but this has not been tested in the tracking studies. Children at or above the 95th percentile for BP demonstrate echocardiographic evidence of increased left ventricular mass and other hemodynamic abnormalities as well as abnormal electrocardiographic (ECG) findings (50). Racial differences compound the problem; black children, for example, have higher systemic vascular resistance and respond to a high-salt diet to a greater degree than white children (9).

Obesity and fitness are important factors that modify arm blood pressure measurements in children and further complicate interpretation of blood pressure readings. There appears to be an inverse relation between fatness on the one hand and fitness or physical activity on the other (51). The reader is referred to the Report on the Second Task Force on Blood Pressure Control in Children–1987 (52) for more information. The range of blood pressures in normal children from birth to 18 years of age are illustrated in Figures 10–15 and Tables 9 and 10. An algorithm for identifying children with high blood pressure is illustrated in Figure 16 (52).

Accurate and reproducible blood pressures can be obtained in the office setting (Fig. 17) (53). It is very important for primary care physicians to take careful BP measurements on all children and repeat BP determinations at various stages of their development. Only in this way is it possible to identify children at risk for developing hypertension. Once identified, we can try to alter favorably the course of essential hypertension and decrease morbidity and mortality in later life. The first-line treatment of essential hypertension is alteration of lifestyle factors such as diet and weight control, exercise, and reduction of stress. The pharmacologic treatment of systemic hypertension is beyond the scope of this chapter. In general, the antihypertensive drugs used for children are the same as those used for adults (52). The drugs of choice are those that are effective and have minimal side effects. Children do not tolerate unpleasant adverse reactions and are less likely than adults to continue with a drug regimen that makes them feel badly.

E. Physical Activity and Physical Fitness

Sedentary lifestyle is frequently cited as a risk factor for CHD (54,55). Unfortunately, no hard data from randomized trials prove a direct relationship between increased physical activity or a state of high physical fitness and reduced morbidity and mortality from CHD. Very persuasive epidemiologic studies relate increased physical activity with decreased mortality from CHD as well as decreased all-cause mortality (56,57). However, it has not been proven that regular exercise resulting in increased physical fitness has a direct negative influence on the pathogenesis of coronary atherosclerosis. Although this topic is discussed thoroughly in Chapter 12, a brief interpretation of the existing data is offered as an argument to encourage more physical activity in children.

It is likely that a sedentary lifestyle is an important coronary risk factor because of the known effects of physical activity and aerobic fitness on lipid metabolism. Studies in this area suggest that levels of physical activity resulting in increased aerobic capacity are associated with more normal blood levels of total cholesterol, lower levels of LDL cholesterol, and increased levels of HDL cholesterol (58–60). These changes occur in association with decreased body fat and increased lipo-

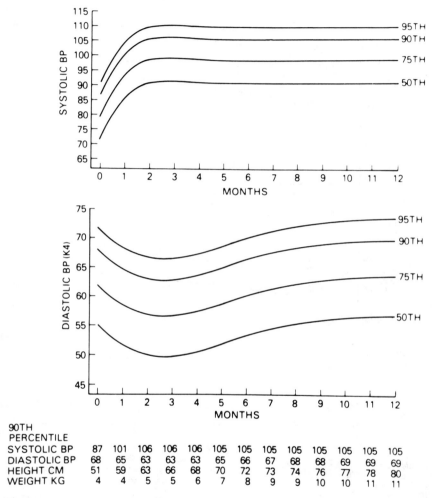

90TH PERCENTILE												
SYSTOLIC BP	87	101	106	106	106	105	105	105	105	105	105	105	105
DIASTOLIC BP	68	65	63	63	63	65	66	67	68	68	69	69	69
HEIGHT CM	51	59	63	66	68	70	72	73	74	76	77	78	80
WEIGHT KG	4	4	5	5	6	7	8	9	9	10	10	11	11

Figure 10 Age-specific percentiles of BP measurements in boys, birth to 12 months of age; Korotkoff phase IV (K4) used for diastolic BP. (Data from Ref. 52.)

protein lipase activity, which probably is responsible for the increased availability of free fatty acids (FFA) for aerobic metabolism. Skeletal muscles of aerobically fit adult males contain two to four times the mitochondrial mass (and thus aerobic enzymes) of sedentary controls (61). Thus, aerobically fit adult males should be able to metabolize carbohydrate and FFA more efficiently than sedentary males. If people with hereditary hyperlipidemias are excluded from this argument,

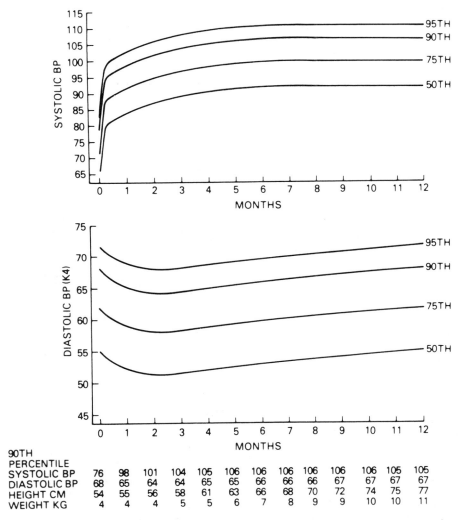

90TH PERCENTILE												
SYSTOLIC BP	76	98	101	104	105	106	106	106	106	106	106	105	105
DIASTOLIC BP	68	65	64	64	65	65	66	66	66	67	67	67	67
HEIGHT CM	54	55	56	58	61	63	66	68	70	72	74	75	77
WEIGHT KG	4	4	4	5	5	6	7	8	9	9	10	10	11

Figure 11   Age-specific percentiles of BP measurements in girls, birth to 12 months of age; Korotkoff phase IV (K4) used for diastolic BP. (Data from Ref. 52.)

normal adults have a limitation on how much dietary fat they can consume without producing obesity and contributing to the atherosclerotic process. In animal experiments involving primates and nonprimates, atherosclerosis and CHD can be produced by atherogenic diets excessively rich in saturated fats and cholesterol. This suggests a "dynamic equilibrium" between food intake and the capacity

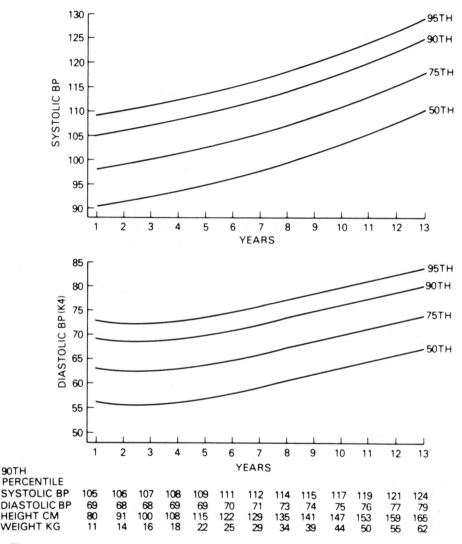

90TH PERCENTILE													
SYSTOLIC BP	105	106	107	108	109	111	112	114	115	117	119	121	124
DIASTOLIC BP	69	68	68	69	69	70	71	73	74	75	76	77	79
HEIGHT CM	80	91	100	108	115	122	129	135	141	147	153	159	165
WEIGHT KG	11	14	16	18	22	25	29	34	39	44	50	55	62

Figure 12 Age-specific percentiles of BP measurements in boys, 1–13 years of age; Korotkoff phase IV (K4) used for diastolic BP. (Data from Ref. 52.)

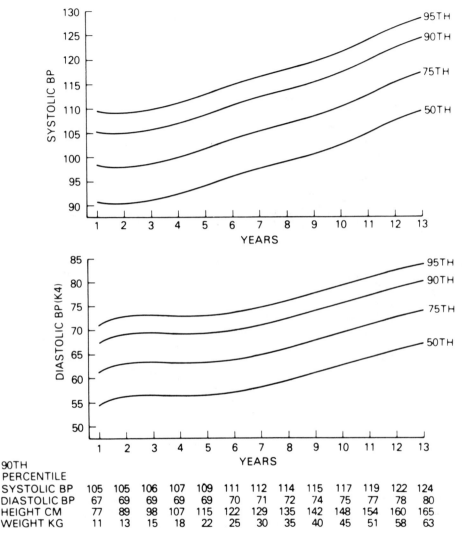

90TH PERCENTILE													
SYSTOLIC BP	105	105	106	107	109	111	112	114	115	117	119	122	124
DIASTOLIC BP	67	69	69	69	69	70	71	72	74	75	77	78	80
HEIGHT CM	77	89	98	107	115	122	129	135	142	148	154	160	165
WEIGHT KG	11	13	15	18	22	25	30	35	40	45	51	58	63

Figure 13 Age-specific percentiles of BP measurements in girls, 1–13 years of age; Korotkoff phase IV (K4) used for diastolic BP. (Data from Ref. 52.)

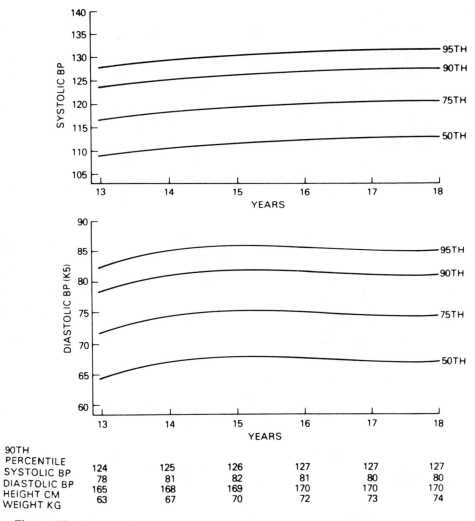

90TH PERCENTILE						
SYSTOLIC BP	124	125	126	127	127	127
DIASTOLIC BP	78	81	82	81	80	80
HEIGHT CM	165	168	169	170	170	170
WEIGHT KG	63	67	70	72	73	74

Figure 14 Age-specific percentiles of BP measurements in boys, 13–18 years of age; Korotkoff phase V (K5) used for diastolic BP. (Data from Ref. 52.)

to utilize the food substrate. Many other factors act on this equilibrium, some of which are known risk factors such as cigarette smoking and androgenic steroids, and others are proposed but still controversial (stress, neuroendocrine factors). It has been conclusively demonstrated not only in nonprimate mammals but also in primates fed an atherogenic diet (62) that regular exercise significantly decreases the morbidity and mortality from atherosclerosis.

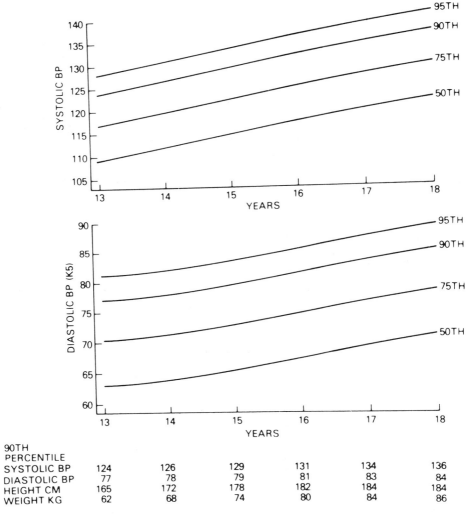

90TH PERCENTILE						
SYSTOLIC BP	124	126	129	131	134	136
DIASTOLIC BP	77	78	79	81	83	84
HEIGHT CM	165	172	178	182	184	184
WEIGHT KG	62	68	74	80	84	86

Figure 15 Age-specific percentiles of BP measurements in girls, 13–18 years of age; Korotkoff phase V (K5) used for diastolic BP. (Data from Ref. 52.)

Although data in humans are circumstantial, they are compelling enough for us to accept tentatively a sedentary lifestyle as a risk factor for CHD in adults. Sedentary is a relative term. How much physical activity is enough? One only has to look back to our ancestors' lifestyles during the previous two centuries, or study "primitive" people in this century, to realize that "civilized" humans are very

Table 9 Definitions of Hypertension

Term	Definition
Normal BP	Systolic and diastolic BPs <90th percentile for age and sex
High normal BP[a]	Average systolic and/or average diastolic BP between 90th and 95th percentiles for age and sex
High BP (hypertension)	Average systolic and/or average diastolic BPs ≥95th percentile for age and sex with measurements obtained on at least three occasions

[a]If the BP reading is high-normal for age but can be accounted for by excess height for age or excess lean body mass for age, BP is considered normal.
Source: Data from Ref. 53.

sedentary. Our ancestors may have had short life spans with early deaths from infections, epidemics, or war, but atherosclerosis was most likely very rare; their daily activity was far greater than that of present day "healthy" humans. In fact, it is likely that the only segment of our civilized society that is as physically active as our ancestors are our children.

It is not surprising that blood lipid profiles of children are usually normal, that is, for a given population or ethnic group. Children tend to have high HDL with

Table 10 Classification of Hypertension by Age Group

Age group	Significant hypertension (mmHg)	Severe hypertension (mmHg)
Newborn		
7 days	Systolic BP ≥ 96	Systolic BP ≥ 106
8–30 days	Systolic BP ≥ 104	Systolic BP ≥ 110
Infant (<2 yr)	Systolic BP ≥ 112	Systolic BP ≥ 118
	Diastolic BP ≥ 74	Diastolic BP ≥ 82
Children (3–5 yr)	Systolic BP ≥ 116	Systolic BP ≥ 124
	Diastolic BP ≥ 76	Diastolic BP ≥ 84
Children (6–9 yr)	Systolic BP ≥ 122	Systolic BP ≥ 130
	Diastolic BP ≥ 78	Diastolic BP ≥ 86
Children (10–12 yr)	Systolic BP ≥ 126	Systolic BP ≥ 134
	Diastolic BP ≥ 82	Diastolic BP ≥ 90
Adolescents (13–15 yr)	Systolic BP ≥ 136	Systolic BP ≥ 144
	Diastolic BP ≥ 86	Diastolic BP ≥ 92
Adolescents (16–18 yr)	Systolic BP ≥ 142	Systolic BP ≥ 150
	Diastolic BP ≥ 92	Diastolic BP ≥ 98

Source: Data from Ref. 52.

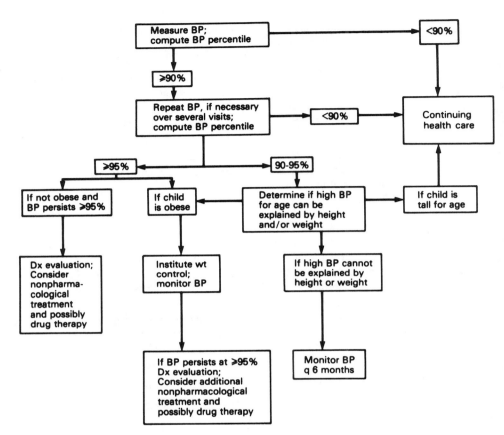

Figure 16   Algorithm for identifying children with high BP. Note: whenever BP measurement is stipulated, the average of at least two measurements should be used. (Data from Ref. 52.)

normal LDL and total cholesterol lipid profiles. Studies of the effects of exercise on blood lipoproteins in children are usually not well controlled for diet and other risk factors such as weight and cigarettes. Nevertheless, some studies have correlated regular aerobic exercise in children with increases in HDL cholesterol (63). However, prospective studies in which diet and weight are controlled have not shown significant changes in blood lipoproteins in children after an aerobic exercise program that effectively improved working capacity (64).

A study of weight training in adolescent boys demonstrated favorable alterations of blood lipids. The study group showed lower LDL, increased HDL, and increased HDL/total cholesterol compared to the control group (65). Rowland in 1985 reviewed all studies in children that evaluated HDL cholesterol changes with exercise and training (66). He concluded that while athletic children may have higher HDL cholesterol than inactive controls, prospective controlled studies did not reveal significant increases in HDL cholesterol. Since exercise-induced weight loss has been shown to be an essential element of HDL response (67), differences in blood lipoproteins in more active children and adults may be more related to lower weight and percentage body fat than to selection (68).

A recent study demonstrated that children who watch television more than 2 hours a day are more likely to have elevated serum cholesterol levels (69). The study did not address the children's eating habits (especially "snacking" while watching television). Of the children with serum cholesterol levels greater than 200 mg/dl, 45% were identified by a family history of myocardial infarction, while 78% of this high-cholesterol group were identified by combining family history with a history of watching television more than 2 hours a day. It seems likely that an accurate history of children's physical activity may be another important factor in identifying high-risk children.

It is reasonable to conclude from existing studies that regular exercise and a more physically active lifestyle are beneficial for many reasons. Physical fitness improves cardiovascular function, reduces blood pressure, increases aerobic capacity and endurance, counteracts obesity, reduces platelet aggregation with facilitation of fibrinolysis, counteracts depression, and improves self-image. It therefore seems reasonable to encourage children to be more physically active and to pursue exercise activities that are enjoyable and that they are likely to continue as adults (Table 11). In this way, we can influence the level of physical activity in the adult population and decrease the risks of a sedentary lifestyle.

It should be obvious that decreasing sedentary time and increasing physical activity are best accomplished in the family setting, especially when the parents are themselves actively involved in exercise activities. Primary care physicians have an important role in encouraging all family members to become physically active and maintain these activities for a lifetime.

IV. SUMMARY AND CONCLUSIONS

It is generally accepted by workers in the field of cardiovascular medicine that atherosclerosis and coronary heart disease begin in childhood. It is also universally agreed upon that smoking, hypertension, diets rich in saturated fats, cholesterol, and calories, and an abnormal blood lipoprotein profile are very important risk factors for atherosclerosis. It is likely that sedentary living, obesity, and stress are also important risk factors, but the evidence is not as complete, and their importance in prevention is not emphasized as much by leaders in preventive cardiology.

Given the early age of origin and the accepted risk factors for atherosclerosis and given the acceptance of the preventive cardiology approach to reducing risk factors, it is reasonable to apply the principles of preventive cardiology to children.

Table 11 Suggested Plan for Children and Adolescents to Increase Their Physical Fitness

---

Limit sedentary activities
    Limit TV watching to 1 hr/day (2 hr/day on weekends)
    Limit computer games to ½ hr/day (1 hr/day on weekends)
    Walk if possible, rather than be driven
      —to and from school
      —to and from shopping
      —to and from friends' homes
Encourage regular participation in aerobic activities
    Bicycle riding
    Long walks with family and friends
    Swimming and other water sports
    Roller skating, ice skating
    Racquet sports (tennis, squash, badminton, table tennis)
    Basketball, volleyball
    Soccer, touch football
    Ice hockey, field hockey
    Cross-country and downhill skiing
    Aerobic, jazz, and ballet dancing

There are two general approaches to the problem: 1. identifying and treating children at high risk for early CHD, and 2. universal screening and application of preventive cardiology principles to all children. These two approaches are not mutually exclusive.

The first approach is now recommended and implemented in clinical practice. The identification of children at risk is usually accomplished with a careful medical history by the primary care provider. The measurement of total serum cholesterol in children from "high-risk" families will identify 50% of all children with elevated cholesterol levels. The child and the child's family should then receive counseling on diet and other lifestyle risk factors and have serum cholesterol levels evaluated periodically. This can be done in the private clinic or in the specialized lipid clinic found in most medical centers.

What about the other 50% of high-risk children who are not identified by family history? The methods of identifying these children are still controversial. Although the yield is low, there is a gradual movement towards universal cholesterol testing in all children, usually during the preschool physical examination.

The prevalence of children with abnormally high total cholesterol levels is low. Since only a small number of children are identified as being at high-risk for CHD, counseling and treatment, as a public health problem, is a small task.

It is a considerably greater task to address the population at large. Applying risk-lowering principles to all children and families would be a major national undertaking that would require a large budget and commitment of staff from the public health sector, the school systems, and local governments. In the long run, this approach may prove to be very effective not only in reducing the risk and prevalence of CHD but also in reducing health care costs.

The key to a successful prevention campaign is education: educating primary care providers, parents, and children. The Cholesterol Education Program for Physicians is already in progress. Primary care physicians must be competent in the diagnosis and management of hyperlipidemias. Parents need to be educated about the importance of a healthy lifestyle for their children's future. The educational process should begin during prenatal visits and especially during the immediate postpartum period when parents (especially mothers) are most receptive to information that promises to protect their babies.

Educating children through the school system should be very effective in promoting a more healthy lifestyle. Children spend a large part of their day in school every year from 5 to 18 years of age. There is ample opportunity to expose them to health care concepts. To teach this subject effectively, however, we need teachers who are well versed in preventive cardiology and a curriculum appropriate for each age group with enough time allowed for the subject to be taught at intervals throughout the school years. In this way, it should be possible to improve futures lifestyles, particularly with regard to smoking and diet.

The universal approach would also require a larger portion of the educational budget to be devoted to training physical education teachers and to providing adequate facilities for physical activities. The ideal goals for adequate facilities would be for each school to have a swimming pool, tennis courts, soccer fields, and basketball courts. More emphasis needs to be placed on involving the majority of children in sports that are not only aerobic but also are the kind of activities they will continue to enjoy as adults.

ACKNOWLEDGMENT

The author is deeply indebted to Kris Sjoblom for editing and typing the manuscript.

REFERENCES

1. The cholesterol facts. A summary of evidence relating dietary fats, serum cholesterol, and coronary heart disease. A Joint Statement by the American Heart Association and the National Heart, Lung, and Blood Institute. Circulation 1990; 81:1721–33.
2. Sytkowski PA, Kannel WB, D'Agostino RB. Changes in risk factors and the decline in mortality form cardiovascular disease. The Framington Heart Study. N Engl J Med 1990; 322:1635–41.

3. Strong WB. You are a preventive cardiologist: The scope of pediatric preventive cardiology. Editorial. Am J Dis Child 1989; 143:1145.

4. Reisman M. Atherosclerosis and pediatrics. J Pediatr 1965; 66:1–7.

5. Enos WF, Holmes RH, Beyer J. Coronary disease among United States soldiers killed in action in Korea. JAMA 1953; 251:1090–3.

6. McNamara JJ, Molot MA, Stremple JF, Cutting RT. Coronary artery disease in combat casualties in Vietnam. JAMA 1971; 216:1185–7.

7. Strong JP, McGill HC Jr. The natural history of atherosclerosis. Am J Pathol 1962; 40: 37–49.

8. Strong JP, McGill HC Jr. The pediatric aspects of atherosclerosis. J Atheroscler Res 1969; 9:152–66.

9. Newman WP III, Freedman DS, Voors AW, Gard PD, Srinivasan SR, Cresanta JL, Williamson GD, Webber LS, Berenson GS. Relation of serum lipoprotein levels and systolic blood pressure to early atherosclerosis: the Bogalusa Study. N Engl J Med 1986; 314:138–44.

10. Berenson GS, Srinivasan SR, Webber LS, Harsha DW, Wattigney W. Cardiovascular risk factors in children—update on the Bogalusa Heart Study. Primary Cardiol 1990; 16:61–72.

11. Lauer RM, Lee J, Clarke WR. Factors affecting the relationship between childhood and adult cholesterol levels: the Muscatine Study. Pediatrics 1988; 82:309–18.

12. Laskarzewski MS, Morrison JA, deGroot I, Kelly KA, Mellies MJ, Khoury P, Glueck CJ. Lipid and lipoprotein tracking in 108 children over a four-year period. Pediatrics 1979; 64:584–91.

13. Orchard TJ, Donahue RP, Kuller LH, Hodge PN, Drash AL. Cholesterol screening in childhood: does it predict adult hypercholesterolemia? The Beaver County experience. J Pediatr 1983; 103:687–91.

14. Lauer RM, Clarke WR. Use of cholesterol measurements in childhood for the prediction of adult hypercholesterolemia. JAMA 1990; 264:3034–8.

15. The Lipid Research Clinics Program. The Lipid Research Clinics Coronary Primary Prevention Trial results. II. The relationship of reduction in incidence of coronary heart disease to cholesterol lowering. JAMA 1984; 251:365–74.

16. Manninen V, Elo O, Frick H, Haapa K, Heinonen OP, Heinsalmi P, Helo P, Huttunen JK, Kaitaniemi P, Koskinen P, Maenpaa H, Malkonen M, Manttari M, Norola S, Pasternack A, Pikkarainen J, Romo M, Sjoblom T, Nikkila EA. Lipid alterations and decline in the incidence of coronary heart disease in the Helsinki Heart Study, JAMA 1988; 260:641–51.

17. Knuiman JT, Hermus RJJ, Hautvast JGAJ. Serum total and high density lipoprotein (HDL) cholesterol concentrations in rural and urban boys from 16 countries. Atherosclerosis 1980; 36:529–37.

18. Golubjatnikov R, Paskey T, Inhorn SL. Serum cholesterol levels of Mexican and Wisconsin school children. Am J Epidemiol 1972; 96:36–9.

19. Connor WE, Cergueira MT, Connor RW, Wallace RB, Malinow MR, Casdorph HR. The plasma lipids, lipoproteins, and diet of the Tarahumara Indians of Mexico. Am J Clin Nutr 1978; 31:1131–42.

20. Blackburn H, Berenson GS, Christakis G, Christian JC, Epstein F, Feinleib M, Havas

S, Heiss G, Heyden S, Jacobs D, Joosens JV, Kagan A, Kannel WB, Morrison JA, Roberts NJ, Tiger L, Wynder EL. Conference on the health effects of blood lipids: optimal distributions for populations. Workshop Report: epidemiological section. Prev Med 1979; 8:612–78.

21. The Lipid Research Clinics Population Studies Data Book. Vol. I: The Prevalence Study. U.S. Department of Health and Human Services, National Institutes of Health Publication 80–1527, Government Printing Office, July 1980.

22. Cresanta JL, Srinivasan SR, Webber LS, Berenson GS. Serum lipid and lipoprotein cholesterol grids for cardiovascular risk screening of children. Am J Dis Child 1984; 138:379–87.

23. Newman TB, Browner WS, Hulley SB. The case against childhood cholesterol screening. JAMA 1990; 264:3039–43.

24. Garcia RE, Moodie DS. Routine cholesterol surveillance in childhood. Pediatrics 1989; 84:751–5.

25. Griffin TC, Christoffel KK, Binns HJ, McGuire PA, the Pediatric Practice Research Group. Family history evaluation as a predictive screen for childhood hyper-cholesterolemia. Pediatrics 1989; 84:365–73.

26. Gidding SS, Whiteside P, Weaver S, Bookstein L, Rosenbaum D, Christoffel K. The child as proband. High prevalence of unrecognized and untreated hyperlipidemia in parents of hyperlipidemic children. Clinical Pediatrics 1989; 28:462–6.

27. Moll PP, Sing CF, Weidman WH, Gordon H, Ellefson RD, Hodgson PA, Kottke BA. Total cholesterol and lipoproteins in school children: Prediction of coronary heart disease in adult relatives. Circulation 1983; 67:127–34.

28. Consensus Conference. Lowering blood cholesterol to prevent heart disease. JAMA 1985; 253:2080–6.

29. Kimm SYS, Payne GH, Lakatos E, Darby C, Sparrow A. Management of cardio-vascular disease risk factors in children. Am J Dis Child 1990; 144:967–72.

30. Carlson SE, DeVoe PW, Barness LA. Effect of infant diets with different polyunsaturated to saturated fat ratios on circulating high-density lipoproteins. J Pediatr Gastroenterol Nutr 1982; 1:303–10.

31. Friedman G, Goldberg SJ. An evaluation of the safety of a low-saturated fat, low-cholesterol diet beginning in infancy. Pediatrics 1976; 58:655–7.

32. Ford CH, McGandy RB, Stare FJ. An institutional approach to the dietary regulation of blood cholesterol in adolescent males. Prev Med 1972; 1:426–45.

33. Cooper R, Allen A, Goldberg R, Trevisan M, Van Horn L, Liu K, Steinhauer M, Rubenstein A, Stamler J. Seventh-Day Adventist adolescents—life-style patterns and cardiovascular risk factors. West J Med 1984; 140:471–7.

34. Steinberg D. The cholesterol controversy is over. Why did it take so long? Circulation 1989; 80:1070–8.

35. Weidman W, Kwiterovich P Jr, Jesse MJ, Nugent E. Diet in the healthy child. Task Force Committee of the Nutrition Committee and the Cardiovascular Disease in the Young Council of the American Heart Association. Circulation 1983; 67:1411A–4A.

36. Smoak CG, Burke GL, Webber LS, Harsha DW, Srinivasan SR, Berenson GS. Relation of obesity to clustering of cardiovascular disease risk factors in children and young adults. The Bogalusa Heart Study. Am J Epidemiol 1987; 125:364–72.

37. Freedman DS, Burke GL, Harsha DW, Srinivasan SR, Cresanta JL, Webber LS, Berenson GS. Relationship of changes in obesity to serum lipid and lipoprotein changes in childhood and adolescence. JAMA 1985; 254:515–20.

38. Epstein LH, Kuller LH, Wing RR, Valoski A, McCurley J. The effect of weight control on lipid changes in obese children. Am J Dis Child 1989; 143:454–7.

39. The health consequences of smoking: cardiovascular disease. In "A Report of the Surgeon General." 1983. Rockville, Md: U.S. Dept. of Health and Human Services.

40. Craig WY, Palomaki GE, Johnson AM, Haddow JE. Cigarette smoking-associated changes in blood lipid and lipoprotein levels in the 8- to 19-year-old age group: a meta-analysis. Pediatrics 1990; 84:155–8.

41. Cardiovascular risk factors from birth to 7 years of age: the Bogalusa Heart Study. Pediatrics (Suppl.) 1987; 80:767–816.

42. Glantz SA, Parmley WW. Passive smoking and heart disease: epidemiology, physiology, and biochemistry. Circulation 1991; 83 (In Press).

43. Moskowitz WB, Mosteller M, Schieken RM, Bossano R, Hewitt JK, Bodurtha JN, Segrest JP. Lipoprotein and oxygen transport alterations in passive smoking preadolescent children. The MCV Twin Study. Circulation 1990; 81:586–92.

44. Walter HJ, Hoffman A, Vaughan RD, Wynder EL. Modification of risk factors for coronary heart disease. Five-year results of a school-based intervention trial. N Engl J Med 1988; 318:1093–100.

45. Perry CL, Silvis GL. Smoking prevention: behavioral prescriptions for the pediatrician. Pediatrics 1987; 79:790–9.

46. Weitzman M, Gortmaker S, Walker DK, Sobol A. Maternal smoking and childhood asthma. Pediatrics 1990; 85:505–11.

47. Voors AW, Webber LS, Berenson GS. Epidemiology of essential hypertension in youth—implications for clinical practice. Pediatr Clin North Am 1978; 25:15–27.

48. Clarke WR, Schrott HG, Leaverton PE, Connor WE, Lauer RM. Tracking of blood lipids and blood pressures in school age children: the Muscatine Study. Circulation 1978; 58:626–34.

49. Michels VV, Bergstralh EJ, Hoverman VR, O'Fallon WM, Weidman WH. Tracking and prediction of blood pressure in children. Mayo Clin Proc 1987; 62:875–81.

50. Soto LF, Kikuchi DA, Arcilla RA, Savage DD, Berenson GS. Echocardiographic functions and blood pressure levels in children and young adults from a biracial population: the Bogalusa Heart Study. Am J Med Sci 1989; 297:271–9.

51. Gutin B, Basch C, Shea S. Contento I, DeLozier M, Rips J, Irigoyen M, Zybert P. Blood pressure, fitness, and fatness in 5- and 6-year-old children. JAMA 1990; 264:11233–7.

52. Report of the Second Task Force on Blood Pressure Control in Children—1987. Pediatrics 1987; 79:1–25.

53. Park MK, Menard SM. Normative oscillometric blood pressure values in the first 5 years in an office setting. Am J Dis Child 1989; 143:860–4.

54. Astrand P-O. Exercise physiology and its role in disease prevention and in rehabilitation. Arch Phys Rehab 1987; 68:305–8.

55. Powell KE, Thompson PD, Caspersen CJ, Kendrick JS. Physical activity and the incidence of coronary heart disease. Annu Rev Public Health 1987; 8:253–87.

56. Blair SN, Kohl HW III, Paffenbarger RS Jr, Clark DG, Cooper KH, Gibbons LW. Physical fitness and all-cause mortality. A prospective study of healthy men and women. JAMA 1989; 262:2395–401.

57. Paffenbarger RS Jr, Hyde RT, Wing AL, Hsieh C-C. Physical activity, all-cause mortality and longevity of college alumni. N Engl J Med 1986; 314:605–13.

58. Williams PT, Wood PD, Haskell WL, Vranizan K. The effects of running mileage and duration on plasma lipoprotein levels. JAMA 1982; 247:2674–9.

59. Wood PD, Haskell WL, Blair SN, Williams PT, Krauss RM, Lindgren FT, Albers JJ, Ho PH, Farquhar JW. Increased exercise level and plasma lipoprotein concentrations: a one-year randomized controlled study in sedentary, middle-age men. Metabolism 1983; 32:31–9.

60. Thompson PD, Cullinane EM, Sady SP, Flynn MM, Bernier DN, Kantor MA, Saritelli AL, Herbert PN. Modest changes in high-density lipoprotein concentration and metabolism with prolonged exercise training. Circulation 1988; 78:25–34.

61. Saltin B, Gollnick PD. Skeletal muscle adaptability: significance for metabolism and performance. In: Pezchy LD, Adrian RH, Geiger SR, eds. Handbook of physiology, Section 10, Skeletal muscle. Baltimore: Williams and Wilkins, 1983; 555–631.

62. Kramsch DM, Aspen AJ, Abramowitz BM. Reduction of coronary atherosclerosis by moderate conditioning exercise in monkeys on an atherogenic diet. N Engl J Med 1981; 305:1483–9.

63. Nizankowska-Blaz T, Abramowicz T. Effects of intensive physical training on serum lipids and lipoproteins. Acta Paediatr Scand 1983; 72:357–9.

64. Linder CW, DuRant RH, Gray RG, Harkess JW. The effects of exercise on serum lipid levels in children. Clin Res (abstr) 1979; 27:797A.

65. Fripp RR, Hodgson JL. Effect of resistive training on plasma lipid and lipoprotein levels in male adolescents. J Pediatr 1987; 111:926–31.

66. Rowland TW. Exercise and atherosclerosis in children and adolescents. Cardiovasc Rev Rep 1985; 6:851–7.

67. Williams PT, Wood PD, Krauss RM, Haskell WL, Vranizan KM, Blair SN, Terry R, Farquhar JW. Does weight loss cause the exercise-induced increase in plasma high density lipoproteins? Atherosclerosis 1983; 47:173.

68. Krauss RM. Exercise, lipoproteins, and coronary artery disease. Circulation 1989; 79:1143–5.

69. Hei TK, Gold KV, Ququndah PY, Wong ND. A comparison of television viewing habits and family history of myocardial infarction as cholesterol screening indicators in children. Circulation (abstr) 1990; 82(III):227.

6

The Periodic Health Evaluation with Emphasis on Cardiovascular Risk Assessment

TED D. ADAMS
The Fitness Institute
LDS Hospital
and University of Utah
Salt Lake City, Utah

JOHN H. HOLBROOK
University of Utah School of Medicine
Salt Lake City, Utah

In a recent "Position Statement," The American Heart Association (1) stated:

> "The American Heart Association (AHA) takes the position that prevention is the *greatest need* in cardiovascular medicine. The association is committed to the belief that many cardiovascular diseases, particularly atherosclerotic disease, can be *prevented*." (*italics* added)

Undergirding this position statement is the effective inclusion and management of preventive patient services: periodic medical screening, lifestyle counseling, and immunizations and chemoprophylaxis. When these preventive services are systematically integrated into patient care, the physician and the patient have greater assurance that 1. all has been done to minimize early death and disability, 2. identification and planned modification of individual risk factors have been implemented, and 3. counseling about healthy lifestyle practices in an effort to alter personal health behaviors has been addressed.

This chapter discusses recommendations for systematically incorporating preventive services for the apparently healthy patient population in an office practice. The cornerstone of these recommendations, the periodic health examination (PHE), will be reviewed with attention given to individualizing the PHE to the

105

patient's age, gender, and risk. The assessment of cardiovascular risk, an integral component of the PHE, will also be carefully delineated. The background and scientific basis for the PHE will be addressed, including the critical need to integrate into the PHE lifestyle counseling topics such as physical activity, nutrition, and preventing injuries and sexually transmitted diseases. The future demand to computerize preventive services will also be discussed.

I. BACKGROUND

The concept of period health screening and health maintenance is not new. As early as the turn of the century medical professionals were beginning to advocate this notion. In the year 1900 an oculist by the name of G.M. Gould introduced the need for periodic health examinations (2,3). While addressing the American Medical Association, he said:

> Based on the fact actually felt by every physician, that a series of systematized periodic examinations of patients apparently well would often reveal beginning diseases, prevent future illnesses, and increase the vital values of life, everyone can prevail upon patients, students and members of his family to undergo the necessary tests. . . . It is the catching sight of the forerunning indication of disease, the symptom of a symptom, the functional beginning of organic abnormalism, that a large deal of progress lies.

Approximately 20 years later, in the early 1920s, the American Medical Association and the Metropolitan Life Insurance Company, convinced of the long-term health benefits of an annual check-up, officially supported the periodic examination of asymptomatic people (4,5). For almost 50 years the endorsement by the American Medical Association to have an annual medical "check-up" became a household word. Following World War II, and as early as 1955, multiphasic testing for various types of cancer began to be introduced (4). The American Dental Society also became very active in encouraging regular dental check-ups.

During the 1970s the need for an annual check-up began to be questioned by physicians and other medical scientists. These concerns were largely the result of an increased awareness of costs, a greater involvement by patients regarding their expectations of medical care, and an improved methodology to examine the basis for various health procedures (6–10). Major efforts were undertaken to analyze periodic medical screening data and to make recommendations to practicing physicians regarding the type and frequency of screening tests. Criteria generally used in analyzing periodic medical evaluation data have included the following

1. Whether the disease (or condition) significantly affects the person's life span or quality of life
2. Whether treatment of the disease, before symptoms occur, will reduce the impact of the disease and prolong life span

3. Whether adequate treatment is available if the disease or condition is discovered
4. Whether the screening procedures for the disease are both acceptable to the patient and can be performed at a reasonable cost
5. Whether the treatment administered during the nonsymptomatic phase of the disease will be "superior to that obtained by delaying treatment until symptoms appear"
6. Whether enough people are affected by the disease or condition to justify the screening costs (10–12)

The first efforts to survey adult health maintenance and make recommendations regarding preventive services were made by Frame and Carlson in 1975 (11–14). They developed preventive screening guidelines for 36 selected diseases based upon incidence and prevalence of disease, progression of disease (with and without treatment), risk factors for disease, and the overall availability of screening tests. Their recommendations also suggested that tests used for screening apparently healthy individuals be based upon age and gender. In 1986, Frame updated these recommendations for primary care physicians (15–18).

Perhaps the most noted analysis was conducted by a large Canadian medical task force in 1979, referred to as the Canadian Task Force on the Periodic Health Examination. Similar to Frame and Carlson's adult maintenance approach, this group of medical specialists, clinicians, and scientists recommended that the popular annual physical examination be abandoned, suggesting instead that physicians use a periodic testing approach based on age and sex-specific recommendations (19). This group identified 78 major medical conditions that were affecting Canadians and had the potential of being prevented. The task force recommended a number of health protection packages based on conditions thought to be preventable at each stage of life. The content and frequency of testing of these packages varied with age and gender (19). Not only did the task force propose that individuals follow a periodic health examination rather than a routine annual check-up, but it also suggested that some tests traditionally performed as part of the routine examination be eliminated. For example, it recommended that routine chest x-rays and electrocardiograms be discontinued. With updates in 1984, 1986, and 1988, this task force (20–22) continues to review the efficacy and frequency of procedures used for periodic screening. Although the task force analysis was a major contribution in health maintenance, additional important reasons for performing the periodic health examination (Table 1) were not included as part of the developmental criteria of the Canadian Task Force (23).

In 1981, the Medical Practice Committee of the American College of Physicians (ACP) also recommended that the annual physical examination be replaced with periodic preventive clinical services. This committee compared the recommendations of Frame and Carlson (11–14), Breslow and Somers (24), the Canadian

Table 1 Selected Purposes of the PHE

Purpose	Example
Prevent disease	Immunize against infection
Detect asymptomatic disease	Hypertension
Identify risk factors	Hypercholesterolemia
Assess cardiovascular risk ratio	Probability score for developing CHD
Update comprehensive database	Allergic drug reaction
Facilitate patient–physician communication	Review how to reach physician during an emergency
Counsel on unhealthy behavior	Failure to wear seat belts
Promote healthy behavior	Give exercise prescription
Provide data for third parties	Respond to insurance company questionnaire

Source: From Ref. 23, with permission.

Task Force (19), and the American Cancer Society (25) and recommended guidelines for physician use. The ACP has recently updated these recommendations (26). The revised recommendations include the review of preventive guidelines of the United States Preventive Services Task Force and other "well-known authorities" (26).

In 1987, the American Heart Association (AHA) published a Position Statement that set forth the recommendations of the PHE with particular emphasis on the detection of silent coronary heart disease and coronary risk factors (1). Specific AHA recommendations will be considered later in this chapter. Other periodic health examination recommendations have also been published by a number of professional medical organizations and researchers (Table 2).

A significant contribution to the periodic health examination literature was completed in 1989 by the U.S. Preventive Services Task Force. The 20-member task force, commissioned in 1984 by the Assistant Secretary for Health in the

Table 2 Guidelines Sources for PHE

Breslow and Somers (24)	American Cancer Society (25,27,28)
The National Cancer Institute Early Detection Branch (29,30)	The Institute of Medicine (31)
	The American College of Physicians
The Mayo Clinic (32)	(10,26)
The Carter Center—closing the health policy gap (34)	The American Medical Association (33)
	The Henry Ford Hospital (36)
The National Cholesterol Education Program (37)	Holbrook (23,35)

Source: From Ref. 23, with permission.

Department of Health and Human Services, spent 4 years to develop preventive services recommendations for all age groups. Their comprehensive report provides "recommendations for clinical practice on more than 100 preventive interventions—screening tests, counseling interventions, immunizations, and chemoprophylactic regimens—for the prevention of 60 target conditions" (39,40). Scheduled tables have been prepared by the task force outlining the recommended preventive interventions for all age groups and risk categories. In addition to recommendations regarding immunizations and clinical screening tests, the task force emphasized the vital role of physicians in counseling patients to improve personal health behaviors relating to cigarette smoking, physical activity, nutrition, injuries, and sexually transmitted diseases.

A careful review of the various guidelines presented by these clinical investigators and medical agencies reveals a lack of agreement pertaining to what interventions should be included in the PHE and how often these components should be provided. In large degree the controversy stems from the sparsity of adequate research for validating recommendations. Despite some disagreement regarding preventive services recommendations, there is a clear consensus that a periodic health evaluation should be the principal component of the healthy patient's clinical care, with a major emphasis on preventing disease and promoting health (23). Moreover there is almost complete unanimity among clinicians regarding the need to identify or evaluate cardiovascular risk factors for the purpose of preventing or controlling coronary heart disease. There is also general agreement that the PHE should be streamlined based on age, gender, and risk, and include personal health behavior counseling.

II. SCIENTIFIC BASIS

Despite the increasing popularity of medical screening, only one long-term prospective study has been conducted to assess the periodic health examination. This study, initiated in 1964, involved over 10,000 members of the Kaiser Foundation Health Plan (7,41). These participants were randomly assigned to two groups: a control group and a group receiving regular periodic health examinations (the periodic health examinations included more comprehensive and expensive medical tests than those recommended for current use). Results after 11 years of follow up showed that the periodic health check-up group had lower death rates from potentially preventable causes in the 35–54 year age group, and in this group there was a cost savings of $2100 per male participant (6–8). Similar savings were not found, however, in women and younger men. This study also revealed a trend towards earlier detection of colon cancer and reduced mortality from hypertension and colorectal cancer in those participating in the periodic health examination. Medical tracking of participants has now extended for over 16 years (41).

The most comprehensive analysis of existing scientific evidence on the PHE and preventive intervention services has been compiled by the U.S. Preventive Services Task Force (39,40). A very thorough review of the risk factors associated with cardiovascular disease and the relative risk ratios of these factors has also been documented by Grundy and colleagues (1). The National Cancer Institute's Early Detection Branch has carefully examined the scientific evidence associated with cancer screening (29,30). These references, coupled with the recent ACP recommendations (26), serve as invaluable resources for primary care physicians.

Although long-term prospective studies of the efficacy of the PHE are few, several prospective and cross-sectional scientific investigations have been conducted to assess the health benefits of cardiovascular risk factor identification and intervention (1,23). These studies have focused primarily on cigarette smoking, blood pressure, hypercholesterolemia, body weight and body fat, plasma glucose, physical activity, and behavioral characteristics (1).

The identification of cardiovascular risk factors in the healthy population and the implementation of risk intervention strategies have been clearly demonstrated to reduce morbidity and mortality. More detailed information on the beneficial health impact of coronary risk assessment and intervention is found in other chapters of this book.

III. CONTENT

A. Health Questionnaire

A well-organized health questionnaire can make it easier to obtain a comprehensive health history of the patient and allow the physician more time to interact with the patient in discussing particular issues gleaned from the questionnaire. The suggested contents of this questionnaire are listed in Table 3. A detailed health questionnaire with an emphasis on CHD prevention is included as Appendix 1 at the end of this chapter. It is recommended that the questionnaire be mailed to the patient before the initial office visit and that the completed questionnaire be reviewed by the physician before seeing the patient.

If possible, the questionnaire should be designed to facilitate easy computer entry. Commercially developed computerized patient files are now available for medical office use and in the future, standardized (in-depth) health questionnaires may become available to help streamline patient record keeping.

B. Initial and Interim Assessments

The initial patient visit should be as thorough as possible to generate a comprehensive database (35). The American Heart Association recommends that patients be asked about a history of "rheumatic fever, heart murmur, hypertension, anemia, and the use of drugs, tobacco, alcohol, and medications," and that the physician make detailed inquiry regarding the patient's family history for "heart disease,

Table 3 Recommended Contents of the Health Questionnaire

General information
  Demographic data, past physicians, medical insurance information
Past medical history
  Past illnesses, hospitalizations, operations, procedures
  Medications, drug reactions, allergies
  Information on heart disease, stroke, hypertension, hypercholesterolemia, diabetes, and
    their treatments
  Current medical problems
Review of systems
  Chest discomfort, dyspnea, palpitations, syncope
Lifestyle history
  Cigarette smoking, alcohol consumption, dietary history, physical activity habits, psy-
    chological data
  Occupational/environmental exposures
Family history
  Early familial coronary heart disease (see Chap. 4)
  Early familial cancer

hypertension, hyperlipidemia, stroke, peripheral vascular disease, heart murmur, diabetes mellitus, and congenital heart disease" (1). The initial interview is an excellent opportunity to stress the important concept that the patient assume a greater responsibility for his or her health (39) and follow a periodic health matrix based upon age, gender, and individual risk. In addition the initial interview provides an opportunity to discuss further the patient's current personal health practices. Data should be obtained regarding sleep patterns, dietary and exercise habits, substance abuse, seat belt usage, and sexual practices. The patient's social environment should also be assessed, including relationships with spouse, family members, friends, and co-workers, and the patient's perception of daily stress. Attention should be given to identifiable coronary risk factors and cancer risk factors. If the history suggests the need for greater patient surveillance, plans for additional follow-up should be made at this time.

The interim history is not as time consuming to take as the initial history and should concentrate on significant events since the previous visit (23). This visit promotes patient/physician rapport and might permit especially sensitive personal information such as alcohol and other drug use or sexual behavior to be discussed (23). Table 4 highlights data that can be included as part of the interim visit.

It is important to become familiar with the leading causes of mortality and morbidity associated with various age groups in order to ask age-specific questions during the interim visit. In particular, the 10 leading causes of death among the age groups 25–44 years and 45–64 years are listed in Table 5 (42).

Table 4 Interim History

Elicit new signs or symptoms
Obtain interval past history
  Hospitalizations
  Visits to other physicians
  Medications
  Allergic reactions
  Accidents
  Occupational and environmental exposures
  Unhealthy behavior
  Diet
  Exercise
  Sexual practices
  Contraception
  Social history
  Family history
Review and update problem list
Review screening tests and immunization checklist

Source: From Ref. 23, with permission.

Careful inspection of Table 5 suggests the need to focus on cancer and cardiovascular risk factors among both age groups, to inquire about seat belt usage and smoking in both groups, and to assess life stress and sexual practices among the younger group (25–44 years). The patient should be made aware of the leading causes of death in his or her age group. Because many of these causes of death are

Table 5 Ten Leading Causes of Death Among Adults According to Age

Ages 25–44	Ages 45–64
1. Accidents (vehicular and other)	1. Malignant neoplasms
2. Malignant neoplasms	2. Diseases of the heart
3. Diseases of the heart	3. Cerebrovascular diseases
4. Suicide	4. Accidents (vehicular and other)
5. Homicide and legal intervention	5. Chronic obstructive lung disease
6. Acquired immune deficiency syndrome	6. Chronic liver disease and cirrhosis
7. Chronic liver disease and cirrhosis	7. Diabetes mellitus
8. Cerebrovascular disease	8. Suicide
9. Pneumonia and influenza	9. Pneumonia and influenza
10. Diabetes mellitus	10. Homicide and legal intervention

related to lifestyle issues, this information can help convince patients that they are responsible for their own health and well-being. The leading causes of death can serve as a motivational tool and a springboard for discussing positive lifestyle changes such as improving dietary and exercise habits, and performing periodic cancer screening. The interim visit also serves as a vehicle for following the periodic health matrix, which may include a physical examination, other screening tests, and immunizations.

C. Basic Physical Examination

The basic physical examination contains maneuvers *basic* to all ages (Table 6) and *specific* components that are justified on the basis of age and risk. The traditional or basic physical examination can generally be performed by an experienced physician in 10–15 min (23).

As delineated in Table 6, this examination facilitates screening for several clinical disorders including cancer of the breast, testicle, thyroid, oral cavity, skin, prostate, lymphatics, and rectum (23). During the examination, the patient can be instructed on how to perform self-examination of the breasts, skin, oral cavity, and testicles. Providing instruction during the examination reduces the potential anxiety felt by the patient and at the same time heightens patients' interest in their own health maintenance. Specific maneuvers performed in addition to those in Table 6 should be included if the patient's age, history, or physical examination warrant inclusion. The American Heart Association Task Force suggests that during the physical examination careful attention be given to the cardiovascular system (Table 7) (1).

Although different recommendations exist regarding the frequency of a periodic physical examination, we suggest the following schedule for apparently healthy individuals: every 5 years for ages 19–29, every 4 years for ages 30–39, every 3 years for ages 40–49, every 3 years for ages 50–59, and yearly for ages 60 and older.

D. Laboratory/Diagnostic Procedures

Wide variation of opinion exists regarding what laboratory/diagnostic procedures should be included as part of a periodic health maintenance program. A thorough literature review of the principal clinical screening tests has been completed by the U.S. Preventive Services Task Force (39,40). In addition, the National Cholesterol Education Program Committee has published a detailed report on the detection, evaluation, and treatment of hyperlipidemia in the adult (37).

In many instances little if any research data exist either to support or refute the inclusion of specific laboratory tests. When there is insufficient data supporting a particular screening test, it is generally not recommended for routine use. To date however, conclusive evidence exists supporting the need to screen for breast

Table 6 Basic Physical Examination

Patient Sitting
1. Inspect general appearance
   Inspect hands, nails, skin, joints
   Palpate, compare and count radial (wrist) pulses
2. Measure blood pressure
3. Inspect face and head
   Test visual acuity
   Inspect conjunctiva and sclera
   Test pupillary reaction to light
   Perform ophthalmoscopy
4. Examine ears, externally and with otoscope
   Inspect nose
   Inspect mouth (gums and teeth)
   Test hearing
5. Test range of neck motion
   Palpate neck for nodes and thyroid
6. Observe chest symmetry with deep breath
   Percuss and auscultate lung fields

Patient Supine
7. Palpate breast and axillary nodes
   Inspect neck veins and palpate carotid arteries
   Inspect and palpate precordium
8. Auscultate heart
9. Inspect and palpate abdomen
   Palpate for liver and spleen
   Palpate inguinal nodes and femoral pulses
10. Inspect legs
    Check for edema
    Palpate dorsalis pedis pulses
    Test plantar flexion reflexes

Patient Sitting
11. Inspect breast for asymmetry, retraction (in women)
12. Test nervous system; wrinkle forehead, show teeth, protrude tongue, test biceps, knee and ankle reflexes

Patient Standing
13. Observe gait
    Examine male genitalia:
        Inspect and palpate penis, epididymis, testes, and inguinal canals for hernia
        Perform rectal and prostate examination

Patient Supine
    Examine female genitalia:
        Inspect external genitalia
        Inspect vaginal vault with speculum
        Palpate vagina, cervix, uterus and ovaries
        Perform rectal examination

Source: From Ref. 23, with permission.

Table 7 Examining the Cardiovascular System

---

1. Evaluation of rate, rhythm, and contour of arterial and venous pulsations.
2. Measurements of blood pressure (both arms) with the patient supine or seated and standing.
3. Examination for carotid bruits.
4. Ocular examination for corneal arcus and changes in the fundus, including arterial narrowing, arteriovenous compression, hemorrhages, exudates, and papilledema.
5. Examination of the heart for rate, rhythm, character of apex impulse, other precordial impulses, heart murmurs, third or fourth heart sounds or gallops, ejection or nonejection clicks; the heart should be examined with the patient both recumbent and standing whenever possible.
6. Examination of the chest for configuration, motion and respiration, presence of rales or transmitted heart murmurs.
7. Examination of the abdomen for bruits, enlarged kidneys, or other organs, and digitation of the aorta.
8. Examination of the extremities for diminution or absence of peripheral arterial pulsations, edema, clubbing, and varicose veins.
9. Examination of the nervous system.

Source: From Ref. 1, with permission.

cancer, cervical cancer, and hypercholesterolemia (23). Recommended laboratory tests that screen for the above disorders include the mammogram, Papanicolaou test, and serum cholesterol measurement. Although the data are not definite regarding recommendations for colorectal cancer screening, on balance the evidence favors periodic screening. Age and frequency recommendations for these tests are considered below. For elderly persons evidence also suggests that periodic visual and hearing tests be performed (39).

Although many physicians include urinalysis, complete blood count, CBC, chemical profile, chest x-ray, and electrocardiogram as routine laboratory components, these procedures are *not* recommended as periodic screening tests (23,39).

E. Immunizations/Vaccinations

Pneumococcal disease and influenza are major causes of death and disability in the United States (43), and tetanus remains a serious threat to inadequately immunized individuals (44). There is general consensus that adults should have a tetanus/diphtheria booster every 10 years; this is especially important for individuals over age 50 (43). People aged 65 and older and younger individuals at increased risk should have a yearly influenza vaccination. Adults aged 65 and older and others at increased risk for pneumococcal infection should also receive a pneumococcal vaccination at least once (43). There is some evidence that among high-risk groups a pneumococcal revaccination should be performed 6 years after the initial vaccination (43).

Individuals who work in health-related jobs where there is frequent exposure to blood or blood products should be counseled regarding the need for hepatitis B vaccine (45–47). Finally women of childbearing age who lack immunity to measles and mumps should receive a measles–mumps–rubella vaccination (23,43). Care should be taken not to administer this vaccine to pregnant patients.

F. Lifestyle Counseling

This component of the periodic health examination has usually received little attention by primary care physicians. Reasons for not providing educational and lifestyle counseling have included 1. the notion that physician's efforts should be primarily devoted to the treatment of illness (39,40), 2. the time spent in educating patients regarding diet, exercise, or smoking cessation may not receive adequate remuneration, and 3. the physician may not be adequately trained in counseling procedures and therefore feel ill at ease in this setting (23).

Regardless of the reasons there is increasing need or expectation for physicians to instruct their patients about healthy lifestyles. In the recent U.S. Preventive Services Task Force guidelines, Dr. Robert Lawrence, chairman of the task force, states the following:

> Primary care clinicians have a key role in screening for many of these problems (*referring to heart disease, cancer, accidents, etc.*) and immunizing against others. Of equal importance, however is the clinician's role in counseling patients to change unhealthy behaviors related to diet, smoking, exercise, injuries, and sexually transmitted diseases. . . . It is our belief that the "new morbidity" of injuries, infections, and chronic diseases demands a new paradigm for prevention in primary care—one that includes counseling about safety belt use and diet as well as giving immunizations and screening for cancer (39,40). (italics added)

Studies have verified that physicians have a significant impact influencing patients' personal health behaviors and habits such as using seat belts or smoking cessation (23). It is anticipated that increasing numbers of physicians will align themselves with allied health professionals such as nutritionists and exercise specialists, who are trained to instruct patients in changing unhealthy behaviors.

G. Cardiovascular Risk Profiles

In conjunction with lifestyle counseling, risk profiles for coronary heart disease should be calculated and discussed with the patient. A risk profile is the probability of developing clinical coronary heart disease in a defined period of time according to specific risk-factor characteristics. Care should be taken to choose a probability equation based on sound epidemiologic evidence. An AHA coronary risk profile has recently been published by Anderson et al. (48). This risk profile uses equations designed to estimate the patient's 5 and 10 year CHD risk. These equations have several advantages over previously published risk profiles (48) (see Table 8).

Equations for use in predicting CHD risk (equations include systolic or diastolic blood pressure values) are detailed in the recently published AHA article, and an easy to use point-scoring table (incorporating only systolic blood pressure values) has been developed for predicting CHD risk for 5 and 10 year periods (see Table 9) (48). The risk profile can help teach patients about their personal coronary heart disease (CHD) risk and it can also be a strong motivational tool for encouraging lifestyle change. The risk ratio can provide an opportunity to explain to the patient the concept of multiple risk factors working synergistically to increase risk in an exponential fashion.

An example of using the risk profile is instructive. Consider a 54-year-old man who smokes cigarettes and has the following additional risk factors: total cholesterol level of 292 mg/dl; high-density lipoprotein (HDL) cholesterol 34 mg/dl; systolic blood pressure 154 mmHg; nondiabetic; and without left ventricular hypertrophy. According to the risk profile prediction chart (Table 9), this patient has a 19% and a 33% probability for 5 and 10 year CHD risk, respectively. If he were to make lifestyle changes sufficient to lower his cholesterol to 220 mg/dl, raise his HDL cholesterol to 40 mg/dl, reduce systolic blood pressure to 130 mmHg, and quit smoking, his new risk profile would be a 6% and 13% probability for CHD for 5 and 10 years, respectively, representing an astounding 60% decrease in the probability of developing clinical heart disease.

Table 9 also incudes the average 10-year risk for men and women ages 30–74 years. This table indicates that the probability for CHD for a 54-year-old man is 14%. In the example above, the initial probability risk of 33% (10 year) can be compared with the average 10 year risk of 14% to help the patient understand the important need to reduce his significantly increased risk for CHD.

When one is using coronary risk ratios, the patient should be informed that the value is only a probability score and that a low value does not ensure that a cardiac event will not occur or that a high score will inevitably lead to clinical heart disease. Anderson and colleagues have cautioned users of the risk profile regarding the following important points: 1. all risk factors should have been measured

Table 8   Advantages of the Recently Published AHA Coronary Risk Profile

---

Components of the profile are "objective and strongly independently related to CHD."
Components can easily be measured by simple office procedures and laboratory results.
The data base is larger, more recent, and includes additional data for the over 60 population.
HDL-cholesterol is included as part of the equations.
Both the original Framingham cohort population data and the second-generation study data
   (the Framingham Offspring Cohort) have been combined.

Table 9 Framingham Heart Study Coronary Heart Disease Risk Prediction Chart

1. Find points for each risk factor

Age (female) (yr)				Age (male) (yr)				HDL cholesterol			
Age	Points	Age	Points	Age	Points	Age	Points	HDL	Points	HDL	Points
30	−12	41	1	30	−2	48–49	9	25–26	7	67–73	−4
31	−11	42–43	2	31	−1	50–51	10	27–29	6	74–80	−5
32	−9	44	3	32–33	0	52–54	11	30–32	5	81–87	−6
33	−8	45–46	4	34	1	55–56	12	33–35	4	88–96	−7
34	−6	47–48	5	35–36	2	57–59	13	36–38	3		
35	−5	49–50	6	37–38	3	60–61	14	39–42	2		
36	−4	51–52	7	39	4	62–64	15	43–46	1		
37	−3	53–55	8	40–41	5	65–67	16	47–50	0		
38	−2	56–60	9	42–43	6	68–70	17	51–55	−1		
39	−1	61–67	10	44–45	7	71–73	18	56–60	−2		
40	0	68–74	11	46–47	8	74	19	61–66	−3		

Total cholesterol (mg/dl)				Systolic blood pressure (mm Hg)				Other factors	Points	
Chol	Points	Chol	Points	SBP	Points	SBP	Points		Yes	No
139–151	−3	220–239	2	98–104	−2	150–160	4	Cigarette smoking	4	0
152–166	−2	240–262	3	105–112	−1	161–172	5	Diabetes		
167–182	−1	263–288	4	113–120	0	173–185	6	Male	3	0
183–199	0	289–315	5	121–129	1			Female	6	0
200–219	1	316–330	6	130–139	2			ECG-LVH	9	0
				140–149	3					

2. Add points for all factors

$$\overline{(Age)} + \overline{(Total\ chol)} + \overline{(HDL)} + \overline{(SBP)} + \overline{(Smoking)} + \overline{(Diabetes)} + \overline{(ECG\text{-}LVH)} = \overline{(Total)}$$

Note: Minus points subtract from total.

3. Look up risk corresponding to point total

Points	Probability (%) 5 yr	10 yr	Points	Probability (%) 5 yr	10 yr	Points	Probability (%) 5 yr	10 yr	Points	Probability (%) 5 yr	10 yr
≤1	<1	<2	9	2	5	17	6	13	25	14	27
2	1	2	10	2	6	18	7	14	26	16	29
3	1	2	11	3	6	19	8	16	27	17	31
4	1	2	12	3	7	20	8	18	28	19	33
5	1	3	13	3	8	21	9	19	29	20	36
6	1	3	14	4	9	22	11	21	30	22	38
7	1	4	15	5	10	23	12	23	31	24	40
8	2	4	16	5	12	24	13	25	32	25	42

4. Compare with average 10-year risk

Age (yr)	Probability (%) Women	Men	Age (yr)	Probability (%) Women	Men	Age (yr)	Probability (%) Women	Men
30–34	<1	3	45–49	5	10	60–64	13	21
35–39	<1	5	50–54	8	14	65–69	9	30
40–44	2	6	55–59	12	16	70–74	12	24

HDL, high-density lipoprotein; SBP, systolic blood pressure; ECG-LVH, left ventricular hypertrophy by electrocardiography.
Source: From Ref. 48, with permission.

when using the equations, 2. those individuals who have a significant family history for CHD should be advised of the need for greater surveillance of their risk factors than those without a genetic basis for CHD, 3. the equations may not facilitate accurate probability scores for individuals who have "extremely elevated risk factors," and 4. the probability scores may not be predictive when used among population groups who have a very low or a very high incidence rate of CHD (48,49).

IV. IMPLEMENTATION

Implementation of the PHE requires careful consideration of what preventive services should be recommended for the patient and how the services are to be integrated into clinical practice.

A. Design

Determining what clinical services to provide for patients and at what interval can be somewhat overwhelming; there are hundreds of preventive services recommendations derived from many agencies and clinical researchers.

We recommend using the U.S. Preventive Services guidelines, which include age-specific charts that carefully outline recommended screening, counseling, and immunizations (39,40). The age-specific charts identify high-risk groups and describe the high-risk categories. The leading causes of death for each age group have been catalogued, along with a listing of disorders that clinicians should be alerted to but are not generally recommended as a periodic screening component (these disorders are appropriately titled, "Remain Alert For"). A sample copy of a periodic health examination age-specific chart is included in Appendix 2 at the end of this chapter.

These guidelines can easily form the basis for preventive services, and, based upon clinical judgement, modifications of the recommended services can be made. Additional useful references are the cancer screening document produced by the National Cancer Institute's (NCI) Early Detection Branch (29,30) and the Preventive Care Guidelines compiled by the American College of Physicians (26). The NCI report identifies recommendations for cancer screening and carefully outlines the rationale and basis for including these recommendations. As previously stated, the ACP guidelines compare and contrast preventive services guidelines from several well-known sources. The cardiovascular risk factor evaluation guidelines published by the American Heart Association are particularly useful in focusing on coronary heart disease screening (1).

In many instances the U.S. Preventive Services Task Force Guidelines do not include certain screening procedures because the research findings are inconclusive regarding the benefits derived from the procedures. For example, breast self-examination is not specifically recommended, and the task force concludes that due to insufficient data they do not recommend that current practices be changed. Many of the more traditional recommendations, such as screening for colorectal cancer, are either omitted by the U.S. Preventive Services Task Force or the procedure is listed in the "high-risk group" category only.

In light of the obvious differences existing in screening recommendations, clinical discretion remains an integral component in the design of preventive services in the office setting. It is sometimes helpful to differentiate preventive services that should be performed by the patient, such as self-examinations and lifestyle pursuits, and procedures to be performed by the physician.

There is considerable controversy regarding the need for resting and exercise electrocardiograms (ECG). The AHA Task Force recommends a resting ECG be obtained on healthy adults at ages 20, 40, and 60 years (1) and the American College of Cardiology (ACC) recommends that all adults have a baseline 12-lead ECG at an unspecified age, and repeated every 5 years (50). Contrary to the AHA and the ACC guidelines, the U.S. Preventive Services Task Force and a number of other reviewers have stated that a resting ECG is not necessary (15,51–54). Recommended guidelines for exercise ECG testing are discussed in Chapter 12.

B. Delivery

Decisions regarding the delivery of PHE services should include the following questions: What health questionnaire data should be included to initiate the patient's PHE program? How will the data be collected and stored? How will patients be reminded of when preventive services are to be performed? How can the patient be encouraged to participate more fully in the PHE process? What allied health professionals, if any, should be involved in the delivery of preventive services? What are the financial implications of increasing preventive services from the patent's and the physician's standpoint?

1. *Questionnaire Data*

The health questionnaire should obviously include information necessary to establish a patient file and an initial database. The questionnaire should provide a listing of all preventive services that will be part of the PHE and a place for the patient to indicate which of these procedures have previously been performed and when the service was rendered. Questions should also be included to help the physician identify high-risk groups. See Table 3 for recommendations regarding the contents of the health questionnaire.

The patient should be encouraged to be accurate and thorough when completing the questionnaire: once the questionnaire is completed only a minimal amount of time will be required to update the document at future visits. The patient should also retain a copy of this questionnaire to facilitate revision of personal data.

2. *Tracking and Reminder Systems*

Manual PHE tracking and reminder systems have been designed recently. It is unfortunate that many physicians and office staff fail to utilize these forms and, as a result, many of the recommended screening procedures are not performed. Several studies have looked at ways to improve compliance among physicians and patients participating in the PHE (55–58). This research suggests that reminders in the patient chart, flowsheets, cues on computerized patient records, patient-held minirecords, and other forms of feedback can be used to enhance physicians' and patients' use of preventive services.

Several computerized tracking/reminder systems are now available for commercial use. Physicians interested in purchasing these programs should strongly consider whether the system can incorporate the patient billing system and if the program facilitates one-time data entry. If these criteria are not included with the computerized system, the likelihood of maintaining strong compliance will be significantly reduced. By integrating the billing system, patient services can easily be tracked and reminder letters for upcoming preventive services can be sent. When the computerized system incorporates one-time data entry, significant time and cost reduction is possible.

Some clinics are gradually converting the paper patient chart to a completely electronic chart. The computerized records facilitate storage of all patient/physician interactions such as progress notes, past medical history, problems lists, and preventive maintenance procedures. The automated medical chart can also incorporate tracking and reminder systems. It is anticipated that additional software development in this area will prove beneficial to the overall implementation of preventive services.

3. *Patient Involvement*

All physicians involved in PHE should be encouraged to educate and remind patients that they are largely responsible for their own health. This emphasis is especially important with the expanding body of research relating personal health behaviors to health outcomes.

In an effort to persuade patients to participate in their longitudinal health care needs, we have recently developed an age- and sex-specific screening matrix for the patient and stressed the need to follow recommended health checks as they would follow the necessary maintenance requirements with their automobiles (59). This personalized health "owners manual" is designed in such a way that the patient is encouraged first to develop a working relationship with a primary care physician who is willing to follow the PHE philosophy. The health manual then recommends lifestyle activities or clinical procedures that should be performed on a daily, monthly, or periodic basis. Patients are also encouraged to participate in lifestyle counseling topics such as accident prevention and substance use, and to work closely with their physicians to recognize high-risk conditions. Patients are also asked to record when health maintenance activities or interventions take place. We believe strongly that patients can and will respond favorably to the notion of being active participants in their health care program. Appendix 3 illustrates a sample health check chart for a 50–59-year-old patient.

4. Allied Professionals

There are an increasing number of health specialists trained to assist patients with exercise, nutrition, weight management, and stress management needs. Some primary care physicians have chosen to utilize these health professionals to provide additional lifestyle counseling services to their patients. Based upon the patient's individual requirements, the time necessary for effective lifestyle counseling may be more appropriately spent by an allied health professional such as a nutritionist, nurse, exercise specialist, or social worker. On the other hand, the physician usually has the greatest impact upon the patient who needs to make a behavioral change. Accordingly, the primary care doctor should remain actively involved in recommending appropriate lifestyle change and then determine whether more specific or detailed counseling by a health specialist is necessary.

5. Financial Consequences

At the present time the pluralistic nature of the health care system in the United States provides only a minimal amount of financial reimbursement for outpatient preventive services (23). For this reason careful planning should be made by physicians to ensure that, where possible, preventive services be incorporated into routine clinical encounters (23). Efforts by the health industry, both private and government sectors, are being taken to incorporate greater insurance coverage for preventive maintenance services. We anticipate that more incentive-related insurance packages will be offered to the public where the preventive services are reimbursed if the patient complies with specified lifestyle recommendations. The arena of insurance coverage for preventive services may experience the greatest degree of change in the decade ahead.

IV. CONCLUSION

In the foreword of *Healthy People 2000: National Health Promotion and Disease Prevention Objectives*, James O. Mason has written

> We can no longer afford *not* to invest in prevention. From the perspective of avoiding human suffering as well as saving wasteful costs for treating diseases and injuries that could have been prevented, the 1990s should be the decade of prevention in the United States (60).

An integral component of the investment in prevention is a reliance upon physicians taking an active role in educating their clientele regarding the need to 1. become an active partner in health maintenance and promotion: to take greater responsibility for their own health, 2. participate in periodic health examinations that include careful screening for risk factors, 3. participate in healthy lifestyle behaviors such as physical activity and diet, and change unhealthy behaviors such as smoking and high-risk sexual activities. To accomplish these aims effectively, physicians need to design, implement, and manage delivery of the periodic health evaluation. Physicians may also be required to gain additional competency in the areas of assessing risk and providing patient counseling.

REFERENCES

1. Grundy SM, Greenland P, Herd A, Huebsch JA, Jones RJ, Mitchell JH, Schlant RC. Cardiovascular and risk factor evaluation of healthy American adults. Circulation 1987; 75(6):1340A–62A.
2. Charap MH. The periodic health examination: genesis of a myth. Ann Intern Med 1981; 95:733–5.
3. Gould GM. A system of personal biologic examination: the condition of adequate medical and scientific conduct of life. JAMA 1900; 35:134–8.
4. Battista RN, Beaulieu MD, Feightner JW, Mann KV, Owen G. The periodic health examination: Part 3. An evolving concept. Can Med Assoc J 1984; 130:1288–92.
5. Emerson, H. Periodic medical examination of apparently healthy persons. JAMA 1923; 81:1376–81.
6. Collen MF. Periodic health examinations. Why? What? When? How? Primary Care 1976; 3(2):197–204.
7. Dales LG, Friedman GD, Collen MF. Evaluating periodic multiphasic health checkups: a controlled trial. J Chron Dis 1979; 32:385–404.
8. Collen MF, Dales LG, Friedman GD. Multiphasic check-up evaluation study: 4. Preliminary cost benefit analysis for middle-aged men. Prev Med 1973; 2:236–46.
9. Lawrence RS, Mickalide AD. Preventive services in clinical practice: designing the periodic health examination. JAMA 1987; 257(16):2205–7.
10. Medical Practice Committee, American College of Physicians. Periodic health examination: a guide for assessing individual preventive health care in the asymptomatic patient. Ann Intern Med 1981; 95:729–32.
11. Frame PS, Carlson SJ. A critical review of periodic health screening using specific screening criteria. Part 1: Selected diseases of the respiratory, cardiovascular, and central nervous systems. J Fam Pract 1975; 2:29–36.
12. Frame PS, Carlson SJ. A critical review of periodic health screening using specific screening criteria. Part 2: Selected endocrine, metabolic, and gastrointestinal diseases. J Fam Pract 1975; 2:123–9.
13. Frame PS, Carlson SJ. A critical review of periodic health screening using specific screening criteria. Part 3: Selected diseases of the genitourinary system. J Fam Pract 1975; 2:189–94.
14. Frame PS, Carlson SJ. A critical review of periodic health screening using specific screening criteria. Part 4: Selected miscellaneous diseases. J Fam Pract 1975; 2: 283–9.

15. Frame PS. A critical review of adult health maintenance. Part 1: Prevention of atherosclerotic diseases. J Fam Pract 1986; 22(4):341–6.
16. Frame PS. A critical review of adult health maintenance. Part 2: Prevention of infectious diseases. J Fam Pract 1986; 22(5):417–22.
17. Frame PS. A critical review of adult health maintenance. Part 3: Prevention of cancer. J Fam Pract 1986; 22(6):511–20.
18. Frame PS. A critical review of adult health maintenance. Part 4: Prevention of metabolic, behavioral, and miscellaneous conditions. J Fam Pract 1986; 23(1):29–39.
19. Canadian Task Force on the Periodic Health Examination. The periodic health examination. Can Med Assoc J 1979; 121(3):1193–254.
20. Canadian Task Force on the Periodic Health Examination. The periodic health examination, 1984 update. Can Med Assoc J 1984; 130:1278–85.
21. Canadian Task Force on the Periodic Health Examination. The periodic health examination, 1986 update. Can Med Assoc J 1986; 134:721–9.
22. Canadian Task Force on the Periodic Health Examination. The periodic health examination, 1988 update. Can Med Assoc J 1988; 138:617–26.
23. Holbrook JH. Periodic health examination for adults. In: Stults BM, Dere WH, eds. Practical care of the ambulatory patient. Philadelphia: W. B. Saunders, 1989:416–22.
24. Breslow L, Somers AR: The lifetime health-monitoring program. N Engl J Med 1977; 296:601–8.
25. Eddy D. American Cancer Society. Report on the cancer-related health check-up. CA 1980; 30:194–240.
26. Hayward RSA, Steinberg EP, Ford DE, Roizen MF, Roach KW. Preventive care guidelines: 1991. Ann Intern Med 1991; 114:758–83.
27. Holleb AI. Guidelines for the cancer-related checkup: five years later (editorial). CA 1985; 35:194–5.
28. Holleb AI. Survey of physicians' attitudes and practices in early cancer detection. CA 1985; 35:197–213.
29. National Cancer Institute—Early Detection Branch, Division of Cancer Prevention and Control. Working guidelines for early detection: rationale and supporting evidence to decrease mortality. National Cancer Institute publication, 1987.
30. Smart C. Cancer screening and early detection. In: Cancer medicine, 3rd ed. Philadelphia: JB Lippincott, 1992.
31. Fielding JE. Preventive services for the well population, in Healthy people: the Surgeon General's report on health promotion and disease prevention—background papers. DHEW (PHS) publication No. 79-55071A. Washington, DC: Government Printing Office, 1979: 277–306.
32. Douglas BE. Examining healthy patients: how and how often: Mayo Clin Proc 1981; 56:57–60.
33. American Medical Association Council on Scientific Affairs. Medical evaluations of healthy persons. JAMA 1983; 249:1626–33.
34. White CC, Tolsma DT, Haynes SG, McGee D. Cardiovascular disease. In: Amler RW, Dull HB, eds. Closing the gap: the burden of unnecessary illness. New York: Oxford University Press, 1987:43–54.
35. Holbrook JH. Personal health maintenance for adults. West J Med 1984; 141(6):824–31.

36. Bridges JD, Killip T, Krane NK, et al. Recommendations for care of the asymptomatic patient. Henry Ford Hosp Med J 1983; 31:95–100.
37. National Cholesterol Education Program Committee. Highlights of the report of the expert panel on detection, evaluation, and treatment of high blood cholesterol in adults, 1987. PHS publication no. (NIH)88-2926:1–8.
38. Sox HC. Common diagnostic tests: use and interpretation. Philadelphia: American College of Physicians, 1987.
39. Report of the U.S. Preventive Services Task Force. Guide to clinical preventive services, 1989.
40. U.S. Preventive Services Task Force. Guide to clinical preventive services: an assessment of the effectiveness of 169 interventions. Baltimore: Williams and Wilkins, 1989.
41. Friedman GD, Collen MF, Fireman BH. Multiphasic health checkup evaluation: a 16-year follow-up. J Chron Dis 1986; 39(6):453–63.
42. Advance report of final mortality statistics, 1987. Monthly vital statistics report: final data from the National Center for Health Statistics 1989. 38(5):19.
43. Report of the U.S. Preventive Services Task Force. Adult immunizations. In: Guide to clinical preventive services, 1989.
44. Frame PS. A critical review of adult health maintenance: Part II. Prevention of infectious diseases. J Fam Pract 1986; 22(5):417–22.
45. Report of the U.S. Preventive Services Task Force. Screening for hepatitis B. In: Guide to clinical preventive services, 1989.
46. Changing patterns of groups at high risk for hepatitis B in the United States. MMWR 1988; 37:429–32, 437.
47. Report of the U.S. Preventive Services Task Force. Counseling to prevent human immunodeficiency virus infection and other sexually transmitted diseases. In: Guide to clinical preventive services, 1989.
48. Anderson KM, Wilson PWF, Odell PM, Kannel WB. An updated coronary profile: a statement for health professionals. Circulation 1991; 83(1):356–62.
49. McGee D, Gordon T. The results of the Framingham study applied to four other US-based epidemiologic studies of cardiovascular disease, in Kannel WB, Gordon T, eds. The Framingham study: an epidemiological investigation of cardiovascular disease, section 31. US Dept of Health, Education, and Welfare publication No. 76-1083. Bethesda, MD: US Government Printing Office, 1976.
50. Resnekov L, Fox S, Selzer A, et al. Task Force IV: use of electrocardiograms in practice. Am J Cardiol 1978; 41:170–5.
51. Report of the U.S. Preventive Services Task Force. Screening for asymptomatic coronary artery disease. In: Guide to clinical preventive services, 1989.
52. Canadian Task Force on the Periodic Health Examination. The periodic health examination: 1984 update. Can Med Assoc J 1984; 130:2–15.
53. Goldberger AL, O'Konski M. Utility of the routine electrocardiogram before surgery and on general hospital admission: critical review and new guidelines. Ann Intern Med 1986; 105:552–7.
54. Estes EH. Baseline screening electrocardiogram: an opposing view. J Fam Pract 1987; 25:395–6.

55. Davidson RA, Fletcher SW, Retchin S, Duh S. A nurse-initiated reminder system for the periodic health examination: implementation and evaluation. Arch Intern Med 1984; 144:2167–70.

56. Chambers CV, Balaban DJ, Carlson BL, Ungemack JA, Grasberger DM. Microcomputer-generated reminders: improving the compliance of primary care physicians with mammography screening guidelines. J Fam Pract 1989; 29(2):273–80.

57. McDonald CJ, Hui SL, Smith DM, Tie McCabe GP. Reminders to physicians from an introspective computer medical record: a two-year randomized trial. Ann Intern Med 1984; 100:130–8.

58. McDowell I, Newell C, Rosser W. Computerized reminders to encourage cervical screening in family practice. J Fam Pract 1989; 28(4):420–4.

59. Adams TD, Fisher AG, Yanowitz FG. Maintaining the miracle. Provo, UT: Vitality House Inc., 1991.

60. Department of Health and Human Services. Healthy People 2000: National health promotion and disease prevention objectives. US Department of Health and Human Services, Public Health Service, 1990, Conference Edition.

APPENDIX 1: HEALTH ASSESSMENT AND MEDICAL HISTORY QUESTIONNAIRE

(The material contained within this questionnaire has been used by permission of the Cardiovascular Genetics Research Clinic, University of Utah School of Medicine, and the Fitness Institute at LDS Hospital. Questions on physical activity are adapted in part from the "Harvard Alumni Health Questionnaire," used by permission of Dr. Ralph Paffenbarger. The psychological information is from "Mending the Body, Minding the Mind" and is used by permission of Dr. Joan Borysenko, Ph.D.) Source: From Ref. 59, with permission.

1. GENERAL INFORMATION

A. PERSONAL

Name: _____ (Last) _____ (First) _____ (Middle)   Sex: _____

Date of Birth: _____ (Month) _____ (Day) _____ (Year)   Age: _____

Address: _____

Phone: _____ (Home) _____ (Work)

Marital Status:
☐ Single ☐ Married ☐ Divorced ☐ Widowed ☐ Separated

Total Number of Children: (including adopted) _____

Race:
☐ Caucasian ☐ Black ☐ Asian ☐ Hispanic ☐ Other

Education: (Check highest level attained)
☐ Grade School ☐ Jr. High ☐ High School ☐ College ☐ Graduate School

Occupation: _____

Blood Type: _____   What is your Rh Type: _____

B. MEDICAL COVERAGE

Carrier(s) or Provider(s) including Medicare:
_____
_____

Policy or Identification Number(s):
_____
_____

Name of Policy Holder:
_____
_____

Employer and Address:
_____
_____

(Note: When visiting your doctor, please take insurance/Medicare forms with you.)

C. DOCTORS

Primary Care: _____   Eye: _____
Address: _____ Phone: _____   Address: _____ Phone: _____
Specialist: _____   Dentist: _____
Address: _____ Phone: _____   Address: _____ Phone: _____
Specialist: _____   Dentist: _____
Address: _____ Phone: _____   Address: _____ Phone: _____

2. MEDICAL HISTORY

A. MEDICAL ILLNESS

Have you ever been told BY A DOCTOR that you suffer from any of the following health problems?

	Do you suffer (Yes/No)	AGE AT 1st DIAGNOSIS. Age	Have you taken prescription medication for this health problem? (Yes/No)	Have you ever been hospitalized for this health problem? (Yes/No)	Have you ever had any special tests performed for this health problem? (Yes/No)
1. Heart Attack (Myocardial Infarction [MI], Coronary Thrombosis)	☐ ☐		☐ ☐	☐ ☐	☐ ☐
2. Angina Pectoris	☐ ☐		☐ ☐	☐ ☐	☐ ☐
3. Rheumatic or other Heart Disease Please list: _____	☐ ☐		☐ ☐	☐ ☐	☐ ☐
4. Stroke	☐ ☐		☐ ☐	☐ ☐	☐ ☐
5. High Blood Pressure	☐ ☐		☐ ☐	☐ ☐	☐ ☐
6. High Blood Pressure during Pregnancy only	☐ ☐		☐ ☐	☐ ☐	☐ ☐
7. High Blood Cholesterol or Triglycerides, and/or Low HDL	☐ ☐		☐ ☐	☐ ☐	☐ ☐
8. Diabetes	☐ ☐		☐ ☐	☐ ☐	☐ ☐
9. Cancer	☐ ☐		☐ ☐	☐ ☐	☐ ☐

Do you currently have or have you ever had any of the following: (please indicate the year)

10.___ anemia	15.___ malaria	20.___ mumps	25.___ varicose veins or phlebitis
11.___ asthma	16.___ jaundice or hepatitis	21.___ polio	26.___ venereal disease
12.___ chickenpox	17.___ measles	22.___ scarlet fever	27. Other: _____
13.___ hemorrhoids	18.___ liver disease	23.___ thyroid disease	
14.___ hives	19.___ mononucleosis	24.___ typhoid	

HEART DISEASE

28. If you answered "Yes" to Number 1 (**Heart Attack**), circle any of the following that apply:

a. Hospitalized for _____ days.

b. Was placed in a Coronary or Intensive Care Unit.

c. Experienced chest pain for one hour or more.

Please circle any of the following terms used by your doctor to describe your situation:

1 - Coronary thrombosis
2 - Myocardial infarction (MI)
3 - Congestive heart failure
4 - Unstable angina
5 - Other: _____

29. If you had **other heart problems**, circle any of the following that apply:

a. Congestive heart failure
b. Rheumatic heart disease
c. Congenital heart disease
d. Atrial fibrilation
e. Paroxysmal atrial tachycardia (PAT)
f. Premature ventricular contractions (PVC)
g. Other heart rhythm problems
h. Cardiomyopathy (diseased heart muscle)
i. Pulmonary heart disease
j. Any heart murmurs
k. Any heart valve problems (stenosis, regurgitation, etc.)
l. Other: _____

STROKE

30. If you answered "Yes" to Number 4 (**Stroke**), circle any of the following that apply:

a. My muscles suddenly became weak or paralyzed on one side of my body.
b. I suddenly had difficulty talking.
c. I suddenly had partial or complete loss of vision in one eye.
d. I fainted or passed out (usually not due to a stroke).
e. I was hospitalized for _____ days.
f. Some of the above problems were still present to some degree several months after the stroke.
g. Other: _____

HIGH BLOOD PRESSURE

31. If you answered "Yes" to Number 5 or 6 (**High Blood Pressure**), circle any of the following that apply:

a. Currently take prescription medication for high blood pressure.
b. Previously took prescription medication for high blood pressure, but stopped taking it on my own.
c. Previously took prescription medication for high blood pressure, but my doctor told me to stop.
d. Only had high blood pressure when I was pregnant.
e. Do not take prescription medication, but the doctor follows my high blood pressure (see doctor regularly to check blood pressure).

HIGH BLOOD CHOLESTEROL

32. If you answered "Yes" to Number 7 (**High Blood Cholesterol**, etc.), circle any of the following that apply:

a. Has your blood cholesterol ever been measured ? Yes ☐ No ☐ Date: _____
b. My highest blood cholesterol level was: _____ Date: _____
c. My current cholesterol level is: _____ Date: _____
d. My highest triglyceride level was: _____ Date: _____
e. My current triglyceride level is: _____ Date: _____
f. My lowest HDL level was : _____ Date: _____
g. My current HDL level is: _____ Date: _____
h. Medication has been prescribed by my doctor for my high blood lipids.

DIABETES

33. If you answered "Yes" to Number 8 (**Diabetes**), circle any of the following that apply:

a. Insulin injections have been prescribed by my doctor for control of my blood sugar.
b. Medication (pills or tablets) have been prescribed for control of my blood sugar.
c. I monitor my urine and/or blood sugar at home as directed by my doctor.
d. A special diet for control of my blood sugar has been prescribed by my doctor.

CANCER

34. If you answered "Yes" to Number 9 (**Cancer**), please answer the following questions:

   a. The type of cancer your doctor said you had: _____

   b. Did you undergo any surgical therapy for this cancer? _____ yes _____ no

   c. Did you have chemotherapy? _____ yes _____ no

   d. Did you have radiation therapy? _____ yes _____ no

B. MEDICAL PROCEDURES

Tests

(indicate previous tests and year performed:)

Tests	Year	Was the test normal ? Yes	No
☐ upper GI X-ray	___	☐	☐
☐ lower GI X-ray	___	☐	☐
☐ gallbladder X-ray	___	☐	☐
☐ proctoscopic exam	___	☐	☐
☐ chest X-ray	___	☐	☐
☐ TB skin test	___	☐	☐
☐ tetanus shot	___	☐	☐
☐ allergy tests	___	☐	☐
☐ complete physical examination	___	☐	☐
☐ electrocardiogram (resting EKG)	___	☐	☐
☐ exercise electrocardiogram (stress test)	___	☐	☐
☐ mammogram	___	☐	☐
☐ pap smear	___	☐	☐
☐ colonoscopy	___	☐	☐

☐ Other X-rays

Year   Kind of X-ray

_____ _____

_____ _____

_____ _____

Operations and Hospitalizations

(Please list past hospitalization and operations/major procedures)

_____ Year: _____

_____ Year: _____

_____ Year: _____

_____ Year: _____

_____ Year: _____

_____ Year: _____

_____ Year: _____

_____ Year: _____

_____ Year: _____

_____ Year: _____

_____ Year: _____

_____ Year: _____

C. MEDICATIONS, DRUG REACTION(S) and ALLERGIES

1. MEDICATIONS

(Please list the medications, vitamins and dietary supplements you take, prescription and non-prescription, even ones taken on an occasional basis.)

Name	When did you start this medication?	How often do you take this medication?	Dose

2. DRUG REACTIONS

(Please list any drug reaction you have had and the year you had this reaction.)

Date

Drug:
Side Effect:

Drug:
Side Effect:

Drug:
Side Effect:

Drug:
Side Effect:

Drug:
Side Effect:

3. ALLERGIES

(Please list the things you are allergic to and any reactions you have had.)

Date

Allergic to:
Side Effect:

Allergic to:
Side Effect:

Allergic to:
Side Effect:

Allergic to:
Side Effect:

Allergic to:
Side Effect:

Allergic to:
Side Effect:

3. REVIEW OF SYSTEMS

A. GENERAL REVIEW

(Check the appropriate boxes:)

- [ ] Do you have an intolerance to heat?
- [ ] Do you have an intolerance to cold?
- [ ] Do you often notice excessive fatigue or exhaustion?
- [ ] Do you have difficulty getting to sleep or staying asleep?
- [ ] Have you noticed any unusual thirst?
- [ ] Are you always hungry?
- [ ] Has your appetite disappeared or decreased?
- [ ] Have you noticed any lymph node swelling?
- [ ] Have you ever been exposed to radiation of head or neck? (other than dental or other diagnostic X-rays)

- [ ] Do you ever feel faint?
- [ ] Do you lose feeling in any part of your body?
- [ ] Have you noticed shaking or trembling?
- [ ] Have you ever had convulsions?
- [ ] Have you had excessive bleeding from a cut?
- [ ] Are you prone to bruise easily?
- [ ] Are you bothered with any skin abnormalities?
- [ ] Do you have any physical handicaps?

B. DIGESTIVE SYSTEM

- [ ] Do you notice any discomfort or pain in your upper abdomen or stomach?
- [ ] Do you have much abdominal gas?
- [ ] If you notice pain or discomfort in your abdomen, is it made worse by eating?
  - Is it made better by eating? [ ] Yes [ ] No
  - Is it improved with antacids? [ ] Yes [ ] No
- [ ] Are you bothered with heartburn, belching or do you have trouble swallowing? (underline which)
- [ ] Are you constipated more than once weekly?
- [ ] Do you have loose bowels for more than one or two days?
- [ ] Have you had any black or bloody stools in the last five years?
- [ ] Have you had any rectal bleeding in the last five years?
- [ ] Are your bowel movements painful?
- [ ] Do you have rectal pain?
- [ ] Do you have a hernia?
- [ ] Do you have hemorrhoids?
- [ ] Have you been told you have diverticulitis?

C. GENITO-URINARY SYSTEM

☐ Do you notice pain or burning when urinating?

☐ Do you have trouble starting to urinate?

☐ Does your urination seem too slow?

How many times per night do you generally urinate? _____

How many times per day do you generally urinate? _____

☐ Do you have frequent urinary tract infections?

☐ Have you had past kidney trouble?

D. MEN

☐ Has the force of urine stream markedly decreased?

☐ Do you notice any dribbling after stopping urination?

☐ Have you noticed any discharge from the penis?

☐ Have you been told you have prostate trouble?

☐ Do your testicles become tender and swollen?

E. WOMEN

☐ Have you noticed any breast lumps?

☐ Have you noticed any discharge from your breasts?

☐ Are your periods regular with normal flow?

☐ Do you ever bleed between periods?

☐ Do you have vaginal itching or discharge?

☐ Have you ever taken birth control pills?

☐ Have you ever taken any hormone
(estrogen or progesterone)replacement therapy?

☐ Have you ever been pregnant? If yes, how may pregnancies? _____

F. EYES, EARS, NOSE, THROAT and MOUTH

☐ Do you wear corrective lenses?

☐ Do you ever notice blurred or double vision?

☐ Are you bothered with eye pains or itching?

☐ Do you have excessive eye watering?

☐ Do you have difficulty hearing?

☐ Do you have ringing in your ears?

☐ Do you often have headaches?

☐ Have you had pain or swelling in your neck?

☐ Do you have sore areas on your gums?

☐ Is your tongue or the inside of your mouth sore?

☐ Do you have frequent stuffiness and drainage from your nose?

☐ Do you frequently notice drainage in the back of your throat?

☐ Are you bothered with nosebleeds?

☐ Is your throat sore or hoarse when you don't have a cold?

G. RESPIRATORY SYSTEM

☐ Do you ever have periods of wheezing?

☐ Do you have a regular cough?

☐ Do you often cough up anything?

☐ Have you ever coughed up blood?

☐ Do you need more than one pillow to sleep?

☐ Do you have or have you had the following?

   ☐ Bronchitis
   ☐ Emphysema
   ☐ Pneumonia

4. LIFESTYLE HISTORY (Personal Habits)

A. CIGARETTE SMOKING

1. Please circle the one that applies:
   a. **Smoker:** Have smoked daily for one year or more.
   b. **Ex-smoker:** Have not smoked for at least one year after having smoked daily for at least one year.
   c. **Non-smoker:** Have never smoked daily for at least one year.

2. If **smoker or ex-smoker**, circle **average** amount and indicate number of years smoked. Choose one only.
   a. Less than one pack a day for _____ years.
   b. About one pack a day for _____ years.
   c. One-two packs a day for _____ years.
   d. Two or more packs a day for _____ years.

3. List the last year in which you smoked _____.

4. Do you smoke cigars? _____ yes _____ no _____ cigars per day?

5. Do you smoke a pipe? _____ yes _____ no _____ bowls per day?

6. Would you like to quit smoking? _____ yes _____ no

7. Do you use smokeless tobacco? _____ yes _____ no

8. On the average, how many hours per day are you exposed to other people's cigarette smoke?
   _____ 0 hours   _____ 5-8 hours
   _____ 1-2 hours   _____ more than 8 hours
   _____ 3-4 hours

B. ALCOHOL CONSUMPTION

1. Do you drink alcoholic beverages (beer, wine, or liquors)? Please circle the one that applies:
   a. No.
   b. Less than once a month.
   c. Once a month or more with an average of:
      1. _____ 12-16 oz. cans of beer per week.
      2. _____ 4-6 oz. glasses of wine per week.
      3. _____ shots, jiggers or mixed drinks per week.

C. DIETARY INFORMATION

1. How would you describe your tendency to lose weight? (If in doubt circle #3.)
   1) Lose weight easily by cutting food intake slightly.
   2) Lose weight with difficulty, even if I cut my food intake greatly.
   3) Average - neither tendency above noticed.

2. What is your current weight? _____ lbs. What is the most you have ever weighed (excluding pregnancy)? _____ lbs.

3. If you feel you need to lose weight, how much weight would you like to lose? _____ lbs.

4. How do you feel about your current weight?
   1) very satisfied
   2) satisfied
   3) not concerned
   4) dissatisfied
   5) very dissatisfied

5. Do you follow any special diet most of the time?
   1) No
   2) Yes, low calorie
   3) Yes, low fat or low cholesterol
   4) Yes, diabetic
   5) Yes, low salt
   6) Yes, other _____

6. In a typical week, how many meals or snacks do you eat away from home?
   1) _____ Breakfast (where) _____
   2) _____ Morning Snack (where) _____
   3) _____ Lunch (where) _____
   4) _____ Afternoon Snack (where) _____
   5) _____ Dinner (where) _____
   6) _____ Evening Snack (where) _____

List of foods high in Cholesterol or Saturated Fat:

Bacon		Sweet Rolls	
Hot Dogs		Butter	
Sausage		Shortening	
Marbled and Fatty Meats		Coconut Oil	
(beef, pork, lamb)		Potato Chips	
Spare Ribs		French Fries	
Fish fried in shortening		Other Fried Foods	
Liver or other organ meats		Lard	
Hamburger		Cream and Ice Cream	
Luncheon Meats		Cheese	
Egg Yolks		Butter Rolls	
Cakes and Pies		Donuts	
Whole Milk		Egg Noodles	

12. If you drink coffee or tea, how do you normally drink it?
   1) black, no cream or sugar
   2) cream, no sugar
   3) cream, one spoon of sugar
   4) cream, two spoons of sugar
   5) cream, three or more spoons of sugar
   6) no cream, one spoon of sugar
   7) no cream, two spoons of sugar
   8) no cream, three or more spoons of sugar

13. During the last week, how many days did you experience difficulty in limiting candy eating?
   1 2 3 4 5 6 7 Zero

14. During the past week, how many days did you experience difficulty in limiting your eating of fatty foods?
   1 2 3 4 5 6 7 Zero

15. During the past week, how many days did you plan what you would eat at the start of the day?
   1 2 3 4 5 6 7 Zero

16. During the past week, how many days did you eat your meals at set times?
   1 2 3 4 5 6 7 Zero

17. During the past week, on how many days did you decide not to eat a snack that you wanted, even though the food was available?
   1 2 3 4 5 6 7 Zero

18. How many carbonated soft drinks do you have in a week?

19. How many are diet drinks?

20. How many of the drinks you consume contain caffeine? (Drinks like Coca Cola, Pepsi, Dr. Pepper, Mountain Dew, contain caffine.)

21. How many cups of hot chocolate do you drink each day?

22. How many cups of water do you drink each day?

23. When was the last time you ate eggs, whole milk, meat or other high cholesterol foods from the above list?
   1) Within the last three meals
   2) A day ago
   3) 2-5 days ago
   4) A week ago
   5) Over a week ago
   6) Over a year ago

24. How often do you eat any of the foods listed above?
   1) 2 or more times a day
   2) Once a day
   3) 2-5 times a week
   4) Once a week
   5) Less than once a week
   6) Almost never

25. In an average month, how may times do you skip:
   1) Breakfast?
   2) Lunch?
   3) Dinner?

List of Salty Foods:

Bacon or Ham	Salted Crackers
Hot Dogs	Seasoning Salts
Sausage	(celery, garlic, onion)
Bologna and Luncheon	Pickles
Meats	Sauerkraut
Chipped or Corned Beef	Boullion
Smoked or Salted Meats	Catsup
Herring, Sardines	Canned Soups
Potato Chips	Dried Soups
Pretzels	Chili Sauce
French Fries	Mustard
Salted Snacks	Olives
(popcorn, nuts, etc.)	Relishes
Sauces (soy, steak, etc.)	Meat Tenderizers

7. How often do you salt your food from a shaker at the dinner table or eat salty foods such as potato chips, bacon, or other foods listed above?
   1) 2 or more times a day
   2) Once a day
   3) 2-5 times a week
   4) Once a week
   5) Less than once a week
   6) Almost never (I'm on a special low salt diet)

8. When was the last time you used a salt shaker on your food or ate one of the salty foods listed above?
   1) Within the last three meals
   2) A day ago
   3) 2-5 days ago
   4) A week ago
   5) Over a week ago
   6) Over a year ago

9. Do you place specific emphasis of high fiber in your diet? ____ yes ____ no

10. How many cups of coffee containing caffeine do you drink in an average day?

11. How many cups of tea containing caffeine do you drink in an average day?

D. PHYSICAL ACTIVITY INFORMATION

1. Are you currently participating in a physical activity program? _____ yes _____ no

2. Please list the type, the frequency and the duration with which you participate in physical activity, that either includes brisk walking, jogging, swimming, gardening, aerobics, stationary cycling, country cycling, carpentry, calisthenics, etc. (please include only the time you are physically active).

Type of physical activity	Number of times per week	Time Spent in each activity session		Number of weeks per year (approximately)
		hours	minutes	

3. If you walk briskly on a regular basis, how many miles do you walk each session? _____ How long does it take you to walk one mile? _____ (minutes).

4. On a usual weekday and a weekend day, how much time do you spend on the following activities

	Usual weekday hours/day	Usual weekend day hours/day
a. Vigorous activity (digging in the garden, strenuous sports, jogging, chopping wood, sustained swimming, brisk walking, heavy carpentry, bicycling on hills, etc.)		
b. Moderate activity (housework, light sports, regular walking, golf, yard work, lawn mowing, painting, repairing, light carpentry, dancing, bicycling on level ground, etc.)		
c. Light activity (office work, driving a car, strolling, personal care, standing with little motion, etc.)		
d. Sitting activity (eating, reading, desk work, watching TV, listening to radio, etc.)		
e. Sleeping or reclining		

5. Have you ever had any chest discomfort brought on by exercise? _____ yes _____ no (If yes, please be prepared to discuss it with the doctor.)

E. PSYCHOLOGICAL INFORMATION

Circle the number, from 0 (never) to 4 (frequently), that represents the degree to which the following thoughts, feelings, and behaviors have bothered you during the past month.

THOUGHTS

	Never	Rarely	Sometimes	Often	Frequently
1. Awfulizing (taking things to their worst possible outcome)	0	1	2	3	4
2. Blaming myself	0	1	2	3	4
3. Blaming others	0	1	2	3	4
4. Difficulty concentrating	0	1	2	3	4
5. Holding grudges	0	1	2	3	4
6. Thinking and rethinking the same situation	0	1	2	3	4
7. Wishing I could "turn my mind off"	0	1	2	3	4
8. Constantly criticizing other people or situations	0	1	2	3	4
9. Worrying	0	1	2	3	4
10. Thinking something is wrong with my mind	0	1	2	3	4
11. Needing to be right	0	1	2	3	4
12. Feeling out of control	0	1	2	3	4

BEHAVIORS

	Never	Rarely	Sometimes	Often	Frequently
1. Nail or cuticle biting	0	1	2	3	4
2. Using tobacco in any form	0	1	2	3	4
3. Taking tranquilizers or "street" drugs to change mood	0	1	2	3	4
4. Drinking alcoholic beverages	0	1	2	3	4
5. Chewing gum or sucking candies	0	1	2	3	4
6. Talking a lot	0	1	2	3	4
7. Crying a lot	0	1	2	3	4
8. Sleeping problems (too much or too little)	0	1	2	3	4
9. Eating problems (too much or too little)	0	1	2	3	4
10. Trouble communicating	0	1	2	3	4
11. Avoiding responsibilities	0	1	2	3	4
12. Too much caffeine	0	1	2	3	4

EMOTIONS

	Never	Rarely	Sometimes	Often	Frequently
1. Afraid of specific places or circumstances	0	1	2	3	4
2. Feeling like a victim	0	1	2	3	4
3. Anxious	0	1	2	3	4
4. Blue	0	1	2	3	4
5. Lonely	0	1	2	3	4
6. Irritable	0	1	2	3	4
7. Wanting to throw things or hit people	0	1	2	3	4
8. Guilty	0	1	2	3	4
9. Feeling unfriendly	0	1	2	3	4
10. Uptight	0	1	2	3	4
11. Hopeless about the future	0	1	2	3	4
12. Wanting to "pull the covers over my head"	0	1	2	3	4
13. Feeling that other people don't like me	0	1	2	3	4
14. Upset over criticism	0	1	2	3	4

F. SEAT BELT USAGE

1. Do you wear seat belts when riding in or driving motor vehicles?

   ____ no   ____ sometimes   ____ usually   ____ always

G. SLEEP

1. How many hours of sleep do you usually get a night? ____ hours

2. How would you best describe your night's sleep?

   ____ restful   ____ difficult to get to sleep

   ____ wake at night and can't get back to sleep

3. Do you take naps during the day on a regular basis?

   ____ yes   ____ no

   If yes, how long is your nap? ____ minutes

5. GENETIC HISTORY

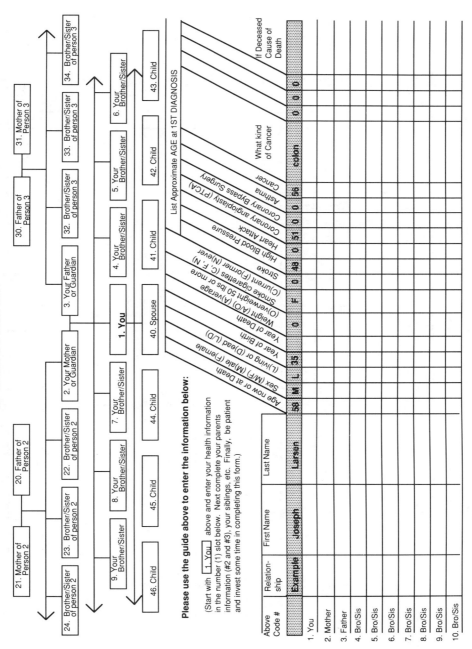

Please use the guide above to enter the information below:

(Start with ☐1. You☐ above and enter your health information in the number (1) slot below. Next complete your parents information (#2 and #3), your siblings, etc. Finally, be patient and invest some time in completing this form.)

Above Code #	Relation-ship	First Name	Last Name	Age now or at Death	Sex (M/F) (M)ale (F)emale	(L)iving or (D)ead (L/D)	Year of Birth	Year of Death	Weight (A/O) (A)verage (O)verweight 50 lbs or more	Smoke cigarettes (C, F, N) (C)urrent (F)ormer (N)ever	Stroke	High Blood Pressure	Heart Attack	Coronary angioplasty (PTCA)	Coronary Bypass Surgery	Asthma	Cancer	What kind of Cancer	If Deceased Cause of Death
Example		Joseph	Larsen	58	M	L	35	0	O	F	0	40	0	51	0	56	0	colon	0 0 0
1. You																			
2. Mother																			
3. Father																			
4. Bro/Sis																			
5. Bro/Sis																			
6. Bro/Sis																			
7. Bro/Sis																			
8. Bro/Sis																			
9. Bro/Sis																			
10. Bro/Sis																			

List Approximate AGE at 1ST DIAGNOSIS

Family tree boxes:
- 21. Mother of Person 2
- 20. Father of Person 2
- 24. Brother/Sister of person 2
- 23. Brother/Sister of person 2
- 22. Brother/Sister of person 2
- 2. Your Mother or Guardian
- 9. Your Brother/Sister
- 8. Your Brother/Sister
- 7. Your Brother/Sister
- 3. Your Father or Guardian
- 30. Father of Person 3
- 31. Mother of Person 3
- 32. Brother/Sister of person 3
- 33. Brother/Sister of person 3
- 34. Brother/Sister of person 3
- 4. Your Brother/Sister
- 5. Your Brother/Sister
- 6. Your Brother/Sister
- 1. You
- 40. Spouse
- 41. Child
- 42. Child
- 43. Child
- 44. Child
- 45. Child
- 46. Child

11. Bro/Sis	12. Bro/Sis	20. Grand-Father	21. Grand-Mother	22. Ant/Unc	23. Ant/Unc	24. Ant/Unc	25. Ant/Unc	26. Ant/Unc	27. Ant/Unc	28. Ant/Unc	30. Grand-Father	31. Grand-Mother	32. Ant/Unc	33. Ant/Unc	34. Ant/Unc	35. Ant/Unc	36. Ant/Unc	37. Ant/Unc	38. Ant/Unc	40. Spouse	41. Son/Dau	42. Son/Dau	43. Son/Dau	44. Son/Dau	45. Son/Dau	46. Son/Dau

APPENDIX 2

Ages 40–64

Schedule: Every 1–3 Years*

Leading Causes of Death:
Heart disease
Lung cancer
Cerebrovascular disease
Breast cancer
Colorectal cancer
Obstructive lung disease

SCREENING

History
Dietary intake
Physical activity
Tobacco/alcohol/drug use
Sexual practices

Physical Exam
Height and weight
Blood pressure
Clinical breast exam[1]
HIGH-RISK GROUPS
 Complete skin exam
  (HR1)
 Complete oral cavity
  exam (HR2)
 Palpation for thyroid nod-
  ules (HR3)
 Auscultation for carotid
  bruits (HR4)

**Laboratory/Diagnostic
Procedures**
Nonfasting total blood cho-
 lesterol
Papanicolaou smear[2]
Mammogram[3]
HIGH-RISK GROUPS
 Fasting plasma glucose
  (HR5)
 VDRL/RPR (HR6)
 Urinalysis for bacteriuria
  (HR7)
 Chlamydial testing (HR8)
 Gonorrhea culture (HR9)
 Counseling and testing for
  HIV (HR10)
 Tuberculin skin test (PPD)
  (HR11)
 Hearing (HR12)
 Electrocardiogram (HR13)
 Fecal occult blood/sig-
  moidoscopy (HR14)
 Fecal occult blood/colon-
  oscopy (HR15)
 Bone mineral content
  (HR16)

COUNSELING

Diet and Exercise
Fat (especially saturated fat), choles-
 terol, complex carbohydrates, fiber,
 sodium, calcium[4]
Caloric balance
Selection of exercise program

Substance Use
Tobacco cessation
Alcohol and other drugs:
 Limiting alcohol consumption
 Driving/other dangerous activities
  while under the influence
 Treatment for abuse
HIGH-RISK GROUPS
 Sharing/using unsterilized needles
  and syringes (HR19)

Sexual Practices
Sexually transmitted diseases; partner
 selection, condoms, anal inter-
 course
Unintended pregnancy and contraceptive options

Injury Prevention
Safety belts
Safety helmets
Smoke detector
Smoking near bedding or upholstery
HIGH-RISK GROUPS
 Back-conditioning exercises (HR20)
 Prevention of childhood injuries
  (HR21)
 Falls in the elderly (HR22)

Dental Health
Regular tooth brushing, flossing, and
 dental visits

**Other Primary Preventive
Measures**
HIGH-RISK GROUPS
 Skin protection from ultraviolet light
  (HR23)
 Discussion of aspirin therapy
  (HR24)
 Discussion of estrogen replacement
  therapy (HR25)

IMMUNIZATIONS

Tetanus-diphtheria (Td)
 booster[5]
HIGH-RISK GROUPS
 Hepatitis B vaccine
  (HR26)
 Pneumococcal vaccine
  (HR27)
 Influenza vaccine (HR28)[6]

**This list of preventive ser-
vices is not exhaustive.**
It reflects only those topics
reviewed by the U.S. Pre-
ventive Services Task
Force. Clinicians may wish
to add other preventive services on a routine basis,
and after considering the
patient's medical history and
other individual circum-
stances. Examples of target
conditions not specifically
examined by the Task Force
include:
 Chronic obstructive pul-
  monary disease
 Hepatobiliary disease
 Bladder cancer
 Endometrial disease
 Travel-related illness
 Prescription drug abuse
 Occupational illness and
  injuries

Remain Alert For:
Depressive symptoms
Suicide risk factors (HR17)
Abnormal bereavement
Signs of physical abuse or
 neglect
Malignant skin lesions
Peripheral arterial disease
 (HR18)
Tooth decay, gingivitis,
 loose teeth

---

*The recommended schedule applies only to the periodic visit itself. The frequency of the individual
preventive services listed in this table is left to clinical discretion, except as indicated in other
footnotes.

1. Annually for women. 2. Every 1–3 years for women. 3. Every 1–2 years for women beginning at age 50 (age 35 for those at increased risk). 4. For women. 5. Every 10 years. 6. Annually.

HR1   Persons with a family or personal history of skin cancer, increased occupational or recreational exposure to sunlight, or clinical evidence of precursor lesions (e.g., dysplastic nevi, certain congenital nevi).

HR2   Persons with exposure to tobacco or excessive amounts of alcohol, or those with suspicious symptoms or lesions detected through self-examination.

HR3   Persons with a history of upper-body irradiation.

HR4   Persons with risk factors for cerebrovascular or cardiovascular disease (e.g., hypertension, smoking, CAD, atrial fibrillation, diabetes) or those with neurologic symptoms (e.g., transient ischemic attacks) or a history of cerebrovascular disease.

HR5   The markedly obese, persons with a family history of diabetes, row omen with a history of gestational diabetes.

HR6   Prostitutes, persons who engage in sex with multiple partners in areas in which syphilis is prevalent, or contacts of persons with active syphilis.

HR7   Persons with diabetes.

HR8   Persons who attend clinics for sexually transmitted diseases, attend other high-risk health care facilities (e.g., adolescent and family planning clinics), or have other risk factors for chlamydial infection (e.g., multiple sexual partners or a sexual partner with multiple sexual contacts).

HR9   Prostitutes, persons with multiple sexual partners or a sexual partner with multiple contacts, sexual contacts of persons with culture-proven gonorrhea, or persons with a history of repeated episodes of gonorrhea.

HR10   Persons seeking treatment for sexually transmitted diseases; homosexual and bisexual men; past or present intravenous (IV) drug users; persons with a history of prostitution or multiple sexual partners; women whose past or present sexual partners were HIV-infected, bisexual, or IV drug users; persons with long-term residence or birth in an area with high prevalence of HIV infection; or persons with a history of transfusion between 1978 and 1985.

HR11   Household members of persons with tuberculosis or others at risk for close contact with the disease (e.g., staff of tuberculosis clinics, shelters for the homeless, nursing homes, substance abuse treatment facilities, dialysis units, correctional institutions; recent immigrants or refugees from countries in which tuberculosis is common (e.g., Asia, Africa, Central and South America, Pacific Islands); migrant workers; residents of nursing homes, correctional institutions, or homeless shelters; or persons with certain underlying medical disorders (e.g., HIV infection).

HR12   Persons exposed regularly to excessive noise.

HR13   Men with two or more cardiac risk factors (high blood cholesterol, hypertension, cigarette smoking, diabetes mellitus, family history of CAD); men who would endanger public safety were they to experience sudden cardiac events (e.g., commercial airline pilots); or sedentary or high-risk males planning to begin a vigorous exercise program.

HR14   Persons aged 50 or older who have first-degree relatives with colorectal cancer; a personal history of endometrial, ovarian, or breast cancer; or a previous diagnosis of inflammatory bowel disease, adenomatous polyps, or colorectal cancer.

HR15   Persons with a family history of familial polyposis coli or cancer family syndrome.

HR16   Perimenopausal women at increased risk for osteoporosis (e.g., Caucasian race, bilateral oophorectomy before menopause, slender build) and for whom estrogen replacement therapy would otherwise not be recommended.

HR17   Recent divorce, separation, unemployment, depression, alcohol or other drug abuse, serious medical illnesses, living alone, or recent bereavement.

HR18   Persons over age 50, smokers, or persons with diabetes mellitus.

HR19   Intravenous drug users.

HR20   Persons at increased risk for low back injury because of past history, body configuration, or type of activities.

HR21   Persons with children in the home or automobile.

HR22   Persons with older adults in the home.

HR23   Persons with increased exposure to sunlight.

HR24   Men who have risk factors for myocardial infarction (e.g., high blood cholesterol, smoking, diabetes mellitus, family history of early-onset CAD) and who lack a history of gastrointestinal or other bleeding problems, and other risk factors for bleeding or cerebral hemorrhage.

HR25   Perimenopausal women at increased risk for osteoporosis (e.g., Caucasian, low bone mineral content, bilateral oophorectomy before menopause or early menopause, slender build) and who are without known contraindications (e.g., history of undiagnosed vaginal bleeding, active liver disease, thromboembolic disorders, hormone-dependent cancer).

HR26   Homosexually active men, intravenous drug users, recipients of some blood products, or persons in health-related jobs with frequent exposure to blood or blood products.

HR27   Persons with medical conditions that increase the risk of pneumococcal infection (e.g., chronic cardiac or pulmonary disease, sickle cell disease, nephrotic syndrome, Hodgkin's disease, asplenia, diabetes mellitus, alcoholism, cirrhosis, multiple myeloma, renal disease or conditions associated with immunosuppression).

HR28   Residents of chronic care facilities and persons suffering from chronic cardiopulmonary disorders, metabolic diseases (including diabetes mellitus), hemoglobinopathies, immunosuppression, or renal dysfunction.

Source: From Refs. 39, 40.

APPENDIX 3*

Ages 50 to 59

• Health Check Table •

**LEADING CAUSES OF DEATH — AGES 50 TO 59
ARRANGED IN ORDER OF INCIDENCE**

Men	Women
Heart Disease	Heart Disease
Lung Cancer	Breast Cancer
Liver Disease and Cirrhosis	Lung Cancer
Strokes	Cancer of Cervix and Uterus
Colon and Rectal Cancer	Strokes
Non-Vehicle Accidents	Colon and Rectal Cancer

A. (GO!) Daily Health Checks

Daily logs or record sheets for Daily Health Checks are located with the expanded sections (see pages listed).

C. [STOP] Yearly or Periodic Health Checks

Record the month and year (e.g. 8/92) when the Health Check is performed and, where appropriate, the value (such as blood pressure, 120/80). Record this information in the column that corresponds with your age at the time the Health Check is performed. (NOTE: M = male; F = female)

		Reference	Frequency	Age 50	Age 51
1	Physical Examination & History (Initial/Interim) (M, F)	page 76	Every 2 years		
2	Cardiac Risk Factor Screening[†] (M, F)	page 79	Every 1 – 2 years		
3	Blood Pressure Screening[†] (M, F)	page 84	Yearly		
4	Digital Rectal Exam[†] (M, F)	page 87	Yearly		
5	Clinical Skin Exam[†] (M, F)	page 92	Every 2 years		
6	Clinical Testicular Exam[†] (M)	page 98	Every 2 years		
7	Examine for Thyroid Nodules[†] (M, F)	page 101	Every 2 years		
8	Clinical Oral Cavity Exam[†] (M, F)	page 103	Every 2 years		
9	Total Blood Cholesterol (M, F)	page 105	Every 5 years		
10	Sigmoidoscopy (M, F)	page 87	Every 3 – 5 years (if first exam is normal)		
11	Blood Stool Test[†] (M, F)	page 87	Yearly		
12	Pap Test/Pelvic Exam[†] (F)	page 109	Every 1 – 3 years[*]		
13	Clinical Breast Exam[†] (F)	page 111	Yearly		
14	Mammogram (F)	page 111	Yearly		
16	Tonometry (M, F)	page 117	Every 2 – 4 years[∞]		
18	Blood Test (CBC, SMAC) and Urinalysis (M, F)	page 119	Optional[§]		
19	Dental Checkup (M, F)	page 132	Yearly		
20	Tetanus-Diphtheria Vaccination (M, F)	page 121	Every 10 years		
23	Height and Weight (M, F)	page 76	Yearly		

[†] These health checks are often performed in concert with a periodic physical examination.
[*] Pap test every 1 – 3 years, following two initial negative Pap tests.
[∞] This recommendation is by the American Academy of Ophthalmology.

B. (STOP) Monthly Health Checks

Record the day and month (d/m) when these Health Checks are performed. (NOTE: M = male; F = female)

(1) Breast Self-Exam (F) ....page 111 ....

d/m	d/m	d/m	d/m	d/m	d/m

(2) Skin Self-Exam (M, F) ....page 92 ....

d/m	d/m	d/m	d/m	d/m	d/m

(4) Oral Cavity Self-Exam (M, F) ....page 103 ....

d/m	d/m	d/m	d/m	d/m	d/m

Age 52	Age 53	Age 54	Age 55	Age 56	Age 57	Age 58	Age 59

§ Routine blood tests (CBC, SMAC) and urinalysis are generally not recommended by most adult health maintenance organizations. The frequency of performing this health check is left to the discretion of you and your physician. *Continued next page*

D. ⟨YIELD⟩ Lifestyle Counseling

Review the Lifestyle Counseling information every one to three years and record the date.

	mo / yr	mo / yr	mo / yr
⟨1⟩ Substance Use .... page 123 ..			
⟨2⟩ Injury Prevention .... page 127 ..	mo / yr	mo / yr	mo / yr
⟨3⟩ Dental Health .... page 132 ..	mo / yr	mo / yr	mo / yr
⟨4⟩ Preventing Sexually Transmitted Diseases ..... page 135 ..	mo / yr	mo / yr	mo / yr
⟨5⟩ Preventing Low-Back Injury .... page 138 ..	mo / yr	mo / yr	mo / yr
⟨6⟩ Choosing a Doctor .... page 142 ..	mo / yr	mo / yr	mo / yr
⟨7⟩ Choosing a Health Care Plan .... page 144 ..	mo / yr	mo / yr	mo / yr
⟨8⟩ Assessing Genetic and Environmental Risk ... page 147 ..	mo / yr	mo / yr	mo / yr
⟨9⟩ Proper Sleep Hygiene .... page 149 ..	mo / yr	mo / yr	mo / yr

E. ⟨WARN-ING⟩ High-Risk Health Checks

The frequency of these tests should be based on your medical history and other individual circumstances (see specific pages listed below).

1 Fasting Plasma Glucose .... page 152	14 Injuries in the Elderly .... page 127
2 Urinalysis for Bateriuria .... page 153	15 Prevention of Childhood Injuries .... page 127
3 Hearing Screening .... pages 115, 154	16 Hepatitis B Vaccine .... page 162
4 Colonoscopy .... pages 87, 154	19 Pneumococcal Vaccine .... page 121
5 Resting Electrocardiogram .... page 79	20 Influenza Vaccine .... page 121
6 Exercise Electrocardiogram .... page 79	21 Auscultation for Carotid Bruits .... page 164
8 Tuberculin Skin Test .... page 156	22 Chlamydial Test .... page 165
9 Bone Mineral Content .... page 157	23 Gonorrhea Culture .... page 166
10 Estrogen Replacement .... page 157	24 VDRL (Syphilis Screen) .... page 166
11 Osteoporosis Risk .... page 157	25 Testing for AIDS Virus (HIV) .... page 167
12 Aspirin Therapy .... page 159	27 Prostate Specific Antigen Test .... pages 87, 168

When additional High-Risk Health Checks are recommended, use this space to record pertinent information.

Recommended Health Check	Date	Date	Date	Comments
1.				
2.				
3.				
4.				
5.				
6.				
7.				
8.				
9.				
10.				
11.				
12.				
13.				
14.				
15.				
16.				
17.				
18.				

REMAIN ALERT FOR SIGNS IN SELF AND OTHERS:

Depression	page 67
Suicide Risk Factors	page 67
Abnormal Bereavement	page 67
Signs of Physical Abuse or Neglect	page 127
Peripheral Arterial Disease	page 83
Possible Skin Cancer	page 92
Tooth Decay, Gingivitis, Loose Teeth	page 132

Source material for this *Health Check Table* has included:
- The "Age-Specific Charts" of the U.S. Preventive Services Task Force (USPSTF);
- The cancer screening recommendations of the National Cancer Institute and the American Cancer Society;
- The screening test guidelines of the American College of Physicians;
- The periodic health evaluation guidelines by Dr. John H. Holbrook;
- The National Cholesterol Education Program Committee;
- Other medical organizations and medical scientists as set forth in the references of this book.

Source: From Ref. 59, with permission.

7

Nutrition and the Prevention of Coronary Heart Disease

ARTHUR S. LEON and TERRYL HARTMAN

School of Public Health
University of Minnesota
Minneapolis, Minnesota

I. INTRODUCTION

Behavioral practices common in industrialized Western societies appear to be strongly and causally related to the development of coronary heart disease (CHD) and other prevalent medical disorders, including obesity, hypertension, hyperlipidemias, non-insulin-dependent or type II diabetes mellitus, atherothrombotic cerebral strokes, certain types of malignancies, gallstones, and osteoporosis. Contributing behaviors for these medical conditions include dietary habits, physical inactivity, and cigarette smoking. Dietary practices interact with physical activity to have a significant impact on the metabolic and physiological risk factors for atherosclerosis listed in Table 1. The goals of this chapter are to identify the influence of common dietary practices and associated sedentary lifestyle on physiological and metabolic maladaptations contributing to risk of CHD; to provide the rationale for modifying these unhealthy dietary practices and for promoting physical activity as cornerstones for CHD prevention; to provide the clinician with assessment instruments and intervention strategies suitable for use in a medical practice, and; to provide a management approach for modification of nutritionally related risk factors with emphasis on correction of blood lipid disorders and obesity.

Table 1 Physiological and Metabolic Risk Factors for Coronary Heart Disease Affected by Diet and Physical Activity

Body weight/adiposity	Glucose–insulin dynamics
Blood lipid/lipoprotein profile	Blood coagulability
Blood pressure level	

II. DIETARY FACTORS CONTRIBUTING TO ATHEROSCLEROSIS

A. Obesity

The high prevalence of obesity in the United States (20–50% of the population depending on the survey, measurement method, and standard employed) results from a combination of low levels of on-the-job and leisure-time physical activity and an abundance of easily accessible food with a high energy density (2). An insidious progressive weight gain is especially common during the middle years of life (3). This is generally associated during this period of life with a reduction in food energy intake, but a still greater decline in energy expenditure on-the-job and during leisure-time.

The independent contributions of obesity and weight gain after physical maturity to risk of CHD mortality have been demonstrated by a number of large-scale, long-term, prospective, observational studies, particularly the Framingham Study (4); however, other prospective studies have found either no independent relationship or a U-shaped relationship between overweight and CHD rates (5). Nevertheless, there is strong consistent evidence that obesity indirectly affects risk of CHD by its contributions to blood lipid abnormalities and blood pressure elevation, and by the induction of abnormalities in glucose-insulin dynamics, including increased cell insulin resistance, hyperinsulinemia, glucose intolerance, and type II diabetes (1). These conditions respond promptly and impressively to weight reduction achieved by diet, increased physical activity, or a combination of the two interventions.

There also has accumulated a substantial body of evidence indicating that certain subgroups of people with obesity are at excess risk of CHD compared to the average obese person. An abdominal preponderance of fat (i.e., the so-called "middle-aged spread" or "pot belly") in obese men, and especially women, appears more likely to be associated with physiological and metabolic risk factors for CHD, greater risk for cardiovascular disease and type II diabetes, and premature mortality compared to other obese people (6,7). A regional excess of body fat in the abdominal area can be documented by the finding of a waist/hip circumference greater than 1.0 in men and above 0.8 or 0.9 in women. The waist girth is taken in the erect position at the level of the umbilicus with the individual breathing normally; the hip circumference is measured at the level of the superior iliac crest. Abdominal adipose tissue appears to be morphologically and metabolically different from adipose tissue at other body sites, but how these differences alter risk factors for CHD requires further research (7).

B. Blood Lipid and Lipoprotein Levels

It is now firmly established that plasma concentrations of total cholesterol and its principal carrier low-density lipoprotein (LDL) are potent risk factors for CHD. Severity of coronary atherosclerosis and risk of initial and recurrent CHD events are directly related to levels of total and LDL cholesterol (8–10). LDL is involved in the insudation of cholesterol into the arterial wall and formation of atheromas. The rate of major CHD events in prospective epidemiologic studies shows a continuous, graded increase of about 2% for each 1% increase in total plasma cholesterol above 180 mg/dl (4.67 mmol/L). The rate of CHD events was demonstrated in the Lipid Research Clinics' (LRC) Coronary Primary Prevention Trial (CPPT) to decline 2% for each 1% reduction in plasma cholesterol concentration (primarily reflecting a reduction in level of LDL cholesterol) by diet and a cholesterol-lowering drug in middle-aged men with hypercholesterolemia (11). In the CPPT, CHD risk was reduced most substantially in participants maintaining the highest plasma high-density lipoprotein (HDL) cholesterol levels (12). An inverse relationship between plasma levels of HDL cholesterol and death from cardiovascular disease was also evident in the LRC Program's Prevalence Study (9), which included 8,825 middle-aged men from 10 North American communities. A substantially greater risk of CHD mortality was found at the 10-year follow-up of those men with initial low HDL cholesterol levels (<35 mg/dl) who had pre-existing evidence of CHD than in those who were disease-free at baseline. This study illustrates the independent contribution of HDL cholesterol to severity of atherosclerosis and risk of initial and recurrent CHD events. Furthermore, in the Framingham Study for every 10 mg increment in HDL cholesterol there was an approximate 50% lower risk of initial CHD events (13). In addition, in The Helsinki Heart Study (14) a 34% greater reduction in 5-year incidence of CHD was observed in middle-aged men with hypercholescholesterolemia who received a combination of diet and a cholesterol-lowering drug, gemfibrozil, compared to those receiving diet and placebo. The combination therapy was associated with an average decrease of 8% in plasma total cholesterol levels. Based on the 2:1 association cited above, only a 16% decline in CHD events would be expected from this degree of cholesterol reduction. It is postulated that an accompanying 10% mean increase in plasma HDL cholesterol level in the treatment group probably accounted for the greater than expected reduction in rate of CHD events. The antiatherogenic role of HDL appears to be related to its ability as a cholesterol scavenger to remove cholesterol from tissues, including atheromas, and transport it in the form of fatty acid esters to the liver for catabolism to bile salts.

Dietary habits profoundly influence plasma total and LDL cholesterol levels.

The most potent dietary influence on LDL cholesterol is the percentage of daily energy intake from saturated fat. This is well documented by cross-cultural population comparisons of saturated fat intake with blood cholesterol levels and CHD rates, such as provided by the Seven Countries' Collaborative Study (15). Confirmation of this triangular relationship between diet, blood cholesterol levels, and severity of atherosclerosis has been provided by animal experiments, including those in nonhuman primates (16). Quantification of the effect of type and quantity of dietary lipid intake on blood cholesterol levels has come from human metabolic ward isocaloric feeding studies (17,18). Percentage of food energy from saturated fatty acids has the largest measurable impact on blood total and LDL cholesterol levels of any known dietary lipid. The blood cholesterol-enhancing effect of dietary cholesterol is much less potent than that of saturated fatty acids and is related to total food energy intake. In contrast, increasing the percentage of daily energy intake from omega-6 polyunsaturated fatty acids (PUFA) contained in large quantities in certain vegetable oils lowers blood cholesterol levels; however the power of PUFA to reduce cholesterol levels is about half that of an equal reduction in intake of saturated fatty acids (SFA) expressed in percentage of daily energy intake. Replacing percentage calories from SFA with monounsaturated fatty acids has been reported either to have no effect on serum cholesterol levels (17,18) or a cholesterol-lowering effect equal to that of omega-6 PUFA (19).

The effects of omega-3 PUFA fatty acids found in fish oils on blood lipids will be discussed later in this chapter along with their effect on blood coagulation, since this appears to be their most important potential site of antiatherogenic activity.

Weight changes also profoundly affect blood lipid levels. Weight gain increases levels of plasma total and LDL cholesterol, as well as very-low-density lipoproteins (VLDL) and triglycerides while reducing HDL cholesterol levels (1). Hyperinsulinemia, which often accompanies weight gain related to cell insulin resistance, seems to contribute to these blood lipid changes. Weight loss has the opposite effect of weight gain on these blood lipid and lipoprotein levels, particularly in men.

Water-soluble constituents of dietary fiber, such as pectins and certain gums, also may have a slight cholesterol-reducing effect, probably by promoting fecal elimination of cholesterol in the form of bile salts and neutral steroids of cholesterol origin (21).

Since HDL is a lipid scavenger, a high intake of dietary fat and cholesterol usually physiologically increases plasma HDL levels, while a diet low in fat and cholesterol generally lowers HDL cholesterol levels along with plasma levels of the other lipoprotein cholesterol fractions (22). The threshold for reduction of plasma HDL cholesterol level appears to be a dietary fat level less than 20% of daily energy requirements, and this appears to be counteracted by partial substitution of monounsaturated fats for saturated fats (23).

Populations who consume very little SFA or are vegetarians have low plasma levels of HDL cholesterol along with low levels of total and LDL cholesterol (24,25) and almost nonexistent CHD. This illustrates the critical relationship of plasma LDL cholesterol level independent of HDL cholesterol level to the occurrence of CHD. Plasma HDL cholesterol concentration is also directly related to intake of alcohol (22,26) and levels of physical activity and physical fitness (27,28), and it is inversely impacted by cigarette smoking (29).

The effect of exercise on levels on HDL cholesterol and other blood lipids has been extensively reviewed (27,28). The postulated principal mechanism for the usual increase in HDL cholesterol levels with exercise conditioning appears to be through stimulation of lipoprotein lipase activity (LPL). HDL formation is believed to be increased with exercise by the accelerated clearance of VLDL and triglycerides from the blood through lipolytic activity of LPL. Thus, it appears that in order to optimize a patient's blood lipid and lipoprotein profile a combination of dietary changes, loss of excess body weight, regular exercise, and smoking cessation are required. Dietary changes to optimize blood lipid/lipoprotein levels consist of a modest reduction in total and saturated fat and cholesterol intake with substitution of energy from complex carbohydrates in place of fat calories and an equal percentage of calories from saturated, monounsaturated, and PUFA. Comprehensive lifestyle changes have been recently demonstrated to bring about regression of even severe angiographically demonstrated coronary atherosclerosis after only 1 year without use of lipid-lowering drugs (30). More details on dietary management of hyperlipidemia are provided later in this chapter.

C. Blood Pressure Effect

Blood pressure level, another major risk factor for atherosclerosis and CHD, also is influenced by diet and body weight and to a lesser extent by exercise habits. Severity of atherosclerosis and risk of myocardial infarction and strokes, progressively increase with levels of both systolic and diastolic blood pressure (31). Several landmark clinical trials have provided conclusive proof of reduced cardiovascular events with treatment of even mild diastolic hypertension. Dietary factors believed to increase blood pressure levels are a high intake of sodium and perhaps low dietary levels of potassium (from fruits and vegetables) and calcium (from dairy and plant sources), excess body weight, and alcohol consumption (1,32). It was recently demonstrated, however, that potassium supplements do not contribute to blood pressure reduction in hypertensive patients on a low sodium diet (33). Nevertheless, experimental data suggest a possible vasoprotective effect of potassium administration independent of blood pressure reduction (34). A high intake of SFA and a low ratio of PUFA to SFA also have been reported to be associated with increased blood pressure levels, perhaps through altered prostanoid synthesis (35). Furthermore, it has recently been demonstrated that administration of omega-3 PUFA (i.e., eicosapentaenoic or EPA and docosahexaenoic acid or DCA) found in fish oils can reduce blood pressure levels in patients with essential hypertension, but this observation remains to be confirmed and the dose–response relationship better defined (36).

It also is well known that a transient reduction in levels of blood pressure occurs with acute dynamic exercise and persists for several hours postexercise, apparently related to peripheral vasodilatation (37). Chronic dynamic exercise involving large muscle groups also may have a modest systolic and diastolic blood pressure-reducing effect (on the average about 10 mmHg for each), with weight reduction often a contributing factor (37,38). The feasibility of multifactorial nonpharmacologic intervention, including weight loss, reduced sodium and alcohol intake, and regular exercise for prevention and treatment of mild hypertension has been demonstrated by clinical trials (39,40).

D. Diabetes Mellitus

Diabetes mellitus is another important promoter of atherosclerosis and a potent risk factor for CHD and other serious cardiovascular disorders (41,42). Epidemiologic studies indicate that obesity is the principal causative factor for non-insulin-dependent or type II diabetes and that physical inactivity is another important contributor (41). Diet, exercise, and weight management also appear to play important preventive and therapeutic roles in type II diabetes, which is much more common than type I diabetes in North America (43,44). Peripheral cell insulin resistance, glucose intolerance, and hyperinsulinemia can be induced experimentally by overeating and development of obesity, but they also can be demonstrated after only a few days of bed rest (41,42). Furthermore, a decrease in physical activity and associated weight gain are important contributors to glucose intolerance and peripheral insulin resistance commonly associated with aging in affluent societies. A strong link also seems to exist between peripheral insulin resistance, hyperinsulinemia, and hypertension (45). A diet low in complex carbohydrates and high in fat also may adversely affect glucose tolerance (5). Thus, it appears that a combination of maintenance of proper weight or the loss of excess body fat, a reduction in dietary intake of SFA with an associated increase in complex carbohydrates, and regular dynamic physical activity may act in concert to help prevent type II diabetes. These dietary and physical activity recommendations are particularly important for individuals with a family history of diabetes and/or a concentration of adipose tissue in the abdominal region because of the associated excess risk of type II diabetes (6,7).

Acute moderate-intensity, prolonged dynamic exercise (30–60 min or more duration) has been demonstrated to lower blood glucose levels for up to 48 hr in both nondiabetic and diabetic individuals through increased glucose uptake by participating skeletal muscles (42). This is accompanied by a temporary improvement in insulin sensitivity and reduced blood glucose levels or diabetic drug dosage requirements in diabetic patients. These effects are potentiated by regular exercise training through promotion of increased cell insulin receptor activity and beneficial skeletal muscle hemodynamic and metabolic adaptations (42). However, the principal beneficial long-term interactive effects of diet and regular physical activity on the prevention and therapy of type II diabetes appear to be through their contributions to weight management and fat loss, since with cessation of exercise, other beneficial adaptive effects on glucose-insulin dynamics regress within a week.

E. Blood Coagulation

As discussed in Chapter 2, interactions among the arterial wall endothelial cells, lipoproteins, and blood platelets are postulated to be involved in both the development and subsequent progression of coronary atherosclerosis and thrombosis (46). Diet and exercise alter platelet function and blood coagulability, and thereby affect severity of atherosclerosis and risk of coronary thrombosis, myocardial infarction, and sudden cardiac death (1).

The influence of dietary fat intake on platelet function and thrombosis is currently not as well understood as its effect on blood lipids and lipoproteins. The type of fatty acids in the diet apparently can alter platelet aggregability and vascular reactivity through their influence on synthesis of prostaglandins and related compounds in platelets and arterial endothelial cells (47,48). Although the evidence is not yet conclusive, it appears that a high intake of SFA and/or a low dietary PUFA to SFA ratio can promote platelet aggregation and synthesis of a prostaglandin called thromboxane A_2 (TXA_2). TXA_2 promotes both platelet aggregation (the initial step in blood coagulation) and constriction of vascular smooth muscle. Dietary omega-6 PUFA promotes production of both TXA_2 by platelets and another prostaglandin, prostacyclin (PGI_2), by arterial endothelial cells. PGI_2 has the opposite effect on platelet and vascular smooth muscle reactivity as TXA_2. It reduces platelet aggregation and promotes vascular arterial smooth muscle relaxation, resulting in vasodilatation including the coronary arteries. The other class of PUFA, the omega-3 type, promotes synthesis of a prostacyclin derivative that has similar antiplatelet aggregation and vasodilatory properties to PGI_2. In addition, this type of fatty acid promotes platelet synthesis of an alternative prostaglandin to TXA_2, which does not cause platelet aggregation nor blood vessel constriction. The end result of increased omega 3-PUFA consumption is reduced platelet aggregation in response to usual physiological stimuli, resulting in reduced blood coagulability as manifested by an increase in bleeding time. Although it is unknown at this time whether such changes induced by ingestion of omega-3 PUFA can protect against vascular disease, there is a strong suspicion that they may (49). This is because aspirin has a similar effect on blood coagulability and bleeding time and has proven beneficial in reducing vascular thrombosis. Both plant and animal food sources of omega-3 PUFA exist. Green leafy vegetables and seed oils (particularly canola and soybean oils) are rich in alpha-linolenic acid, which can be converted by the body to EPA and DCA. EPA and DCA are abundant in fatty fish, particularly those from cold northern oceans such as mackerel and salmon. As previously mentioned, preliminary evidence suggests that these fatty acids may have a blood-pressure-lowering effect (36). In addition, fish oils have proven effective in the treatment of hypertriglyceridemia by reducing levels of its principal carrier in the fasting state, VLDL (47,48). However, the effects of ingestion of omega-3 PUFA on plasma total and LDL cholesterol levels are more variable, with an increase in LDL cholesterol a possibility. In addition, the quantity of omega-3 PUFA necessary for the physiological and metabolic effects described above makes it impractical to obtain from food sources and would require dietary supplementation with fish oil or EPA and DCA. It is concluded that the potential usefulness of omega-3 PUFA in the prevention and management of CHD, their optimal amounts, long-term safety, and specific dietary advice or supplementation required for possible CHD protection all remain to be elucidated more clearly. In the meantime, it is prudent to increase the use of plant sources of omega-3 PUFA and consume fish several times per week in place of red meat.

Both acute and chronic exercise also affect platelet aggregation and blood coagulation, as well as fibrinolysis (50–52). A temporary increase in platelet aggregation and blood coagulability accompanies heavy physical exertion; however, this hypercoagulable state is counteracted by an increase in fibrinolytic activity. Exercise training appears to diminish the increased blood coagulability during acute physical exertion and reduces the sensitivity of platelets to the action of agonists while maintaining or augmenting reactivity of the clot-dissolving fibrinolytic system (50–52). Thus, endurance exercise conditioning, a reduced intake of SFA, and an increase in PUFA, particularly of the omega-3 variety, may favorably interact to reduce risk of vascular thrombosis and perhaps attenuate the postulated contribution of platelet aggregation to development of atherosclerosis.

III. NUTRITIONAL ASSESSMENT TECHNIQUES

Nutritional assessment techniques relevant to a CHD prevention program that can be used in a physician's office are discussed in this section. These include techniques for the determination of desirable body weight, daily energy requirements, physical activity status, and usual eating pattern and nutrient intake.

A. Desirable Body Weight in Reference to Height

The normal or "desirable" level of body fat from a health standpoint is not known, since the amount of adipose tissue carried by apparently healthy people varies widely. A commonly used standard is based on the usual percentage of body fat at physical maturity (i.e., 14–20% for men and 21–27% for women) (53,54). Based on these standards, men are considered to be borderline fat at 21–24% body fat and obese if more than 25% of their body weight is fat. Women are considered borderline fat at 26–29% body fat and obese if their body fat level exceeds 30%. Since the precise determination of body fat requires sophisticated laboratory techniques that are not widely available, indirect anthropometric measurements based on height and weight measurements (i.e., relative weight determinations) are generally used as a substitute. In fact, most of the available information about the health implications of obesity is based on such measurements rather than on actual body fatness assessments. The term "overweight," or excess of body weight in relationship to height, generally is used as a surrogate for obesity.

Commonly used standards for "desirable" weight for height are the 1959 (55) or the more recent 1983 (56) Metropolitan Life Insurance Tables based on insurance company survival data. The 1983 tables have been criticized because of their higher standard weights for both men and women compared to the 1959 tables, particularly for the shortest people. This is because of concern that the extra weight "permitted" in the 1983 tables may have adverse effects on health. Other criticisms of these actuarial tables as reference standards are that the data are based on an insured population that may not be representative of the population as a whole; the technical quality of the data; and the presence of confounding variables that may affect mortality rates in either direction, particularly the fact that cigarette smokers generally weigh less than nonsmokers and have higher mortality rates. Furthermore, the tables necessitate making judgments about body "frame size" for which there is no generally accepted method. A commonly used compromise is to use as a standard for desirable weight the midpoint of the medium body build for the weight range at a specified height based on the 1959 Metropolitan Life Insurance Table (57,58).

Table 2 shows this median value for weight relative to height for the medium body build for men and women. These median weights approximate the actual 25th percentile of weights for heights for adults in the U.S. population age 17–74 years based on national survey data (59). The "normal" range shown in Table 2 indicates the extremes of weights for large and small frame sizes. The weights become progressively less desirable as they diverge from the median value for each height level. Adults are generally considered significantly overweight if their relative weight for height exceeds the median weight value by 20% or more. Obvious exceptions are athletes who may be overweight because of excess lean skeletal muscle. Likewise, there are some people whose weight is in the normal range for height, even though their body fat exceeds standard levels. In this situation, the extra fat weight is masked by deficient skeletal muscle mass.

Another approach for determining whether a person's weight is appropriate for height, which does not require the use of tables, is to calculate the body mass index (BMI), commonly expressed in the metric system as weight in kilograms (kg)

Table 2 Recommended Weight (lbs) in Relation to Height

Height (in)	Men Median	Men Range	Women Median	Women Range
58	—		102	92–119
59	—		104	94–122
60	—		107	96–125
61	—		110	99–128
62	123	112–141	113	102–131
63	127	115–144	116	105–134
64	130	118–148	120	108–138
65	133	121–152	123	114–142
66	136	124–156	128	114–146
67	140	128–161	132	118–150
68	145	132–166	136	122–154
69	149	136–170	140	126–158
70	153	140–174	144	130–168

divided by height in meters squared (i.e., kg/m^2). BMI has a stronger relationship with body fatness than relative weight for height (58). BMI in kg/m^2 can be calculated from weight (W) in pounds and height (H) in inches as follows:

$W/H^2 \times 703.1$

Based on weight standards in Table 2, the recommended BMI for U.S. men is 21.6 kg/m^2 and for women 21.2 kg/m^2, and the normal BMI range for both men and women is approximately 19–25 kg/m^2. By standards adopted at a recent NIH Consensus Conference (59), men are considered overweight when their BMI equals or exceeds 27.8 kg/m^2 and severely overweight when the BMI equals or exceeds 31.1 kg/m^2. For women these corresponding values are 27.3 and 32.3 kg/m^2.

An additional approach for determining desirable body weight applicable for use in the clinic is to estimate body fatness by measurement of skinfold thickness using standardized calipers at designated sites. Percentage body fat can be estimated from skinfold thickness measurements using validated regression equations (60,61). A desirable body weight goal for a weight reduction program can be determined from this estimate of body fat and the desirable level of lean weight calculated for the individual (60,61). As an example, consider a man weighing 200 lbs with an estimated 30% body fat by skinfold measurements. His total fat weight would be 200 lbs × 0.30 or 60 lbs. His current lean tissue weight would then be 200 minus 60 or 140 lbs. Based on the criterion that a more desirable body composition would be 20% fat and 80% lean tissue (53), his desirable weight would be calculated as follows:

$$\text{Desirable weight} = \frac{\text{lean weight}}{\% \text{ lean tissue}} \times 100 = \frac{140 \text{ lbs}}{80} \times 100 = 175 \text{ lbs}$$

Thus, this man's goal for a weight loss program would be 200 minus 175 or 25 lbs.

B. Determination of Daily Energy Requirements

The energy requirement of an individual is generally defined as the level of energy intake from food that will balance energy expenditures for an individual of desirable body size and composition and level of physical activity required to perform usual occupational activity and recreational pursuits commensurate with good health (62). For children and pregnant or lactating women, the energy requirements also include the energy needs associated with proper growth, deposition of tissues, or secretion of milk at rates consistent with good health. Total energy expenditure is commonly divided into several compartments. These include resting expenditure (REE), the thermic effect of food (TEF), thermogenesis, and energy expenditure during physical activity (62). These components are, in turn, altered by a number of variables, including age, gender, body size and composition, genetic factors, food energy intake, nutritional and physiological state, ambient temperature, and coexisting pathologic conditions.

With the exception of individuals with extremely high physical activity levels, REE makes the largest contribution to daily energy expenditure, usually accounting for 60–75% of daily energy requirements. In the average 70 kg man, REE amounts to approximately 1700 kcal/day and in the average 55 kg woman about 1400 kcal/day (63). A difference in lean body mass in favor of men is the principal contributor to variance in REE between average men and women and between individuals of the same gender, age, height and weight. REE can be estimated by using any of several empirically derived equations. For example, by the Harris and Benedict equations (62):

For women: REE (kcal/24 hr) = 655 + 1.85 × height + 9.56 × weight − 4.68 × age

For men: REE (kcal/24 hr) = 665 + 5.03 × height + 13.75 × weight − 6.75 × age

where height is in cm, weight in kg, and age in years.

TEF represents the energy cost of digestion, absorption, transport, metabolism, and storage of ingested food. It reaches a maximum about 1 hr after eating and virtually disappears 4 hr after eating. Its magnitude is affected by the energy content and composition of the meal, as well as the nutritional and physical activity status of the individual. Individual variation also appears to exist in TEF due to differences in energy costs when a meal is absorbed and utilized, which may be under genetic influence. These differences may contribute to discrepancies between estimated and actual energy balance (64). TEF is small in relationship to total energy requirements, accounting for 10–15% of daily energy expenditure.

Thermogenesis, or so-called luxus consumption, is another variable component of energy expenditure. It reflects the adaptive conversion of substrate chemical energy apparently by brown adipose tissue to heat in response to cold exposure (nonshivering thermogenesis), excess food intake (dietary-induced thermogenesis), and other stimuli (62). It has been postulated that variability among individuals in efficiency in conversion of energy intake to ATP or fat compared with dissipation as heat by thermogenesis contributes to susceptibility to obesity. This intriguing hypothesis has been around for over 80 years but still remains to be proven (65).

Physical activity is the most variable component of daily energy expenditure. For the average person, it usually contributes about 20–30% of the daily energy requirements. Methodologies for assessing habitual physical activity have recently been reviewed (66,67). The energy cost of this component may be measured by having individuals keep records or diaries of all their physical activities for 1–3 day periods, (including a weekend day), or by a systematic recall of activities for the previous 1 to 2 days or for a "typical" weekday and weekend day. The estimated energy cost of each activity mentioned in the physical activity recall or record can be obtained from tables derived from direct or indirect calorimetry studies (61,68]. An alternative approach is to determine relative activity status by having the patient complete a quantitative physical activity history questionnaire such as the Minnesota Questionnaire (69) or shorter general survey questionnaires. Further discussion of physical activity assessment techniques is found in Chapter 12.

The Food and Nutrition Board of the National Research Council has derived conversion factors for estimating usual total daily energy expenditure for people with different levels of physical activity (63). These are summarized in Table 3. One simply has to multiply these conversion factors by the individual's body weight in kg to obtain an estimate of an individual's daily total energy needs. Examples of various types of job, home, maintenance, sport, and recreational activities making up each of the activity classes in Table 3 (i.e., light, moderate, heavy or very heavy) are shown in Appendix B. To qualify for one of these activity categories, the individual must have a predominance of activities in the given category. Table 4 lists actual estimated average daily energy allowances for Americans of average heights and weights and physical activity levels based on national nutritional survey data (63).

C. Assessment of Dietary Status

A number of techniques are available to help the health professional understand an individual's dietary patterns and practices. Such an understanding is essential for

Table 3 Estimated Energy
Expenditure at Various Levels of
Physical Activity for Men and Women
of Medium Weight (Ages 19–50 Yrs)[a]

Level of Activity	Energy Cost (kcal/kg per day)	
	Men	Women
Light	38	35
Moderate	41	37
Heavy	50	44
Very heavy	58	51

[a]For those over age 50, subtract 300 kcal/day
for men and 200 kcal/day for women.

making nutritional recommendations in order to help the patient reduce excess
weight and other risk factors for CHD. In the next section we will briefly review
some of the more common assessment methods that can be used in a physician's
office. Available food survey methods include food records, a dietary recall,
dietary histories of usual food habits, and food frequency questionnaires. These

Table 4 Average Daily Energy Intakes for People of
Medium Height and Weight and Moderate Physical Activity
Status

Age	Weight (lb)	Height (in)	kcal/kg	kcal/day
Men				
15–18	145	69	45	3000
19–24	160	70	40	2900
25–50	174	70	37	2900
51+	170	68	30	2300
Women				
15–18	120	64	40	2200
19–24	128	65	38	2200
25–50	138	64	36	2200
51+	143	63	30	1900
Pregnancy 1st trimester	+ 0			
2nd trimester	+ 300			
3rd trimester	+ 300			
Lactating	+ 500			

approaches have been reviewed in detail elsewhere (70) and only the highlights are briefly discussed below.

1. Food Record

The food record or diary is one of the most accurate methods for determining food and nutrient consumption, especially if food is weighed before eating and leftovers weighed after eating. A less accurate but more practical alternative is to estimate portion and leftover sizes rather than actually weighing them. However, even with this adjustment this approach remains burdensome for many individuals and may bias normal eating patterns, especially if the food record is maintained for longer than 1 week. Food records also consistently yield lower reported energy intakes than the dietary recall method to be discussed below. With this method, an individual is asked to record all food and beverages consumed for 1–14 days. Compliance is usually better using a 2 or 3 day period than 1 week or longer. The quantities of food eaten usually are estimated by using common household utensils such as cups or measuring spoons for descriptive purposes. For food items such as eggs or slices of bread, a simple count is requested. For prepared foods, the package weight is entered on the food record.

Because of the burden placed on the patient, there is the problem of noncompliance. There also is the need for a health professional skilled in nutrition to review the food record with the patient for completeness. Thus, this method is not commonly used in the clinical setting unless a dietitian or nutritionist is on staff. However, referral to a nutritional professional for this service is an option.

2. Twenty Four Hour Recall

The 24 hr recall is one of the most commonly used methods of dietary assessment. As the name implies, the individual is asked by a nutrition professional to recall all food and beverages consumed over the preceding 24 hr. The recall usually proceeds backwards in time to the previous day. For example, if the recall is initiated at 1 pm, the interview would progress backwards from this time to 1 pm on the previous day. As an alternative, the recall could systematically cover the previous full day, using a midnight to midnight time period. The information is usually obtained by a personal interview using sample measuring instruments and food models to help with judgment of portion sizes. A recall also can be obtained by a telephone interview, although this is a less commonly used method and is less accurate in terms of estimating portion sizes. If the recall is carried out unannounced, the patient does not have the opportunity to modify his or her diet before the interview in order to attempt to please the interviewer or the physician. The great advantage of the 24 hr recall over the food record is that it can be completed in 20–30 min and it requires little effort on the part of the respondent. Since there is a great deal of variation in what people eat from day to day and in different seasons of the year, a single 24 hr recall may not provide a representative picture of usual year-round food and nutrient intake. A much more accurate estimate of usual dietary habits can be obtained when a mixture of three or four weekend and weekday recalls is obtained, especially if they include days from different seasons of the year (71).

3. Diet History

The dietary history is designed to collect detailed data on usual food habits and practices of individuals for extended periods of time, typically a 2 or 3 month period. A complete diet history consists of three distinct components: health history, usual food intake pattern, and frequency of consumption of selected food groups.

The health history section provides details on eating habits, food preferences, and economic and health factors that may affect food choices. This information is useful in interpreting food consumption data and in counseling for specific needs of the individual. The food intake component of the dietary history provides information on the usual meal patterns of the patient. For each of the three meals and usual snack times, the nutrition professional asks the patient what he or she usually eats and the usual portion sizes. If the respondent's usual pattern is different on weekdays and weekends, as is frequently the case, both patterns are recorded. The final component of the dietary history consists of assessing the frequency of consumption of selected food groups. This provides additional information on a broad range of food items and serves as a cross-check of the reported usual dietary pattern.

Although the diet history provides a comprehensive picture of an individual's eating habits, it has several major disadvantages that limit its use in a clinical setting: it takes about an hour to complete, which is much longer than required for a 24 hr dietary recall, it requires a good deal of expertise on the part of the interviewer, and it tends to overestimate food intake compared to the 24 hr recall.

4. Food Frequency Questionnaires

A food frequency survey is a simplified version of the last two components of a diet history. This assessment tool obtains information on the number of times certain food or food groups are consumed over a given period of time from a day to a month or longer. For example, the food questionnaire used in the Second National Health and Nutrition Examination Survey (NHANES-II) included 18 food groups (72). Participants were asked to recall the frequency of consumption of each of the food groups for the 3 month period before the interview. Other questionnaires using as few as four food groups have been reported to yield valuable information. Two commonly used, validated food frequency questionnaires are those of Willett (73) and Bloch (74).

The major advantage of the use of food frequency questionnaires in clinical practice is their simplicity. With proper instructions, they can even be self-administered. Disadvantages include their lack of adequate quantitative data on nutrient intake, and that they may not be appropriate for use with certain ethnic groups whose diet habits differ greatly from the general population. However, in general they do provide relatively accurate information about a patient's eating pattern and they are useful for monitoring dietary changes during nutritional intervention.

Figure 1 provides an example of a short dietary frequency questionnaire reported to be a useful clinical tool for the clinical office for pinpointing nutritional problems related to CHD risk: the Three-Minute Dietary Assessment Questionnaire (75). Another short questionnaire specifically targeted for assessment of total fat, saturated fat, and dietary fiber intake was recently published by Kristal et al. (76).

5. Determination of Nutrient Content from Food Records or Recalls

The data from quantitative dietary survey measurements must be converted from food items into nutrients. This usually is accomplished by the use of food

Category	Specific Questions
Meal frequency	How many meals do you eat per day? How many are prepared at home? Do you know how to select a low-fat diet when eating out?
Meat intake	How many of your weekly meals include beef, pork, lamb, or veal? Do you know what the leaner cuts of meat are? Is the portion you usually eat larger than the palm of your hand or a deck of cards? Do you eat poultry with the skin? How often do you eat organ meats? Hot dogs? Sausage?
Egg yolks	How many egg yolks do you eat per week? Have you tried egg substitutes or just using egg whites?
Dairy	What kind of milk do you drink (whole, 2%, skim)? How often? Do you eat cheese? What kinds (high or low-fat)? How often? Low-fat? How often? Ice cream?
Fats	Do you eat baked goods (doughnuts, cakes)? Do you know what kinds of fat they contain?
Cooking	Do you cook with any kinds of fat (lard, butter, liquid oil)? Do you use butter, margarine, or salad dressings at the table? Low fat?
Snacks	Do you eat candy bars? Chips?
Alcohol	How many drinks do you have per week? (1 drink = 1 oz. liquor, 1 can beer, 1 4 oz. glass of wine.)
Salt	Do you salt food when cooking? At the table? Do you like salty foods: pickles, olives, chips, convenience foods? Do you use spices in seasoning? Salt substitutes?

Figure 1   Three minute dietary assessment. (Adapted from Ref. 75.)

composition tables from the U.S. Department of Agriculture (77). A more sophisticated method, which is being increasingly employed, is the use of special computer software programs such as the Nutrient Calculating System (NCS) developed at the University of Minnesota's National Nutritional Coding Center (Minneapolis, MN), used in NHANES-III. The NCS permits direct entry of foods into a microprocessor without prior coding. Nutritional information obtained usually includes daily intake of energy, protein, carbohydrates, fat, types of fatty acids, dietary fiber, vitamins, and minerals. The values are generally compared for adequacy with standards such as those of the National Academy of Sciences' (NAS) Recommended Dietary Allowances (RDA) (63). When the RDA are being used to judge nutritional adequacy, one should remember that they represent population standards and tend to exaggerate nutritional needs of individuals for most nutrients, with the exception of energy.

IV. NUTRITIONAL COUNSELING GOALS

Nutritional counseling goals elaborated on in this section include guidelines for meeting energy needs and RDA for essential nutrients, weight reduction and maintenance, management of blood lipid abnormalities and other risk factors as well as practical considerations in food choices, reading food labels, cooking methods, and a list of nutritional educational materials and sources.

A. Meeting Energy and Nutrient Requirements

The food-energy needs of the individual should be determined and explained in relationship to age, resting energy requirements, and physical activity status. If the patient's weight is within the desirable range for his or her height, and the individual is only moderately active, the food energy intake requirements called for in Table 4 will generally suffice at least initially. A blend of proper food choices required to obtain all of the key nutrients in recommended amounts can be obtained by encouraging the use of appropriate number of choices from the basic food groups. This so-called food exchange system is a simple way of providing a variety of foods with a high probability that the diet will be nutritionally adequate. This system calls for a proper number of choices from the basic food groups: bread, cereals, and other starchy foods; milk and dairy products; protein choices (or meat–legume group); the vegetable group; fruit choices. A sixth food group called the "fats, sweets, and alcohol group" consists of high-energy, low-nutrient-density nonessential foods (e.g., butter, margarine, vegetable oils, honey, syrups, refined sugar, and alcoholic beverages). There are no minimum servings required of this last group and these foods may be omitted entirely by those who need to limit energy intake. Others may use them in moderation to complement food selections from the five major groups. Most nutrition books provide food exchange lists for various types of diets (e.g., Shils and Young [78]). Below are described choices from each of the five major food groups appropriate for an individual on a "heart healthy" cholesterol-lowering diet and the usual number of servings required from each group to meet the RDA for essential nutrients.

The bread-cereal group includes all grain and grain products made of wheat, rice, oats, barley, and rye used in the form of breads, breakfast cereals, and pastries. Usual recommendations are for at least four daily servings from this group. A typical serving may include a slice of whole grain bread, a cup (1 oz) of oatmeal, a half cup of rice, a cup of ready-to-eat cereal, a ½ cup of pasta, or ½ cup of flour.

Food choices from the milk–dairy product group for someone on a cholesterol-lowering diet are low-fat, skimmed, or partially skimmed milk and milk products. These include milk used as a beverage or in food preparation, natural and processed cheeses, yogurt, or frozen desserts. The usual recommended number of daily servings from this group are: for children, three servings/day; for adolescents, three; for adults, two; for pregnant women, three; and for lactating women, four.

A typical serving from this group would consist of a cup (8 oz) of 2% fat milk; 1 oz of cheddar cheese; a ½ cup of low fat cottage cheese; 4 oz of low- or no-fat fruit-flavored yogurt or 8 oz of plain yogurt; or ½ cup of reduced fat ice cream, ice milk, or low- or no-fat frozen yogurt.

The modified meat–legume group includes well-trimmed, lower-fat cuts of red meat (beef, veal, pork, or lamb); poultry without the skin; fish or shellfish; eggs (limited to two or three egg yolks/week); legumes (such as beans, peas, and lentils), or nuts. A minimum of two servings per day is recommended from this group. This should include several meatless days per week and fish several times per week. A serving could consist of 2 oz of cooked lean red meat, poultry, or fish, an egg, ½ cup of cooked dry beans, ½ cup of nuts, or 4 tablespoonfuls of peanut butter.

The vegetable group includes all fresh, canned, or frozen vegetables (except high-protein beans and peas included in the meat–legume group). Recommendations call for two or more servings daily from this group including a green leafy vegetable. Examples of a serving are a small salad, 1 cup of shredded cabbage or other vegetables, 1 ear of corn, or ½ of a plain boiled potato.

The fruit group includes all fresh, canned, frozen, and dried fruit. Two or more daily servings from this group are recommended, which should include a daily citrus selection to meet vitamin C requirements. A serving may include 1 whole fresh fruit, ½ cup of cooked fruit, or ½ cup of juice.

In addition, the total daily intake of sodium chloride should be limited to 6 g or less. This includes reducing the use of salt in cooking and avoiding its addition to foods at the table, and the use of salty or salt-processed or preserved foods sparingly. Alcohol consumption should be limited to the equivalent of 1–2 oz or less of pure alcohol per day. This is the equivalent of two cans of beer, two small glasses of wine, or one to two average cocktails. Pregnant women and people with hypertriglyceridemias should avoid alcoholic beverages completely.

B. Weight Reduction and/or Maintenance

Weight reduction is recommended for those who are substantially over the desirable levels (Table 2), especially when the BMI is greater than 30 kg/m^2, excessive body fat is demonstrated by skinfold measurements, and abdominal distribution of fat is predominant. The presence of other risk factors for CHD adversely affected by body weight is another strong indication for weight reduction.

When weight reduction is required, it is necessary first to determine the individual's usual food energy intake. This can be accomplished by repeated 24 hr recalls, as previously discussed. An alternative approach is to have the patient maintain a dietary record for a minimum of 3 days, 1 of which should be a weekend day.

A desirable body weight for height can be estimated from Table 2 or more accurately from percentage body fat, as previously described. The required weight loss then is calculated by subtracting the desirable weight from the patient's actual weight. It also is important to assess motivation and the patient's ability to modify his or her food habits prior to prescribing dietary changes. On the basis of the individual's medical needs and food-related behaviors, a weight loss of either 1 or 2 lbs per week is generally considered a reasonable and safe goal (79). To lose 1 lb per week it is necessary to reduce 500 kcal daily from baseline energy intake or to increase physical activity by 500 kcal daily or, still better, to combine dieting and an increase in physical activity to create a 500 kcal per day energy deficit. These values are doubled for a 2 lbs per week weight loss. These recommendations for energy deficits are based on the following calculations:

1 lb of body fat = 454 g
1 g of body fat yields 7.7 kcal
454 g of body fat yields 454 g/lb × 7.7 kcal/g = 3496 kcal per lb of body fat (or about 3500 kcal).

If 3500 kcal is divided into 7 days, a reduction of 500 kcal/day is required to lose 1 lb of body fat. This, of course, is only a general estimate and there is a great deal of variability in responsiveness to energy restriction, necessitating individualized adjustments during the weight reduction program. It is desirable, especially in cases of gross obesity, to have the patient consult a nutritional professional to help plan and assist with the weight reduction plan.

Other general recommendations for a safe weight loss and lifelong maintenance program include the following (79):

1. Increase physical activity both as part of the daily routine and by adding a structured exercise program following guidelines elaborated upon in Chapter 12.

2. Reduce intake of energy-dense foods rich in fats, oils, or simple sugars, as well as alcohol intake while maintaining an adequate blend of required nutrients.

3. The energy intake should not be reduced lower than 1200 kcal/day and 2 lbs per week should be the maximum rate of weight loss.

4. The diet should consist of food acceptable to the dieter from the viewpoints of his or her culture, habits and taste, food cost, and ease of food acquisition and preparation.

5. Behavioral modification techniques described in Chapter 11 are helpful to identify and eliminate problem eating practices, for example, snacking while watching television.

6. Newly acquired physical activity and eating practices should be reinforced and maintained indefinitely.

C. Management of Blood Lipids and Other Nutritionally Related Risk Factors

A multidisciplinary NAS Committee on Diet and Health has proposed dietary recommendations to reduce blood cholesterol levels and the risk of CHD and other diet-related chronic diseases (80). These are directed to healthy American adults and children and are to be used in conjunction with the RDA to achieve "an optimal and desirable dietary pattern for maintenance of good health." The guidelines that follow are those relevant to prevention of CHD, hypertension, type II diabetes and its complications, and other chronic nutritionally related diseases. They are consistent with earlier ones proposed by the American Heart Association (81), the American Medical Association (82), the Senate Select Committee on Nutrition (83), and the National Cholesterol Education Program (NCEP) (8).

These guidelines call for the following general changes in the usual American eating pattern. Total fat intake should be reduced to 30% or less of calories from the usual current levels of about 37–40% of calories. The SFA intake should make up 10% or less of daily energy intake, the same as for PUFA and monounsaturated fatty acids, and the intake of cholesterol should be less than 300 mg/day (the usual cholesterol content of a typical egg yolk is 250 mg). Additional reductions in total fat, SFA, and cholesterol intake are believed to confer still greater benefits. It is recommended that fat, SFA, and dietary cholesterol intake be reduced by appropriate substitutions in the meat–legume and milk–dairy product food groups as shown in Table 5. For example, use fish, poultry without skin, lean meats, and legumes in place of animal flesh, and low- or nonfat dairy products as previously outlined. In addition more cereal and grain products, vegetables, and fruits should

Table 5 Recommended Dietary Modifications to Lower Blood Cholesterol Levels

Food Group	Choose	Decrease
Fish, chicken, turkey, and lean meats	Fish, poultry without skin, lean cuts of beef, lamb, pork, or veal, shellfish	Fatty cuts of beef, pork, organ meats, cold cuts, hot dogs, bacon, sausage
Skim and low-fat milk, cheese, yogurt, and dairy substitutes	Skim or 1% fat milk, buttermilk	Whole milk: regular, evaporated, condensed; cream, half and half, most nondairy creamers, whipped toppings
	Nonfat or low-fat yogurt	Whole-milk yogurt
	Low-fat cottage cheese	Whole-milk cottage cheese
	Low-fat cheeses, farmer or pot (labeled 2–6 g fat/oz)	All natural cheeses (blue, cheddar, Swiss), cream cheese or "light cream cheese"
		Sour cream or "light sour cream"
	Sherbet, sorbet	Ice cream
Eggs	Egg whites or substitutes	Egg yolks
Fruits and vegetables	Fresh, frozen, canned	Vegetables prepared in sauces (butter, cream)
Breads and cereals	Homemade baked goods made with unsaturated oils, angel food cake, low-fat crackers or cookies	Commercial baked goods (pie, cake, doughnuts), high-fat crackers or cookies
	Rice, pasta	Egg noodles
	Whole grain breads and cereals (whole wheat, rye, multigrain, etc.)	Breads in which eggs are the major ingredient
Fats and oils	Baking cocoa	Chocolate
	Unsaturated vegetable oils (corn, olive, rapeseed, safflower, sesame, soybean, sunflower)	Butter, coconut oil, palm oil, lard, bacon, fat
	Mayonnaise, salad dressing made from unsaturated oils, low-fat dressings	Dressings made with egg yolk
	Seeds and nuts	Coconut

Source: Adapted from Ref. 81.

be used to meet energy requirements. Oils, solid fats, egg yolks, and fried foods should only be used in limited amounts.

These recommendations are intended for all Americans over age 2 years, but are especially important for those whose blood total cholesterol levels are greater than 200 mg/dl and LDL levels above 130 mg/dl, and especially if there is clinical evidence of CHD or two or more risk factors present, including male gender (8).

Suggested incremental dietary steps to achieve the goals of reducing elevated levels of blood total and LDL cholesterol levels and maintaining lower levels are described below.

Information should be provided about the relative risk for CHD and the need for dietary modification to reduce blood cholesterol level and risk of CHD. The patient should know that a reduced-fat diet is the key element of a CHD-prevention program, and that recommendations for changes in eating patterns are permanent and desirable for everyone in the family over age 2 years. The importance of a reduction in excess weight should also be stressed not only because it helps normalize the blood lipid profile but also because of the additional beneficial effects on other risk factors for CHD. An increase in habitual physical activity should be part of the plan for weight management, as well as to improve the blood lipid profile, reduce elevated blood pressure, risk of type II diabetes and CHD, and to improve quality of life.

Assess the patient's usual dietary habits by methods previously described in this chapter.

Determine and modify problem areas in the patient's eating pattern including reducing major dietary sources of SFA and cholesterol. The NCEP suggests a two-step dietary approach to lower total and LDL cholesterol levels. The NCEP goals for the step-one diet are essentially the same as recommended by the NRC's Committee on Diet and Health (80). The NCEP step-two diet is recommended if the step-one diet fails to achieve a satisfactory reduction in plasma cholesterol levels. The step-two diet calls for a further reduction in total and saturated fat intake. Energy from fat is reduced to 28% of total calories, with less than 7% of total calories from SFA. In addition, a dietary cholesterol intake of less than 200 mg/dl per day is recommended.

To avoid overwhelming the patient, it is suggested that dietary changes be introduced gradually to achieve the above goals, targeting usually only one or two concerns at a time with practical suggestions made for appropriate changes. Except for those patients with extremely high blood total and LDL cholesterol levels, it is appropriate to take as long as 6 months to institute gradually all desirable dietary modifications. Consultations are advised with a nutritional consultant or dietitian for problem cases. Practical tips for food selection and preparation of a "heart healthy" eating style designed to be nutritionally sound and highly palatable are provided later in this chapter.

Individualize dietary instructions for each patient. Some patients are intimi-dated by detailed literature, while others want to read and learn as much as possible. It is helpful to have both simple and more complicated literature on hand to satisfy the needs of all patients. Examples of printed materials available through a number of sources are listed at the end of this chapter. The NHLBI's and the NCEP's publications are not copyrighted, and may be reproduced without permission.

Schedule a follow-up visit within 6 weeks of initiating a step-one diet to recheck the patient's blood cholesterol levels and evaluate compliance with the advised dietary modifications. Many patients will respond favorably after only a few dietary changes, and will simply require routine follow up visits to re-evaluate blood cholesterol levels periodically. Other patients may have had difficulty adhering to their new eating pattern. These, in particular, may benefit from consultation with a nutrition professional. Patients should constantly be reassured that lifestyle changes take time and dedication.

Continue to re-evaluate blood cholesterol levels periodically to demonstrate interest in the patient's condition and to encourage compliance or further changes. Blood cholesterol levels should be measured at least every 3 months until the goal has been achieved and then at appropriate intervals thereafter for an indefinite period of time. Patients whose plasma LDL-cholesterol levels remain high (>160 mg/dl) despite adequate dietary therapy should be considered for lipid-lowering drug treatment, particularly if they have evidence of CHD or have several other risk factors. At least 6 months of intensive dietary therapy and counseling should be carried out before lipid-lowering drug therapy is begun. However, in patients with severe baseline elevations of plasma LDL cholesterol (> 190 mg/dl), a briefer trial of dietary therapy is indicated before drug therapy is begun or it may be necessary to initiate diet and drug therapy concurrently.

D. Practical Considerations in Food Choices

According to the most recent USDA Nationwide Food Consumption Survey, total fat intake in the United States is currently estimated as contributing 37% of total calories and saturated fat 13–14% of total calories. Reducing fat as an energy source to 30% of calories translates to the consumption of about 50 g fat for someone with a 1500 calorie/day intake, and 67, 83, and 100 g of fat for individuals with 2000, 2500, and 3000 calorie/day intakes, respectively. Most people do not wish to count grams of fat every day but prefer instead sample eating plans or guidelines. Tables 6 and 7 provide sample eating plans at different energy levels for step-one and step-two diets developed by the American Heart Association using the food exchange system previously described (81). In addition, NCEP has developed simplified guidelines showing which food choices meet the dietary recommendations designed to lower blood cholesterol (8).

As previously indicated, the most effective approach to reduce blood cholesterol levels is to reduce intake of SFA. SFA are found in animal products, with highest amounts in marbled red meats, high fat dairy products, and in tropical oils. Coconut oil and palm oil are vegetable oils that have high concentrations of SFA,

Table 6 Sample Eating Plans for Step One Diets

Food Group	Daily Portions			
	2500 calories	2000 calories	1600 calories	1200 calories
Meat, poultry, and seafood	6 oz.	6 oz.	6 oz.	6 oz.
Eggs, whole	3/week	3/week	3/week	3/week
Dairy products	4	3	3	2
Fats and oils	8	6	4	3
Bread, cereal, pasta, and starchy vegetables	10	7	4	3
Vegetables	4	4	4	4
Fruit	5	3	3	3
Optional foods	2	2	2	0

which raise blood cholesterol levels (i.e, palmitic, myristic, and, to a lesser extent, lauric acids) and should be avoided. Poultry (with the skin removed), fish, and shellfish are animal products that contain less of these cholesterol-raising SFA. Below are listed specific recommendations for "heart-healthy" food selections, food preparation techniques, and suggested upper limits in amounts for each of the major food groups.

1. *Meat and Poultry Selection*

Animal flesh consumption should be limited to 6 oz or less per day. A deck of cards serves as a good visual guide to illustrate a 3 oz portion of meat. This limitation on meat consumption reduces intake of SFA and of dietary cholesterol found only in animal products. Although dietary cholesterol has a much smaller effect on blood

Table 7 Sample Eating Plans for Step Two Diets

Food Group	Daily Portions			
	2500 calories	2000 calories	1600 calories	1200 calories
Meat, poultry, and seafood	6 oz.	6 oz.	6 oz.	6 oz.
Eggs, whole	1/week	1/week	1/week	1/week
Dairy products	3	2	2	2
Fats and oils	8	7	5	3
Bread, cereal, pasta, and starchy vegetables	10	8	5	4
Vegetables	5	4	4	4
Fruit	7	4	3	3
Optional foods	2	2	2	0

cholesterol level than SFA, an additional 100 mg of dietary cholesterol per 1000 kcal of energy intake generally raises plasma LDL cholesterol levels about 8–10 mg/dl (84). On the other hand, some foods may be high in dietary cholesterol but low in SFA. Such is true with shellfish. Furthermore, earlier analytical methods for cholesterol gave falsely high values for cholesterol in shellfish because of interference by the presence of noncholesterol sterols (85). Shellfish and fish are lower in SFA than red meat or poultry. In addition, shellfish and cold water fatty fish, such as mackerel, salmon, and herring are rich in omega-3 PUFA, which reduce blood coagulability, elevated levels of plasma triglycerides, and perhaps blood pressure level as previously mentioned. However, large dosages of these PUFA found in fish oil supplements are not routinely recommended since they can markedly prolong bleeding time and may actually increase plasma LDL cholesterol levels (86). As previously mentioned, current recommendations are for the consumption of fish at least twice a week as part of a cholesterol-reducing regimen.

Red meat choices should be limited to lean cuts, such as trimmed round, sirloin, chuck, loin cuts of beef or extra-lean ground beef, trimmed veal, pork tenderloin, or leg or loin of lamb. Meats graded as "prime" are the richest in fat and should be avoided. "Choice" has less marbling while "good" grades are the lowest in fat and therefore, are better "heart-healthy" selections than the so-called "better grades" of red meats.

Processed meats such as cold cuts, sausage, frankfurters, and bacon are all high in SFA, cholesterol, as well as sodium, and should be avoided as much as possible. Organ meats including liver, kidneys, and brain are very high in cholesterol and should be only eaten occasionally. Chicken, Cornish game hen, and turkey are low in SFA, especially when cooked and eaten without the skin. Ground turkey or chicken can be substituted in place of ground beef in most recipes.

2. Dairy Products

Dairy products are important sources of calcium and should not be eliminated from the diet. Skim or 1% milk is preferable to whole milk, which is about 4% fat. Low-fat cheeses, such as cottage, farmer, or part-skim mozzarella are better choices than hard cheeses like Swiss, American, and cheddar. Cream cheese is also high in fat: about 37% by weight. Low- or no-fat yogurt or cottage cheese may be substituted for sour cream in dips and salad dressings, while skimmed evaporated milk can often be used as a replacement for heavy cream. Buttermilk is actually made from low-fat milk and can be used in baking. Low-fat frozen milk and low-fat frozen yogurt are good dessert substitutes for ice cream.

3. Eggs

The step-one diet permits three eggs per week while only one per week is recommended on the step-two diet. An acceptable replacement for food recipes calling for eggs is to use two egg whites in place of one egg, since all of the cholesterol found in eggs is in the yolk. Commercial egg substitutes that do not contain yolks are also available.

4. Bread, Cereals, Pasta, Rice, Dried Peas and Beans

These foods are high in complex carbohydrates and protein and low in SFA and make good substitutes for fatty animal products. Be aware that sauces and dressings used in the preparation of certain recipes can greatly add to the fat content of the meal. Commercially prepared products containing these foods often contain a significant hidden source of SFA. It is therefore important to carefully read the food labels to determine their fat content and sources. Complex carbohydrate foods also are good sources of water-soluble dietary fiber, which may have a modest independent cholesterol-reducing effect.

5. Fruits and Vegetables

Both fruits and vegetables are low in fat, contain no cholesterol, and are rich in vitamins, minerals, and fiber. Avocados and olives are two exceptions that are high in fat and calories. Instead of using salt or butter to season vegetables, herbs, spices, wine vinegar, and lemon juice may be used. Salads marinated in oil or fruits combined with whipped cream are high in fat.

6. Fats and Oils

Butter, hard margarines, lard, and beef fat are high in SFA. Hydrogenated vegetable oils vary in their saturated fat content, and it is best to read the labels to choose those that have higher levels of unsaturated than saturated fat. Liquid vegetable oils that are high in unsaturated fats and low in SFA like safflower, sunflower, corn, olive, sesame, soybean, and canola oil should be used in cooking and in salad dressings. Canola and soybean oils also are good sources of the omega-3 PUFA-containing form of linolenic acid, which the body can convert to EPA and DCA. Soft margarines made from PUFA-rich oils are appropriate substitutes for butter or hard margarines. Peanut oils and peanut butter are higher in SFA than the vegetable oils listed above and should only be eaten in small amounts. Tropical vegetable oils, high in SFA are contained in many commercial products, such as nondairy coffee creamers, sour-cream substitutes, and whipped toppings as well as commercial baked goods and many cold cereals. Careful label reading is required to detect and avoid such products.

7. Miscellaneous Foods

Nuts, chips, doughnuts, microwave popcorn, and snack crackers tend to be high in fat, calories, and salt. Better choices for snack foods are fruit, raw vegetables, air-popped popcorn, graham crackers, bagels, and english muffins.

E. Reading Food Labels

Reading food labels is an invaluable tool in managing any type of diet and, in particular, a cholesterol-lowering diet. Many packaged foods provide nutrition information on their labels. The ingredients are listed in descending order by weight. Therefore, if a fat high in SFA is one of the first three ingredients, that product should be restricted in amounts and not eaten on a regular basis. More and more food labels also are including the amounts of SFA, PUFA, total fat, and cholesterol among the information on nutrients per serving. Calories from fat per serving can be determined by multiplying grams of fat by 9 calories/g. It also is important to note the serving size according to the manufacturer.

Consumers should be alert for misleading labeling practices. Foods labeled "30% fat" may be 30% fat by weight rather than by total calories. For example, in a hot dog, 30% fat by weight is equivalent to 80% of calories. The terms light, lean, and less fat do not necessarily mean these foods are low in fat, but that they are simply lower in fat than similar products; however, a number of baked goods have been reformulated to lower the fat content with excellent results. Particularly misleading are some foods labeled as containing "no fat" or "no cholesterol," which are vegetable products that never had any to begin with. Other deceptive labeling techniques include the use of statements such as "contains one or more of the following oils," followed by a list of both saturated and unsaturated fats or specifies the use of a "vegetable oil," which commonly is a tropical oil high in SFA. In such cases, there is currently no way of knowing which type of oil was used. Thus, it is best to avoid foods with an unspecified vegetable oil on the label. The FDA is currently in the process of revising labeling regulations. We hope that this will result in a more consumer-friendly labeling system that is more helpful to individuals trying to eat more healthily.

F. Cooking Methods

Before cooking red meats it is desirable to trim all visible fat. Broiling, roasting, or baking red meat without added fat allows the fat to drip off, so it can be discarded. Other preparation methods that require little or no fat include steaming, baking, or stir-frying in small amounts of an acceptable vegetable oil. Many foods can be fried using vegetable spray to coat the pan to prevent sticking or in place of oil for browning foods. Soups or stews made with meat or poultry can be prepared ahead of time and chilled in the refrigerator. The fat on the surface can be skimmed off later.

G. Dining Out

Many Americans eat a large proportion of their meals away from home. It is possible to enjoy eating out and still limit calories, fat, and sodium intake, depending on what is ordered and appropriate portion sizes. Menu descriptions that include words like buttered, fried, breaded, creamed, with gravy, scalloped, rich, or au gratin signal a high fat content. Foods prepared by smoking, pickling, in broth, with soy sauce, marinated, or barbecued are high in sodium. Conversely, terms such as grilled, roasted, poached, or steamed generally indicate a lower fat content. A common misleading practice is the so-called "diet plate" that often consists of a beef patty, cottage cheese, a hard-cooked egg, and crackers. This "light meal" typically weighs in at over 600 calories and is high in fat and cholesterol.

Some menu selections fit particularly well in a diet reduced in fat and sodium. For instance, fresh fruit or vegetables for an appetizer, a lettuce salad ("light on the dressing" or with the dressing served on the side), baked or broiled chicken served as the entree, steamed vegetables, and baked potatoes (avoiding butter and sour cream toppings). The diner also should not be afraid to ask about portion sizes, ingredients, preparation methods, or to make special requests for dressings or sauces "on the side." Most reputable restaurants will usually do their best to handle special requests.

Even fast foods selections are improving. Many fast food restaurants now offer salad bars and lower-fat items, such as baked potatoes. Recently Burger King and MacDonalds starting experimenting with substituting vegetable shortening in place of beef fat for preparation of their french fries. One's best bet in a fast food restaurant is to choose simply prepared items and avoid sauces, deep-fried foods, milkshakes (unless they are specified as low fat), cheeseburgers, and deep-fried fish. Fried fish sandwiches with cheese and tartar sauce are even higher in SFA and cholesterol than a simple hamburger.

H. Results Expected from a Cholesterol-Lowering Diet

There is considerable variability in responsiveness to reduced SFA and cholesterol intake. Genetic factors play a role in determining blood cholesterol levels, and the extent to which the level can be lowered. In general, the higher the blood cholesterol level and the more SFA in the baseline diet, the greater the response that can be expected from a cholesterol-lowering diet. Over time most individuals are able to reduce their blood cholesterol levels by as much as 30–55 mg/dl on a cholesterol-reducing diet (80). A small percentage of people may not be able to lower their blood cholesterol level significantly even after carefully following a progressive cholesterol-lowering diet for 6 months or more. Anticholesterolemic drug therapy may then have to be used in conjunction with, but not as a replacement, for a diet low in SFA and cholesterol.

I. The Role of Registered Dietitians/Nutritionists

A registered dietitian or qualified nutritionist can provide considerable help in making dietary assessments and helping the patient to lower intake of calories, saturated fat, cholesterol, and sodium. These professionals have special skills in assessing dietary habits and in providing dietary information individualized to the needs of the patient. Dietitians may be identified through local hospitals, the local or state health department, the local agriculture extension service, and from knowledgeable colleagues. State and district affiliates of the American Dietetic Association also maintain listings of dietitians in their areas, and the Division of Practice of the ADA also will release names of qualified professionals in your area (312-899-0040). Further, as mentioned previously, the NCEP recommends referral to a registered dietitian for patients who require a step-two diet or who are having difficulty following the step-one diet.

V. SOURCES FOR NUTRITION EDUCATION MATERIALS

Human Nutrition Information Service
U.S. Department of Agriculture, HNIS, Room 325 A
6505 Belcrest Road
Hyattsville, MD 20782

National Cholesterol Education Program
National High Blood Pressure Education Program
NHLBI Smoking Education Program
Information Center
4733 Bethesda Avenue, Suite 530
Bethesda, MD 10814
(310) 951-3260

Education Department
National Livestock and Meat Board
444 North Michigan Avenue
Chicago, IL 60611

American Heart Association
National Center
7320 Greenville Avenue
Dallas, TX 75321

Department of Health and Human Services
Food and Drug Administration
Public Health Service
5600 Fishers Lane
Rockville, MD 20857

The American Dietetic Association
216 W. Jackson Blvd.
Chicago, IL 60606-6995

REFERENCES

1. Leon AS. Physiological interactions between diet and exercise in the etiology and prevention of ischemic heart disease. Ann Clin Res 1988; 20:114–20.
2. Anonymous. Hearing before the Senate Select Committee on Nutrition and Human Needs of the United States Senate Ninety-fifth Congress. Diet Related to Killer Diseases, II. Part 2. Obesity. Washington, D.C.: U.S. Government Printing Office 1977; 1–246.
3. Bray GA. The energetics of obesity. Med Sci Sports Exercise 1983; 15:32–40.
4. Hubert HB. The importance of obesity in the development of coronary risk factors and disease: the epidemiologic evidence. Annu Rev Public Health 1986; 7:493–502.
5. Barrett-Connor EL. Obesity, atherosclerosis and coronary heart disease. Ann Intern Med 1983; 103:1010–9.
6. Bjorntorp P. Regional patterns of fat distribution. Ann Intern Med 1985; 103:994–5.
7. Despres J-P, Moorjani S, Lupien PJ, Tremblay A, Nadeau A, Bouchard C. Regional distribution of body fat, plasma lipoproteins and cardiovascular disease. Arteriosclerosis 1990; 10:497–511.
8. National Cholesterol Education Program. Report of the expert Panel on the detection, evaluation, and treatment of high blood cholesterol in adults. Arch Intern Med 1988; 148:36–69.
9. Pekanen J, Linn S, Heiss B, Suchindran CH, Leon AS, Rifkind BM, Tyroler HA. Ten-year mortality from cardiovascular disease in relation to cholesterol level among men with and without pre-existing cardiovascular disease. N Engl J Med 1990; 322:1700–7.
10. Buchwald H, Varco RL, Matts JP, Long JM, Fitch LL, Campbell GS, Pearce MB, Yellin AE, Edmiston WA, Smink RD Jr, Sawin HS Jr, Campos CT, Hansen BJ, Tuna N, Karnegis JN, Sanmarco ME, Amplatz K, Castaneda-Zuniga WR, Hunter DW, Bissett JK, Weber FJ, Stevenson JW, Leon AS, Chalmers TC and the POSCH Group. Effect of partial ileal bypass surgery on mortality and morbidity from coronary heart disease in patients with hypercholesterolemia. Report of the Program on the Surgical Control of the Hyperlipidemias (POSCH). N Engl J Med 1990; 323:946–55.
11. Lipid Research Clinic Program. The Lipid Research Clinics Coronary Primary Prevention Trial II. The relationship of reduction in incidence of coronary heart disease to cholesterol lowering. JAMA 1984; 251:365–74.
12. Gordon DJ, Knoke J, Probstfield JL, Superko R, Tyroler A. High-density lipoprotein cholesterol and coronary heart disease in hypercholesterolemic men: The Lipid Research Clinics Primary Prevention Trial. Circulation 1986; 74:1217–25.
13. Kannel WB. High-density lipoproteins: epidemiologic profile and risk of coronary artery diseases. Am J Cardiol 1983; 52:9B–12B.
14. Frick MH, Elo O, Haapa K, Heinonen OP, Hiensalmi P, Helo P, Huttunen JK, Kaitaniemi P, Koskinen P, Manninen V, Maenpaa H, Malkonen M, Manttari M, Norola S, Pasternack A, Pikkarainen J, Romo M, Sjoblom T, Nikkila Ea. Helsinki Heart Study: primary prevention trial with gemfibrozil in middle-aged men with dyslipidemia. Safety of treatment, changes in risk factors, and incidence of coronary heart disease. N Engl J Med 1987; 317:1237–45.
15. Keys A, Menotti, A, Karvonen MJ, Aravanis C, Blackburn H, Buzine R, Djordjevic

BS, Dontas AS, Fidanza F, Keys MH, Kromhout D, Nedeljkovic B, Pansar S, Seccareccia F, Toshima H. The diet and 15-year death rate in the Seven Countries Study. Am J Epidemiol 1986; 124:403–15.

16. Strong JP, McGill HC Jr. Diet and experimental atherosclerosis in baboons. Am J Pathol 1967; 50:669–90.

17. Keys A, Anderson JR, Grande F. Serum cholesterol response to changes in the diet. Metabolism 1965; 14:747–87.

18. Hegsted DM, McGandy RB, Meyers ML, Stare FJ. Quantitative effects of dietary fat on serum cholesterol in man. Am J Clin Nutr 1965; 17:281–95.

19. Grundy MS. Monounsaturated fatty acids plasma cholesterol, and coronary heart disease. Am J Clin Nutr 1987; 45:1237–42.

20. Amodeo C, Messerli FH. Risk for obesity. Cardiol Clin 1986; 4:75–80.

21. Miettinen TA. Dietary fiber and lipids. Am J Clin Nutr 1987; 45:1237–42.

22. Schlierf G, Lenore A, Oster P. Influence of diet on high-density lipoproteins. Am J Cardiol 1983; 52:178–98.

23. Constant J. Nutritional management of diet-induced hyperlipidemias and atherosclerosis Part III. Ann Intern Med 1987; 8:95–103.

24. Nessel JP, Billinbton T, Smith B. Low density and high density lipoprotein kinetics and sterol balance in vegetarians. Metabolism 1981; 30:941–5.

25. Connor WE, Cerquer MT, Connor RW, Wallace RB, Malinow R, Casdorph HR. The plasma lipids, lipoproteins, and diet of the Tarahumara Indians of Mexico. Am J Clin Nutr 1978; 31:1131–42.

26. Fraser GE, Anderson JR, Foster N, Goldberg R, Jacobs DR Jr, Blackburn H. The effects of alcohol on serum high density lipoprotein (HDL)—a controlled experiment. Atherosclerosis 1983; 46:275–96.

27. Haskell WL. The influence of exercise training on plasma lipids and lipoproteins in health and disease. Acta Med Scand 1986; Supple 711:25–38.

28. Wood PD, Stefanick ML. Exercise, fitness, and atherosclerosis. In: Bouchard C, Shephard RJ, Stephens T, Sutton JR, McPherson BD, eds. Exercise, fitness and health. A consensus of current knowledge. Champaign, Il: Human Kinetics Books, 1990:409–21.

29. Kuller L, Marlahn E, Ockene J. Smoking and coronary heart disease. In: Connor WE, Bristow JD, eds. Smoking and coronary heart disease. Philadelphia: JB Lippincott, 1985:65–83.

30. Orinsh D, Brown SE, Scherwitz LW, Billings JH, Armstrong WT, Ports TA, McLanahan SM, Kirkeeide RL, Brand RJ, Gould KL. Can lifestyle changes reverse coronary heart disease? The Lifestyle Heart Trial. Lancet 1990; 336:129–33.

31. Kaplan NM. Hypertension. In: Kaplan NM, Stamler J, eds. Prevention of coronary heart disease. Philadelphia: WB Saunders, 1983:61–71.

32. Cohen JD. Role of nutrition in management of hypertension. Clin Nutr 1984; 3: 135–38.

33. Grimm RH Jr, Neaton JD, Elmer P, Svendsen KH, Levin J, Segal MJ, Holland L, White LJ, Cleaman DR, Kofron P, LaBountry RK, Crow R, Prineas RJ. The influence of oral potassium chloride on blood pressure in hypertensive men on a low-sodium diet. N Engl J Med 1990, 322:569–74.

34. Kaplan N, Ram CVS. Potassium supplements for hypertension. N Engl J Med 1990; 322:623–24.

35. Puska P, Nissinen A, Vartiainen E, Dougherty R, Mutanen M, Iacon JM, Korhonen JH, Pietenen P, Leino P, Leino L, Morsio S, Huttenen J. Controlled randomized trial of the effect of dietary fat on blood pressure. Lancet 1983; 1:1–10.

36. Bonaa KH, Bjerve KS, Straume B, Gram IT, Thelle D. Effect of eicosapentaenoic and decosahexaneoic acids on blood pressure in hypertension. A population-based intervention trial from the Tromso Study. N Engl J Med 1990; 322:793–801.

37. Hagberg JM. Exercise, fitness and hypertension. In:Bouchard C, Shephard RJ, Stephens T, Sutton JR, McPherson BD, eds. Exercise, fitness and health. Champaign Il: Human Kinetics Books, 1990:455–66.

38. Leon AS. Exercise and risk of coronary heart disease. In: Eckert HM, Montoye HJ, eds. Exercise and health. Champaign IL: Human Kinetics Books, 1984:14–31.

39. Stamler J, Farinaro E, Mojonnier LM, Halls Y, Moss D, Stamler R. Prevention and control of hypertension by nutritional hygienic means. JAMA 1980; 240:1819–23.

40. Stamler R, Stamler J, Grimm R, Dyer A, Gosch FC, Berman R, Elmer P, Fishman J, Van Hell N, Cininelli J, Hoessener R. Nonpharmacologic control of hypertension. Prev Med 1985; 14:336–45.

41. West KM. Epidemiology of diabetes and its vascular lesions. New York: Elsevier, 1978.

42. Leon AS. Exercise for the patient with diabetes mellitus. In: Franklin BA, Gordon S, Timmis GC, eds. Exercise in modern medicine: testing and prescription in health and diseases. Baltimore: Williams & Wilkins, 1987: 131–6.

43. Lipman RL, Schnure JJ, Bradley EM, Lecocq FR. Impairment of peripheral glucose utilization in normal subjects by prolonged bed rest. J Lab Clin Med 1970; 76:221–30.

44. Lipman RL, Raskin P, Love T, Triebwasser J, Lecocq FR, Schnure JJ. Glucose intolerance during decreased physical activity in man. Diabetes 1972; 21:101–7.

45. Black HR. The coronary artery disease paradox: the role of hyperinsulinemia and insulin resistance and implications for therapy. J Cardiovasc Pharmacol 1990; 15 (Suppl 5):S26–28.

46. Steinberg D. Lipoproteins and atherosclerosis: a look back and a look ahead. Atherosclerosis 1983; 3:283–301.

47. Nestal PJ. Polyunsaturated fatty acids (n-3, n-6). Am J Clin Nutr 1987; 45:1161–7.

48. Goodnight SH Jr, Harris WB, Conor WE, Illngworth DR. Polyunsaturated fatty acids, hyperlipidemia, and thrombosis. Arteriosclerosis 1982; 2:87–113.

49. Knapp HR, Reilly LA, Alessandrini P, Fitzgerald GA. In vivo index of platelet and vascular function during fish-oil administration in patients with atherosclerosis. N Engl J Med 19890; 314:937–42.

50. Leon AS. Exercise and coronary heart disease. Hosp Med 1983; 19:38–57.

51. Rauramaa R, Salonen JT, Sappanen K, Salonen R, Venalainen JM, Ihanainer M, Rissanen U. Inhibition of platelet aggregability by moderate-intensity physical exercise: a randomized clinical trial in overweight men. Circulation 1986; 74:939–44.

52. Williams RS, Logue EE, Lewis, JI, Barton T, Slead NW, Wallace AB, Pizza SV. Physical conditioning augments the fibrinolytic response to venous occlusion in healthy adults. N Engl J Med 1980; 302:987–91.

53. Sloan AW. Estimation of body fat in young men. J Appl Physiol 1967; 23:311–5.
54. Sloan AW, Burt JJ, Blyth CS. Estimation of body fat in young women. J Appl Physiol 1961; 17:967–970.
55. Anonymous. Build and blood pressure study, 1959, Vol. 1. Chicago: Society of Actuaries, 1959.
56. Anonymous. 1983 Metropolitan height and weight tables. Stat Bull Metrop Life Insur Co 1984; 64:2–9.
57. Simopoulos AP. Obesity and body weight standard. Annu Rev Public Health 1986; 7:481–92.
58. Bray GA. Definition, measurement, and classification of the syndromes of obesity. In: Gray GA, ed. Obesity. Kroc Foundation symposium on comparative methods of weight control. Westport, CT: Technomic Publishing Co, 1979: 1–14.
59. Van Itallie TB. Health implications of overweight and obesity in the United States. Ann Intern Med 1985; 103:983–8.
60. Pollock ML, Wilmore JH, Fox SM III. Exercise in health and disease. Evaluation and prescription for prevention and rehabilitation. Philadelphia: WB Saunders, 1984: 97–130; 217–228.
61. McArdle WD, Katch PI, Katch VL. Exercise physiology, energy, nutrition and human performance, 2nd ed. Philadelphia: Lea & Febiger, 1946: 483–512; 642–49.
62. Pellett PL. Food energy requirements in humans. Am J Clin Nutr 1990; 51:711–22.
63. Food and Nutrition Board Commission on Life Sciences, National Research Council. Recommended dietary allowances, 10th ed. Washington, D.C.: National Academy Press, 1989; 24–37.
64. Thompson JK, Javie GJ, Lahey BB, Cureton KJ. Exercise and obesity: etiology, physiology, and intervention. Psychol Bull 1982; 91:55–79.
65. Passmore R, Laswood MA. Human nutrition and dietetics. Edinburgh: Churchill Livingstone, 1980: 9.
66. Baranowski I. Validity and reliability of self report measure of physical activity: an information processing perspective. Res Q 1988; 59:314–27.
67. LaPorte RE, Montoye HJ, Caspersen CJ. Assessment of physical activity in epidemiologic research: problems and prospects. Pub Health Rep 1985; 100:131, 146.
68. Leon AS, Fox SM III. Physical activity and fitness. In: Wynder EL, ed. The book of health. A complete guide to making health last a lifetime. New York: Franklin Watts; 1981: 283–341.
69. Taylor HL, Jacobs DR Jr, Schucker B, Knudsen J, Leon AS, De Backer S. A questionnaire for the assessment of leisure time physical activities. J Chron Dis 1978; 31:741–55.
70. Dwyer JT. Assessment of dietary intake. In: Shils ME, Young VR, eds. Modern nutrition in health and disease, 7th ed. Philadelphia: Lea & Febiger, 1988: 887–905.
71. Beaton GH, Milner J, Corey P, McGuire V, Cousins M, Steward E, Deramos M, Hewitt D, Grambsch PV, Kassim N, Little JA. Source of variance in 24-hour dietary recall data: implications for nutrition study design and interpretation. Am J Clin Nutr 1979; 32:2546–59.
72. McDowel A, Engel A, Massey JT, Maurer K. Plan and operation of the Second National Health and Nutrition Examination Survey. 1976–1980. Vital and Health

Statistics Series 1, No. 15. National Center for Health Statistics. Public Health Service, DHHS Pub. No (PHS)81-1317, Washington, DC: Gov't Printing Office, 1981.

73. Willett WC, Sampson L, Stamfer MJ, Rosner B, Bail C, Witschi J, Hennekens CH, Speizer FE. Reproducibility and validity of a semiquantitative food frequency questionnaire. Am J Epidemiol 1985; 122:51–65.

74. Block G, Hartman AM, Dresser CM, Carroll MD, Gannon J, Gardner L. A data-based approach to diet questionnaire design and testing. Am J Epidemiol 1986; 1245:453–69.

75. Stone NJ, Van Horn LV. Controlling cholesterol levels through diet. Postgrad Med 1988; 83:229–42.

76. Kristal AT, Shattack AL, Henry HJ, Fowler AB. Rapid assessment of dietary intake of fat, fiber, and saturated fat: validity of an instrument suitable for community intervention research and nutritional surveillance. Am J Health Promotion 1990; 4:288–95.

77. Consumer Nutrition Division United States Department of Agriculture Human Nutrition Information Service. Composition of Foods. Agriculture Handbook No. 8. Washington, D.C.: Superintendent of Documents, U.S. Gov't Printing Office, 1983.

78. Shils ME, Young VR, eds. Modern nutrition in health and disease, 7th ed. Philadelphia: Lea & Febiger, 1988: 1551–1603.

79. American College of Sports Medicine Position. Statement on Proper and Improper Weight Loss Programs. Med Sci Sports Exercise 1983; 15:ix–xiii.

80. National Research Council. Diet and Health: implications for reducing chronic disease risk. Report of the Committee on Diet and Health Food and Nutritional Board, Commission on Life Sciences. Washington, D.C., National Academy Press; 1989.

81. American Heart Association. Dietary treatment of hypercholesterolemia; a manual for patients. Dallas, TX: American Heart Association, 1988; 1–110.

82. Ulene A. American Medical Association campaign against cholesterol. A program to lower your cholesterol in 30 days. Los Angeles: Alfred A. Knopf, 1989.

83. Select Committee on Nutrition and Human Needs, U.S. Senate. Cambridge, MA: MIT Press, 1977: 1–79.

84. Mattson FH, Grundy SM. Comparison of effects of dietary saturated monounsaturated, and polyunsaturated fatty acids on plasma lipids and lipoproteins in man. J Lipid Res 1985; 26:194–202.

85. King I, Childs MT, Dorsett C, Ostrander JG, Monsen ER. Shellfish: proximate composition, minerals, fatty acids, and sterols. J Am Dietet Assoc 1990; 90:677–85.

86. Sullivan DR, Sanders TAB, Trayner IM, Thompson GR. Paradoxical elevation of LDL apoprotein B levels in hypertriglyceridaemic patients and normal subjects ingesting fish oil. Atherosclerosis 1986; 62:129–34.

APPENDIX 1: LIST OF ACTIVITIES BY RELATIVE INTENSITY LEVELS

Intensity of Activity	Job	Home	Sport or Recreation
Light	Typing Standing Driving	Ironing, sewing Light auto repair Indoor painting	Leisurely walking Softball Bowling Playing a musical instrument
Moderate	Lifting or carrying light objects (up to 5 lbs.) Painting outside of house	Sweeping, mopping, vacuuming Clipping hedge Raking Mowing lawn with power mower Cleaning windows Pushing stroller with child	Brisk walking (on level ground) Shooting baskets Throwing frisbee Leisurely cycling on level ground Swimming laps (easy effort) Weight lifting
Heavy	Construction work Lifting or carrying light objects (5–15 lbs.) Climbing ladder or stairs	Scrubbing floors Shoveling dirt, coal Mowing lawn with nonpower mower Carrying child (5–15 lbs.)	Brisk walking (uphill) Backpacking (on level ground) Brisk cycling on level ground without loss of breath Tennis (doubles) Downhill skiing Swimming laps (moderate effort)
Very heavy	Carry heavy loads such as bricks or lumber Carrying moderate loads up stairs (16–40 lbs.)	Digging ditches Chopping or splitting wood Gardening with heavy tools	Jogging Basketball (in game) Soccer (in game) Backpacking (uphill) Cycling (uphill or racing) Tennis (singles) Cross country skiing Swimming laps (hard effort) Aerobic dancing Circuit training (using a series of Nautilus machines without stopping or running a course)

APPENDIX 2

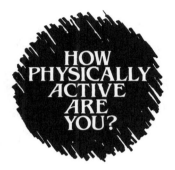

*Are you getting enough of the right kind of exercise
to help reduce your risk factors for heart disease?
This self-assessment will give you a clearer picture
of your physical activity habits along with some
ideas for new activities you may want to try.*

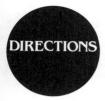

DIRECTIONS

For **each** activity you do on the physical activity charts, circle the number of points for the category that **best** describes the amount of time you spend at that activity in an **average week**.

Write in any additional moderately vigorous or vigorous activities you do at least once a week for at least 20 minutes at a time.

VIGOROUS ACTIVITIES

Note:

Specific activities are classified as **light**, **moderate**, and **vigorous** based on the intensity with which most people do them on the average. Actual levels of intensity may vary greatly among individuals.

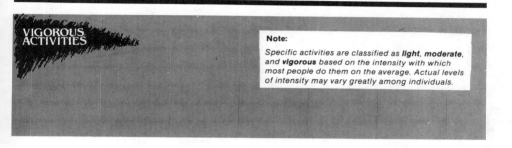

Activity	Once a week for at least 20 minutes at a time	Twice a week for 20-40 minutes at a time	Twice a week for at least 40 minutes at a time	Three times a week for 20-40 minutes at a time	Three or more times a week for at least 40 minutes at a time	
jogging or running	3	4	6	7	9	
swimming	3	4	6	7	9	
aerobic dance	3	4	6	7	9	
jumping rope	3	4	6	7	9	
Other vigorous activities						
_____	3	4	6	7	9	
_____	3	4	6	7	9	**Chart Total**
Column Totals	+	+	+	+	=	

Examples of other vigorous activities: cross-country skiing, running stairs

3

For each chart, record your total points in the lower right-hand corner.

 4

Turn to the back page, fill in your chart totals and bonus points, and add up your total physical activity score.

 5

If you do different activities during different seasons, you may want to figure separate scores for the times when you are **most** and **least** active, for example, summer and winter.

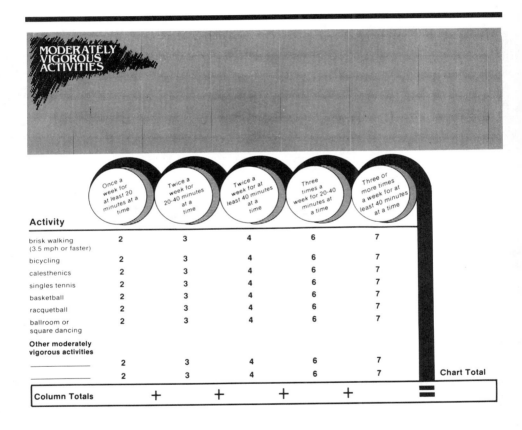

MODERATELY VIGOROUS ACTIVITIES

Activity	Once a week for at least 20 minutes at a time	Twice a week for 20-40 minutes at a time	Twice a week for at least 40 minutes at a time	Three times a week for 20-40 minutes at a time	Three or more times a week for at least 40 minutes at a time	
brisk walking (3.5 mph or faster)	2	3	4	6	7	
bicycling	2	3	4	6	7	
calesthenics	2	3	4	6	7	
singles tennis	2	3	4	6	7	
basketball	2	3	4	6	7	
racquetball	2	3	4	6	7	
ballroom or square dancing	2	3	4	6	7	
Other moderately vigorous activities						
_____	2	3	4	6	7	
_____	2	3	4	6	7	**Chart Total**
Column Totals	+	+	+	+	=	

Examples of other moderately vigorous activities: ice skating, roller skating, water skiing, karate, judo, rowing

Physical Activity Score

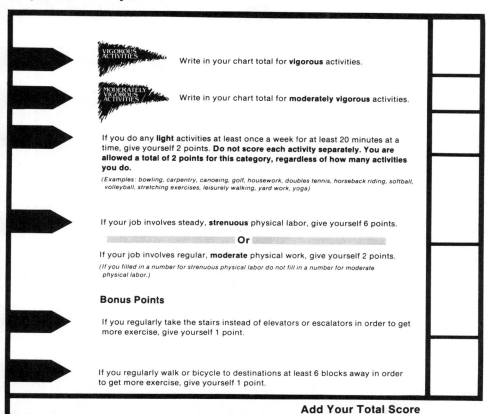

Write in your chart total for **vigorous** activities.

Write in your chart total for **moderately vigorous** activities.

If you do any **light** activities at least once a week for at least 20 minutes at a time, give yourself 2 points. **Do not score each activity separately. You are allowed a total of 2 points for this category, regardless of how many activities you do.**

(Examples: bowling, carpentry, canoeing, golf, housework, doubles tennis, horseback riding, softball, volleyball, stretching exercises, leisurely walking, yard work, yoga)

If your job involves steady, **strenuous** physical labor, give yourself 6 points.

═══════════════ **Or** ═══════════════

If your job involves regular, **moderate** physical work, give yourself 2 points.

(If you filled in a number for strenuous physical labor do not fill in a number for moderate physical labor.)

Bonus Points

If you regularly take the stairs instead of elevators or escalators in order to get more exercise, give yourself 1 point.

If you regularly walk or bicycle to destinations at least 6 blocks away in order to get more exercise, give yourself 1 point.

Add Your Total Score

0-5 Step It Up
If your score is in this range, you are not getting the exercise you need to do the most good for your heart, lungs, and metabolism. You're not alone! Most Americans don't get enough regular exercise. Pick out one or two activities you enjoy and make them part of a regular exercise program. Also, try adding more physical activity to your daily routine by walking and taking the stairs.

6-9 Doing Fine
If your score is in this range, your exercise meets the minimum recommendations for the amount you need to help reduce your risk factors for heart disease. You may benefit even more from more frequent or more vigorous activity. Keep up the good work and spread the word.

10 or higher Going Strong
If your score is in this range, you probably are very active and physically fit. Help your friends and family to be more active, too!

Recommendation: The Heart Health Program recommends a minimum of 30 minutes of moderately vigorous activity at least three times a week.

You can increase your physical activity in three ways:

1. Increase the **frequency** — the number of times a week you exercise.

2. Increase the **duration** — the length of time you spend at your activity.

3. Increase the **intensity** — the effort you put into your activity.

8

Hyperlipidemia: Detection and Treatment

PAUL N. HOPKINS
University of Utah School of Medicine
Salt Lake City, Utah

In the past, physicians in the United States have largely ignored hyperlipidemia. As recently as 1983, only 39% of U.S. physicians believed that reducing elevated plasma cholesterol levels would have a large effect on heart disease. That percentage had increased to 64% in 1986 (1). For every one office visit to a physician for hyperlipidemia in 1986 there were 14 visits for hypertension in the United States. Yet in Japan, where hypertension is more prevalent and hyperlipidemia less common, the ratio was only 1:3. European physicians also treated hyperlipidemia more aggressively than U.S. physicians (2). In a Utah hospital chart survey (conducted in 1978) of 130 women and 152 men who died of coronary heart disease (CHD) prior to age 65 and 55, respectively, 69 were found to have measured total cholesterol levels in the chart exceeding 300 mg/dl, yet for only one-third had hyperlipidemia been listed as a problem (3). Virtually identical results were reported in a New York hospital for patients having serum cholesterol levels greater than 350 mg/dl (4). In a more recent study, among patients with previously unrecognized hyperlipidemia having serum cholesterol levels over 265 mg/dl (6.85 mmol/L), only 22% received any treatment (5). In a California hospital in 1988, 96% of patients with blood pressure >150/90 had a diagnosis and treatment plan recorded for hypertension yet only 17% had diagnosis and treatment plans recorded for serum cholesterol levels greater than 240 mg/dl (6).

Why have physicians as a group remained unmotivated despite convincing evidence that lowering serum cholesterol levels will reduce CHD risk? Perhaps the strongest deterrent to aggressive treatment of hyperlipidemia is lack of effect on total mortality in most of the lipid-lowering trials so far reported. In fact, none of the trials was designed with the power required to detect a reduction in total mortality. This topic will be addressed further. Some of the reluctance to treat hyperlipidemia may be based on beliefs that treatment is difficult or ineffective. Cumbersome definitions of hyperlipidemia or the complexities of lipid metabolism may have discouraged others. Lack of knowledge regarding diet intervention, reluctance to refer patients to a qualified dietitian, and cost of some of the newer, more effective medications may be other impediments. Uncertainty regarding appropriate subgroups for intervention (such as CHD patients, women, and the elderly) may engender ambivalence toward treating abnormal lipids vigorously in many cases. While much remains to be learned, controversy surrounding the lipid hypothesis has, for the most part, been overstated, and authorities have declared, "The cholesterol controversy is over" (7). Indeed, reluctance to treat hyper-lipidemia with appropriate dietary and drug therapy when indicated can no longer be considered a scientifically tenable position despite popular opinion to the contrary (8).

As in any application of medical theory to clinical practice, there is a need for skillful judgment and individualized decision making. This chapter will help to bridge the gap between theory and practice for the clinician. First, some of the scientific background justifying an aggressive approach to treating abnormal plasma lipids will be presented. Second, relevant information emphasizing appro-priate use of medications will be provided to enable the clinician to deal effectively with the individual patient. Details regarding nutritional intervention for preven-tion and treatment of CHD are found in Chapter 7.

I. RISK FACTORS: GENERAL PRINCIPLES

Finding predictable associations between measurable factors and disease occur-rence in populations gave rise to the notion of risk factors. The usefulness of the risk factor concept lies in its extension to preventive measures: by risk factor modification. Patients need to understand that most preventive efforts are a matter of risk reduction, not risk elimination. Furthermore, few interventions can promise a large impact on lifespan (at least for a population) since competing risks of death continue to increase regardless of how low the risk for a single given disease. For example, even though cardiovascular disease accounts for nearly half of all deaths, complete elimination of all cardiovascular disease would probably increase lifespan at birth only 2–8 years (9). For some individuals, however, improvements in longevity may be much greater if serum cholesterol levels are sufficiently high, such as in familial hypercholesterolemia. Untreated, cholesterol levels above 350 mg/dl frequently lead to myocardial infarction (MI) or MI death by the mid or early 40s. Vigorous treatment in such a high-risk individual would predictably add many years of productive life.

An alternative view to risk reduction is expressed in the term "morbidity compression." The goal in this construct of preventive intervention is not to increase lifespan, especially if that increase occurs with no change in the age at onset of disabling diseases. Instead, efforts are directed at delaying the onset of disability. Such an approach is more realistic and in keeping with actual observations from intervention studies. A major benefit from realizing this goal would be a marked reduction in health expenditures for long-term disability. If life was extended without significantly reducing onset of disease and disability, health expenditures might increase dramatically and quality of life diminish (10).

Patients need to have an accurate perception of their own risk. Studies show that individuals are, on average, unrealistically optimistic about their risk until objective measurements and comparisons to the general population are made and presented to them (11–14). Persons at high risk (whether due to a strong family history of coronary heart disease, hypertension, cigarette smoking, diabetes, or a personal history of atherosclerotic cardiovascular disease) will benefit most in terms of absolute risk reduction by treatment of hyperlipidemia (15). This assertion is not surprising since coronary risk factors best fit a multiplicative model (as in the multiple logistic and Cox regression models). Thus, if risk is already high because of the presence of other risk factors, a 50% reduction will result in a much greater absolute risk reduction than if initial risk is low.

To be worthy of efforts at intervention, risk factors must be causally related to disease. Risk factors suggested by epidemiologic studies are strongly suspected of being causal if they meet all of the following criteria, originally proposed by Hill (16).

1. Time Sequence: The risk factor must be present and predictive prior to disease onset.
2. Dose Dependence: Graded increments in risk factor level lead to proportionately higher disease rates.
3. Strength: Risk factors with higher relative risks are more likely to be causal.
4. Consistency: The risk factor consistently predicts disease in multiple studies among a variety of population groups.
5. Independence: The risk factor is still predictive when other, potentially confounding, factors such as age, sex, and other known risk factors are considered.
6. Biological Plausibility and Coherence of Evidence: The risk factor is biologically plausible, including support from animal and laboratory studies of pathogenesis, and all the known facts fit together.

In addition to these tests of causality, the Canadian and U.S. Task Forces evaluating prevention measures add as "grade I" evidence a properly randomized, controlled clinical intervention trial in which treatment of the factor is shown to reduce the incidence of disease. Nonrandomized but otherwise properly controlled trials were considered grade II evidence of causality (17).

As measured by these criteria, serum cholesterol is clearly a major, causal factor in the pathogenesis of atherosclerotic CHD. In fact, for no other CHD risk factor, with the possible exception of cigarette smoking, is there such abundant proof of causality. Some of the epidemiologic evidence for these assertions is presented briefly below. Also a clear understanding of the epidemiology of CHD is necessary to put into perspective individual risks.

II. PROOF OF THE LIPID HYPOTHESIS

Briefly stated, the lipid hypothesis proposes that the positive relationship between serum cholesterol (or low-density lipoprotein [LDL] cholesterol) and CHD seen in epidemiologic studies is causal and that lowering serum cholesterol will result in lower CHD incidence. The relationship between dietary cholesterol and CHD is not directly a part of the lipid hypothesis so stated. Yet much confusion has arisen, especially among the general public, in part because the terms "dietary choles-terol" and "serum cholesterol" are used as if they were synonymous. Clinicians frequently must clarify the difference for patients and point out that dietary cholesterol may have little to do with one individual's initial serum cholesterol level compared to another's (especially in a population where dietary intakes are so similar, as in the United States). About 50% of population variance for serum total cholesterol, LDL cholesterol, triglycerides, and high-density lipoprotein (HDL) cholesterol can be explained by genetic factors (18). Change of serum cholesterol, on the other hand, can be predicted with fair accuracy in individuals after a known change in diet.

A. Animal Studies

Since Virchow found cholesterol in atherosclerotic plaques in 1856 and Anit-schokow induced hypercholesterolemia and atherosclerotic lesions in rabbits by feeding pure cholesterol in 1913, elevated levels of serum cholesterol have been strongly suspected as a major predictor of atherosclerotic cardiovascular disease. After decades of animal research encompassing virtually thousands of experiments, one cardinal fact stands out: higher serum cholesterol levels lead to more severe atherosclerosis. This is true for mice, rats, rabbits, chickens, pigeons, dogs, pigs, macaques, monkeys, and baboons (19,20). Elevated serum cholesterol levels accelerate atherosclerosis in animals whether the hypercholesterolemia is genet-ically determined (as in Watanabe heritable hyperlipidemic rabbits) or achieved by cholesterol feeding (21), increased saturated fat in a cholesterol-free diet (22), a high-sugar diet (23), or a typical American diet (24). In most cases, the atherosclerosis in animal models has somewhat different features than in humans. Nevertheless, cholesterol-fed rabbits subjected to immune injury (25) and pigs bearing a mutation of apolipoprotein B (26), both with only moderate hypercholesterolemia, have atherosclerotic lesions virtually identical to those in humans. Finally, reduction of serum cholesterol in animals by returning to a more natural diet results in regression of atherosclerotic lesions, even when advanced (27,28). Normalizing serum lipids in these animal studies results not only in removal of lipids and (more slowly) excess fibrous tissue from the intima but also a return to normal of previously excessive cell replication (29). There is no reason to believe that human arteries respond differently to hyperlipidemia or its amelioration.

B. Epidemiologic Evidence

The epidemiologic evidence supporting serum total or LDL cholesterol as a risk factor for CHD is voluminous. At least 50 prospective studies have demonstrated a graded, strong, consistent association between increasing serum cholesterol levels and higher coronary disease risk (30). Examples of results from three of these prospective studies are shown in Figures 1–3. Since cholesterol levels were measured before the onset of disease, prospective studies fulfill criteria of appropriate

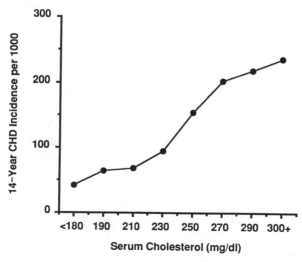

Figure 1 Serum cholesterol as a predictor of new CHD in men and women. The Framingham Study—14 year follow-up. Redrawn from Kannel WB, Am J Cardiol 1976; 37:269.

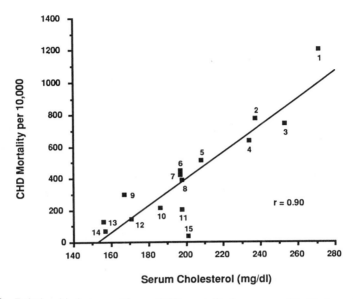

Figure 2   Relationship between 15 year CHD mortality in men age 40–49 at onset—The Seven Country Study. Cohorts: 1–East Finland; 2–US Railroad; 3–West Finland; 4–Zutphen, Netherlands; 5–Rome Railroad, Italy; 6–Montegiorgio, Italy; 7–Crevelcore, Italy; 8–Slavonia, Yugoslavia; 9–Zrenjanin, Yugoslavia; 10–Dalmatia, Yugoslavia; 11–Corfu, Greece; 12–Tanashimara, Japan; 13–Ushibulea, Japan; 14–Velika Krsna, Yugoslavia; 15–Crete, Greece. Data from Keys A, et al, Prev Med 1984; 13:141 and Keys A, et al, Am J Epidemiol 1986; 124:903.

time sequence. In a review of 9 epidemiologic studies that used modern multivariate techniques to establish independence of the measured risk factors (either multiple logistic or Cox regression), the average, independent effect on risk of a 10 mg/dl increase in serum cholesterol was 9.1% (31). This is approximately equivalent to a 2% increase in risk for each 1% increase in serum cholesterol (if baseline is taken as 200 mg/dl), independent of effect from other risk factors. If a serum cholesterol level of 160 mg/dl is taken as the baseline value, relative risks for serum cholesterol values of 200, 240, 300, and 400 mg/dl would be 1.4, 2.0, 3.4, and 8.1, respectively. Indeed, relative risks for cholesterol levels seen in familial hypercholesterolemia (350–550 mg/dl and more) can climb to as much as 30 or more. No other risk factor has such high relative risks attending naturally occurring levels. Biological plausibility is discussed below. Serum total or LDL cholesterol therefore fulfills criteria for suspected causality. The final proof of causality has come more recently through several clinical intervention trials, which are reviewed below.

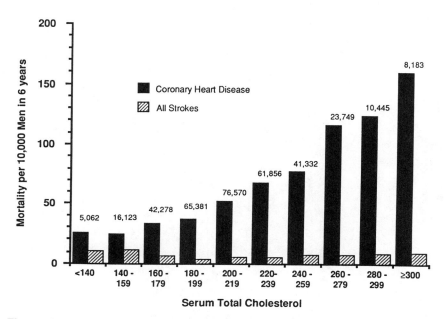

Figure 3 Mortality from coronary heart disease and strokes among 350,979 men followed 6 years from the Multiple Risk Factor Intervention Trial (MRFIT). The number of men in each serum cholesterol category is shown above the bars. Hemorrhagic strokes were actually more common among men with lower serum cholesterol (in the subgroup with diastolic blood pressure >90 mm Hg only) while risk of thrombotic stroke increased progressively with higher serum cholesterol levels. Data from Hiroyasu I, et al, N Engl J Med 1989; 320:904.

Much attention has been focused on the definition of an ideal cholesterol level. Extrapolation of the results from several large angiographic trials in men and women suggests prevalence of significant lesions would reach 0 at a cholesterol level of about 150 mg/dl (see Fig. 4) (32–34). Minimal CHD incidence was also seen in this range in the prospective studies shown in Figures 1–3. Furthermore, in Japan and Puerto Rico, where average serum cholesterol levels were approximately in 160 mg/dl in the past, systolic blood pressure and cigarette smoking were borderline or nonsignificant risk factors for predicting CHD (35). This observation has important clinical implications. Reduction of cholesterol to these lower ranges may protect against the adverse effects of other risk factors, hence the importance of treating hyperlipidemia aggressively in persons at high risk.

From these and other observations, clinically useful ranges of CHD risk based on serum total and LDL cholesterol are presented in Figure 5. Typical ages of onset of CHD are presented with ranges of serum cholesterol. In this figure, HDL cholesterol levels are taken to be average and constant across different total serum

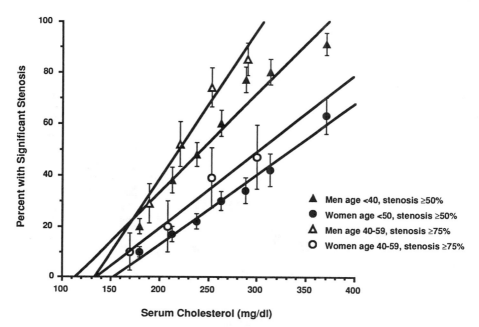

Figure 4 Midpoints of serum cholesterol ranges have been plotted against prevalence of significant stenosis (as defined in figure). Extrapolation of the regression lines to 0 prevalence suggests "ideal" cholesterol levels. Error bars are plus and minus 1 SEM. Each point represents group sizes of 16 to 230 patients. Adapted from references 32–34.

cholesterol ranges. The ranges are purposely broad and overlap. In the protective range, progression of coronary atherosclerosis is greatly retarded and may actually regress. Such low ranges may offer protection against other risk factors and induce regression of already advanced CHD. Levels in the permissive range may not by themselves actively promote atherogenesis, but CHD may progress, especially if other risk factors are present. The promotive range is associated with a steep upturn of CHD risk in population studies, suggesting that mechanisms that actively promote atherogenesis related to LDL cholesterol begin to play an important role. Finally, persons with lifelong serum LDL cholesterol levels in the predictive range (typical ranges for familial hypercholesterolemia and familial defective apolipoprotein B) may be assured with fairly high confidence of early-onset CHD.

In a follow-up of four large Utah familial hypercholesterolemia pedigrees, male heterozygotes having a mean serum cholesterol level of 352 mg/dl were found to have an average age for first MI of 42 years, with coronary death at an average age of 45 years (36). Differences in CHD onset noted in Figure 5 are further justified

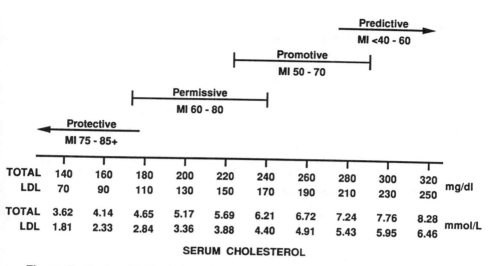

Figure 5 Total and LDL cholesterol ranges with associated effects on atherogenesis, CHD risk, and typical ages for first myocardial infarction (MI).

by a large population study in Western Europe in which average age of first MI decreased by 6–10 years when cholesterol rose from <250 mg/dl to >300 mg/dl (37). These were one-time cholesterol measurements rather than lifelong averages, thus observable effects of serum cholesterol were diluted by random individual variation. (In this same study, smoking >20 cigarettes per day decreased average age of first MI by 8–10 years.) Studies of long-lived individuals typically find LDL cholesterol levels in the protective and permissive ranges (along with moderately high HDL cholesterol) (38,39). Higher HDL levels may play an especially important role in long-lived families and serum total cholesterol levels in the elderly vary widely. Nevertheless, the ranges in Figure 5 provide clinical useful guidelines.

Age is the strongest single risk factor for CHD. Furthermore, the relative risk associated with elevated serum cholesterol levels may decline with age (40). However, the same may be said for all the major CHD risk factors (41). Because CHD incidence rates climb so rapidly with age, even though relative risk associated with elevated cholesterol (and the other risk factors) decline, the absolute excess risk actually increases (42). Prediction into later ages is greatly improved by examining HDL and LDL cholesterol levels together (43). Decreases with age in relative risk associated with serum cholesterol was not seen in men participating in the Honolulu Heart Study (44) or apparently in the Bronx Longitudinal Aging Study (45) and may not, therefore, be a universal phenomenon. Furthermore, age effects on relative risk apply to naive vessels. In coronary artery grafts, atherosclerosis appears to develop more rapidly than in native vessels and the rate of progress is directly related to serum lipids, especially LDL and very-low-density lipoprotein (VLDL) cholesterol (46,47). Therefore, more may be gained by treatment of hyperlipidemia in a patient with a coronary artery bypass graft than in an individual without a graft to protect.

Recent analysis of 30 year follow-up data from Framingham demonstrates greater longevity with lower serum cholesterol levels (48). Nevertheless, a spontaneously falling serum cholesterol level in a patient not attempting lipid reduction is frequently associated with acute or chronic illness (especially colon and other cancers) and may be a harbinger of deteriorating health and poor prognosis generally (49–58). There is no evidence that such observations have relevance to cholesterol intervention, however.

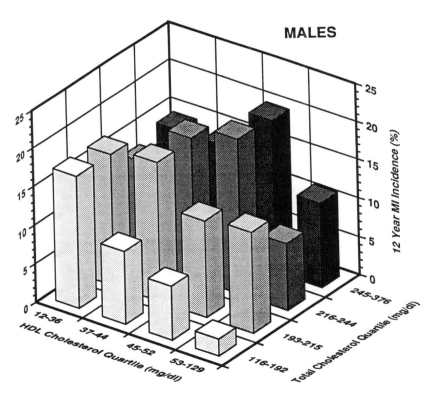

Figure 6 12 year incidence of myocardial infarction in Framingham males age 50–79 according to sex specific HDL and total cholesterol quartiles. Data from Abbott RD, et al, Arteriosclerosis 1988; 8:207.

In addition to serum total or LDL cholesterol, other lipids have been implicated as CHD risk factors. Dyslipidemia refers to any lipid abnormality. Most important clinically are elevated serum triglyceride and low HDL cholesterol levels. HDL cholesterol, in particular, has been consistently demonstrated to be a strong, graded, independent predictor of prospectively determined CHD risk (59,60). The risks associated with low HDL were particularly strong in women in the Framingham Study (Figs. 6 and 7). The ratio of total or LDL/HDL cholesterol was among the best predictors of risk for subsequent coronary disease in the Framingham Study (the linear combination of lipids in a multiple logistic or Cox regression equation is actually slightly better) (61). LDL/HDL cholesterol ratios with associated relative risks are shown in Figure 8 using data from the Framingham study (62). Some have questioned the clinical usefulness of this ratio since HDL choles-

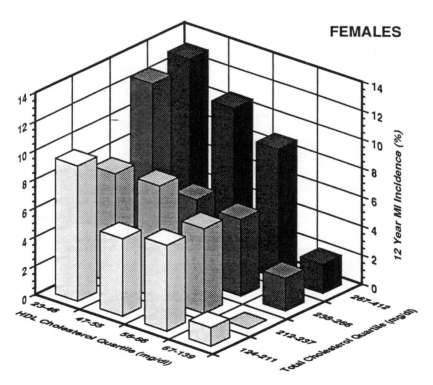

Figure 7 12 year incidence of myocardial infarction in Framingham females age 50–79 according to sex specific HDL and total cholesterol quartiles. Data from Abbott RD, et al, Arteriosclerosis 1988; 8:207.

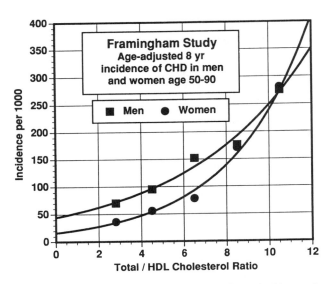

Figure 8   Ratio of plasma total/HDL cholesterol versus 8 year incidence of coronary heart disease (CHD) in older men and women in the Framingham Study. Adapted from Taylor SH, Am J Cardiol 1987; 59:2G.

terol is the most inaccurately measured of the commonly used lipid variables, and, being a relatively small number, when included in the denominator of a ratio could lead to spuriously large deviations from actual risks (63,64). Furthermore, total fat, saturated fat, and dietary cholesterol actually raise HDL cholesterol levels. Populations with low CHD risk, such as vegetarians and a number of non-Western populations eating very little meat or fat, have low LDL cholesterol but also quite low HDL levels and LDL/HDL ratios that may not accurately reflect their much reduced risk (65). Nevertheless, if limitations are recognized, the total or LDL cholesterol/HDL ratio can be a valuable, clinically accessible index of CHD risk.

Lipoprotein(a) (Lp(a)) is a particle composed of apolipoprotein(a) bound by disulfide linkage to the apolipoprotein B moiety of an LDL particle. Levels are almost entirely genetically determined. High levels carry a two to threefold increase risk for premature coronary disease (18). Although Lp(a) is an important determinant of risk, clinical measures are not yet standardized and few data are available regarding intervention (diet is ineffective while niacin and neomycin seem to be the only drugs that significantly affect levels). Optimal approaches to intervention based on Lp(a) levels will have to be based on future studies.

Serum triglyceride levels, when considered in univariate analyses, have consistently been associated with increased CHD risk in case–control, angiographic, and most prospective studies (66). After correction for HDL, however, in most studies the independent risk for triglycerides disappears for men. In Framingham, among the original cohort (67) and in the continuing offspring study (68), elevated triglyceride levels persisted as a significant, independent risk factor in women. Furthermore, high serum triglyceride levels may be an important marker for familial combined hyperlipidemia, a common familial syndrome frequently leading to premature CHD (69). In one study, family risks were evaluated for two groups of individuals with equally elevated triglycerides and normal total cholesterol levels. In the first group, only elevated triglyceride levels were seen in family members (familial hypertriglyceridemia) and prevalence of MI in the 104 family members was low (4%), a value similar to spouse controls. In contrast, in the second group, families displayed a pattern consistent with familial combined hyperlipidemia and prevalence of MI was 10% among 151 relatives: a statistically significant 2.5-fold increased risk (70). The mechanism of triglyceride elevation may be critical for assessing risk. If familial combined hyperlipidemia is due to excess production of VLDL particles and apolipoprotein B, elevated triglycerides may mark an individual family member as a carrier and at high risk (71). In familial hypertriglyceridemia, more often due to a deficit in VLDL removal, the same lipid profile would possibly be benign. In clinical terms, only a complete and accurate family history can differentiate between the two types of patients with elevated triglyceride levels. Finally, elevated triglyceride levels may be a marker for other metabolic disturbances. Thus, increased triglyceride levels are associated with obesity, insulin resistance, increased postprandial lipemia, elevated β-VLDL cholesterol, and hypertension, in addition to the well-known association with lower HDL cholesterol. It is certainly premature to dismiss serum triglyceride levels as a clinically relevant risk factor for CHD.

C. Biological Plausibility

Perhaps some of the delay in a more universal acceptance of the lipid hypothesis was due to incomplete understanding of how dyslipidemia promotes atherosclerosis. Insights into the function of endothelial cells, smooth muscle cells, and monocytes/macrophages have provided further confirmation of the lipid hypothesis. Within days after initiating a high-cholesterol diet in animals (monkeys, rabbits), serum cholesterol becomes markedly elevated due to increased LDL and especially β-VLDL cholesterol (abnormal VLDL and chylomicron remnants). At the same time, changes in endothelial morphology and function occur. These changes result in increased permeability of the endothelium to lipoproteins, especially LDL and β-VLDL, and increased cell turnover (72,73). The endothelium probably plays an important early role in modifying LDL by oxidation of phospholipid polyunsaturated fatty acids, with subsequent breakdown of the phospholipid and modification of apolipoprotein B (74). In response to β-VLDL and oxidized LDL, the endothelium releases a chemoattractant to circulating monocytes causing these cells to adhere to the endothelium and move into the subendothelial space where they are transformed into macrophages (75). Lysolecithin from oxidized lipoproteins is also a chemoattractant for monocytes and inhibits movement of the cells once at the site (73).

When macrophages are stationed within the subintima they imbibe lipoproteins by receptor-specific endocytosis until they are transformed to foam cells. These are cells massively engorged with lipid, primarily cholesterol ester. Native, unmodified LDL are not capable of foam cell formation in vitro, but oxidized LDL, β-VLDL, and proteoglycan-LDL complexes bind to specific (scavenger) receptors and promote foam cell formation (76). Smooth muscle cells can also take up lipoproteins, especially β-VLDL, to become foam cells. During foam cell formation, macrophages release toxic, reactive oxygen metabolites that in turn, may damage overlying endothelium and further promote formation of oxidized lipoproteins (73). Areas of frank desquamation of endothelium appear over areas of foam cell formation (usually after several months of cholesterol feeding in animals). At such denuded sites, platelets may attach and release platelet-derived growth factor (PDGF), which promotes smooth muscle migration and proliferation. Growth factors resembling PDGF are also released from stimulated endothelial cells, smooth muscle cells, and macrophages. Thus, platelets are not mandatory for atherosclerosis progression (77).

Foam cells either egress from the growing atheroma or die, leaving behind a growing collection of extracellular cholesterol ester, free cholesterol, and necrotic debris. The ratio of free cholesterol to other lipids in the subintima increases as lesions progress. This ratio may be an important determinant of cell necrosis associated with free cholesterol crystal formation (78). The lipids and necrotic debris give rise to the gruel in the atheroma's necrotic core. If the fibrous cap (formed from smooth muscle cells) that overlies the atheroma ruptures, exposing the highly thrombogenic necrotic core, platelet-rich thrombi may form and thereby contribute abruptly and dramatically to the stenosis caused by the underlying atheromatous plaque.

In this complex scenario of atherogenesis, lipoproteins play important roles at every step. Most obviously, higher serum levels of LDL and β-VLDL cholesterol increase the deposition of these atherogenic lipoproteins in the arterial wall (79,80). Even if LDL must be modified before becoming directly capable of promoting foam cell formation, higher levels of serum LDL will lead to increased levels of the modified lipoproteins simply because of mass action (73). Very high levels of LDL or β-VLDL may initiate atherogenesis by altering the endothelium, thereby increasing their own permeability through the endothelial barrier, and by promoting monocyte attachment and conversion into macrophages. High serum LDL cholesterol enhances platelet aggregability, thereby potentiating the frequently catastrophic results of thrombosis (81,82). Elevated platelet aggregation in hyperlipidemia returned to normal after LDL reduction with an HMG-CoA reductase inhibitor (synvinolin) (83).

High serum triglyceride levels (and, in some studies, high total cholesterol), are strongly correlated with increased clotting factor activity (mainly factors VII, VIII, and X) (84), and decreased fibrinolytic capacity (primarily because of increased plasminogen activator inhibitor) (85–87). This thrombosis-prone state is largely corrected by treatment of the hyperlipidemia by diet (88), exercise (89), or a fibric acid derivative (such as bezafibrate) (90).

HDL are probably antiatherogenic through multiple mechanisms. The major protective mechanism of HDL is probably its ability to remove cholesterol from macrophages and smooth muscle cells (and other cells), thereby slowing the formation of foam cells. HDL also appears to protect against LDL aggregation and oxidation. HDL levels are also inversely correlated with the degree of postprandial lipemia and may thereby decrease arterial exposure to postprandial remnants and β-VLDL (91).

This brief summary of the last two decades of atherogenesis research points to multiple major roles for serum lipoproteins and provides evidence for the coherence and biological plausibility of the lipid hypothesis.

D. Results from Intervention Trials

The final, and ultimately most convincing, proof of the lipid hypothesis has come from several lipid intervention trials utilizing diet or drugs. The diet intervention trials are reviewed elsewhere in this volume. Perhaps the most convincing evidence that dietary intervention is a practical and important means of preventing CHD came from the Oslo Trial, in which vigorous advice to avoid high-fat foods and to stop smoking was given to hyperlipidemic men. There was a 50% decrease in CHD incidence and a consistent 10% decrease in serum cholesterol levels compared to a randomized control group that received no counseling. Statistical analysis demonstrated that only 25% of the change could be attributed to differences in smoking habits between the advice and control groups (92,93).

Recently, a vigorous lifestyle intervention (vegetarian diet, with <10% calories from fat, with mild exercise, stress management, and smoking cessation) for 1 year resulted in statistically significant, quantitative angiographically assessed coronary atherosclerosis regression ($p < 0.001$) that was proportional to the degree of adherence to the intervention program. Marked reductions in chest pain frequency (by 91%) and severity (by 28%) were also recorded in the intervention group, while symptoms progressed during the 1 year follow-up in the control group. Total cholesterol levels decreased 24% and LDL cholesterol levels 37% from baseline values of 227 mg/dl (5.88 mmol/L) and 152 mg/dl (3.95 mm/L), respectively (94). Thus, vigorous intervention in CHD patients with only mild to moderate elevations in serum cholesterol may be beneficial.

Results of randomized, placebo-controlled drug intervention trials have advanced the status of the lipid hypothesis to virtual certainty. Randomized, primary intervention (subjects initially free of CHD), and secondary intervention (subjects

Table 1　Results of Lipid-Lowering Drug and Surgical Intervention Trials

Trial	Drug, daily dosage	Duration (years)	Number of participants (Rx/Control)	Serum total cholesterol (Rx/Control)	Serum HDL cholesterol (Rx/Control)	CHD rate per 1000 (Rx/Control)
Primary prevention trials						
WHO (205)	Clofibrate, 1.6 g	5	5331/5296	224/244	—/—	31.3/39.3
LRC-CPPT (206)	Cholestyramine, ⩽ 24 g	7	1906/1900	248/276	46.6/45.5	81.3/98.4
LRC-CPPT[a] (207)	Cholestyramine, < 8 g	7	776/1900	269/276	46.3/45.5	99.2/98.4
LRC-CPPT[a] (153)	Cholestyramine, 8–16 g	7	279/1900	253/276	47.0/45.5	75.3/98.4
LRC-CPPT[a] (153)	Cholestyramine, 16–24 g	7	861/1900	230/276	46.3/45.5	67.4/98.4
Helsinki Heart (208)	Gemfibrozil, 1200 mg	5	2051/2030	247/273	51.2/47.0	27.3/41.4
Secondary internvention trials						
Newcastle (209)	Clofibrate, 1.5–2 g	5	244/253	227/253	—/—	234/372
Edinburgh	Clofibrate, 1.6–2 g	6	350/367	227/253	—/—	169/215
CDP (211)	Dextrothyroxine, 6.0 mg	4–5	1083/2715	226/255	—/—	182/165
CDP (212)	Clofibrate, 1.8 g	5–6	1103/2789	235/251	—/—	280/301
CDP (158)	Niacin, 3.0 g	5–6	1119/2789	226/251	—/—	256/301
NHLBI Type II (213)	Cholestyramine, 24 g	5	59/57	256/289	41/39	491/649
CLAS (214)	Colestipol, 30 g plus niacin, 3–12 g	2	94/94	180/232	60.8/44.4	10.6/53.2
Stockholm (215)	Clofibrate, 2 g plus niacin, 3 g	5	279/276	217/251	—/—	293/446
FATS (216)	Colestipol, 30 g plus niacin, 4 g	2.5	32/37	210/254	62/45	31/297
FATS (162)	Colestipol, 30 gm plus lovastatin, 40 mg	2.5	34/37	181/254	50.2/45.3	88/297
POSCH (217)	Partial ileal bypass	9.7	421/417	182/238	41.8/40.2	195/300
Mixed primary and secondary intervention						
Upjohn (218)	Colestipol, 15 g	3	1149/1129	264/283	—/—	16.5/27.5

[a]CHD rates for different packet number groups were based on packet counts taken from a single random visit. Changes in lipids were estimated from reported changes with packet number groups based on average number of packets over several visits (219).

with CHD at baseline) trials of lipid-lowering medications are summarized in Table 1. Also included is a single randomized trial of partial ileal bypass surgery for reducing hyperlipidemia. Virtually all of the trials demonstrated reductions in CHD endpoints and most of these were statistically significant. As shown in Figure 9, the degree of success in preventing CHD events in the treated compared with the control group was largely determined by serum total cholesterol reductions. In that subset of studies in which HDL cholesterol levels were reported, a much better correlation was seen between CHD rate difference (placebo control minus treated) and the difference between the total/HDL cholesterol ratio in placebo vs. treated groups (Fig. 10). Increases in HDL cholesterol, primarily seen with gemfibrozil and niacin treatment, but also, to a limited extent, with cholestyramine in the Lipid Research Clinics (LRC) trial, thus serve to explain discrepancies in expected reductions in CHD rates when decreases in serum total cholesterol only are considered. In the Helsinki Heart Trial, multivariate regression demonstrated that increases in HDL and decreases in LDL cholesterol were the primary determinants for the positive outcome in that study (95). Furthermore, patients with initially low HDL experienced the greatest reduction in CHD rates due to gemfibrozil while patients with initially high HDL did not benefit (96).

Rates in Table 1 are based on clinical CHD endpoints. In the National Heart, Lung and Blood Institute (NHLBI) type II trial, endpoints also included signifi-

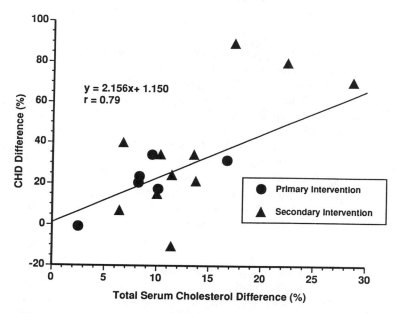

Figure 9 Percent difference (treated versus controls) in CHD incidence versus total serum cholesterol differences in lipid lowering drug intervention studies from Table 1.

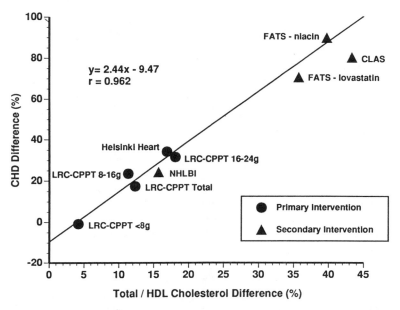

Figure 10 Percent CHD difference in treated versus controls versus percent difference in total/HDL cholesterol ratios. Data from studies in Table 1.

cant increases in angiographically determined atherosclerosis. In the other angiographic trials (Cholesterol Lowering Atherosclerosis Study [CLAS] and Family Atherosclerosis Treatment Study [FATS]) only clinical endpoints, primarily nonfatal MI and CHD death, were included. In most of the trials, only men were studied. Two trials (the Upjohn and Stockholm studies: Table 1) included women who experienced decreases in CHD rates similar in proportion to those in men but because of lower absolute rates, rate reductions were not statistically significant. Women were included with the men in Table 1.

Another important trial in patients with familial hypercholesterolemia was recently reported (97). All subjects were given instructions on diet. The 32 control patients were offered 15 g daily of colestipol but only 14 actually elected to take it regularly. The 40 patients in the intensive intervention group received 30 g colestipol and up to 7.5 g of niacin daily. When lovastatin became available, 16 of the patients took 40–60 mg daily in combination with one or both of the other drugs. Plasma total cholesterol levels decreased 31% (from 378 mg/dl), LDL cholesterol 39% (from 283 mg/dl), and triglycerides decreased 21% (from 133 mg/dl), while HDL cholesterol increased 25% in the aggressively treated group. In comparison, LDL was reduced 12% in the control group while triglycerides and HDL did not change significantly. Angiograms were performed at the beginning and end of the 26 month trial. Stenoses regressed 1.53% in the aggressive treatment group compared to progression by 0.80% in the control group (p = 0.04). Regression was also significant for women considered separately. This was the first trial to demonstrate a statistically significant benefit for women in the treatment of hyperlipidemia.

None of these trials were designed to demonstrate significant decreases in total mortality attributable to lipid lowering (sample sizes were too small). It was not surprising that none of the trials reported any significant decrease in total mortality. Nevertheless, any significant increase in total mortality should send up a "red flag" as a potential indicator of toxicity. In the World Health Organization (WHO) clofibrate trial (Table 2), total (and total non-CHD) mortality was significantly increased in the clofibrate-treated group. Since the results of this trial became known, clofibrate has been abandoned as a first-line agent. This trial illustrates the need for caution in introducing any medication for general use in treating a problem so pervasive as hyperlipidemia. In the Helsinki Heart Trial and the Lipid Research Clinic Coronary Primary Prevention Trial (CPPT) there were nonsignificant increases in violent deaths among persons on active treatment. A careful analysis of each of these deaths failed to reveal any cause and effect relationship attributable to the medications (98). Total mortality was not reported for the most promising trials, namely CLAS and FATS. One would expect the remarkable 70–85% reduction in CHD clinical endpoints reported in these trials to translate into significant reductions in total mortality if the trends were to continue.

The quantitative angiography trials, especially CLAS and FATS, provide the strongest evidence to date in support of the lipid hypothesis. These trials illustrate the need for vigorous, prolonged intervention to achieve a major impact on atherosclerosis progression and offer real hope for regression in many patients. They represent the current state-of-the-art in hyperlipidemia intervention. Details of the FATS trial are provided in Figures 11 and 12.

III. CLINICAL APPROACH TO HYPERLIPIDEMIA AND DYSLIPIDEMIA

A. Definitions and Scope of the Problem

Traditional definitions for dyslipidemia use population percentile cut-offs such as the 90th or 95th percentile. Such definitions are useful for diagnosing familial lipid disorders within a given population and in other situations in which outliers need to be defined. For decisions regarding treatment, however, definitions of dyslipidemia need to be tied directly to CHD risk.

Definitions relevant for preventing CHD have recently been forwarded by the National Cholesterol Education Program (NCEP) (69). A total cholesterol of less than 200 mg/dl or an LDL cholesterol of 130 mg/dl or less is considered desirable (not necessarily ideal). Values of 200–240 mg/dl for total and 130–160 mg/dl for LDL cholesterol are borderline high risk, while higher values are considered high risk. These cutpoints are arbitrary but useful. They correspond roughly to points of inflection in the risk curves from several populations.

Table 2 Lipid Phenotypes and Associated Primary and Secondary Causes with Approaches to Management of Primary Syndromes

Phenotype/criteria	Secondary causes	Primary causes	Management
Type IIa			
Elevated LDL only	Hypothyroidism	Diet induced/sporadic	Low saturated fat, low cholesterol, high soluble fiber diet
Plasma LDL cholesterol:	Cushing's syndrome	Polygenic (mild to severe)	Add bile acid sequestrants
>160 mg/dl in adults	Nephrotic syndrome	Familial combined hyperlipid-emia	Add lovastatin or pravastatin
>130 mg/dl in children	Biliary obstruction (Lp-X)	Familial hypercholesterolemia	Add niacin or gemfibrozil
Normal triglycerides (<200–250 mg/dl)	Anorexia nervosa	Familial defective apo B	
	Acute intermittent porphyria	Familial hyperapobetalipopro-teinemia	
	Lipodystrophy	Sitosterolemia	
	Werner's syndrome		
	Corticosteroids		
Type IIb			
Elevated LDL and VLDL	Cushing's syndrome	Diet induced/sporadic	Low saturated fat, low cholesterol, high soluble fiber diet
LDL cholesterol as above	Nephrotic syndrome	Obesity	Achieve and maintain ideal body weight
Triglycerides >200–250 mg/dl (or age and gender specific 90–95th percentile)	Uremia	Familial combined hyperlipo-proteinemia	Exercise
	Sexual ateliotic dwarfism		Niacin or gemfibrozil
	Drugs: corticosteriods, ana-bolic steroids, cyclosporin		Add bile acid sequestrant with cau-tion (can raise triglycerides)
			Lovastatin or pravastatin

Type	Secondary causes	Primary causes	Treatment
Type III β-VLDL present Ratio of *measured* VLDL cholesterol to plasma triglycerides ≥ 0.30 with plasma triglycerides >150 mg/dl *plus* either: Apo E 2-2 phenotype, or Significant β-VLDL band on gel or paper electrophoresis	Hypothyroidism Monoclonal gammopathies (both usually aggravating factors rather than causative factors) Systemic lupus erythematosus	Familial dysbetalipoprotein-emia Hepatic lipase deficiency	Achieve and maintain ideal body weight Exercise Low saturated fat, low cholesterol, high soluble fiber diet Niacin or gemfibrozil Add lovastatin or pravastatin Consider estrogen replacement in females
Type IV Elevated VLDL only Triglycerides as for IIb LDL cholesterol <type II criteria. No fasting chylomicronemia	Diabetes mellitus Hypothyroidism Stress (emotional stress, extensive burns, sepsis) Acute hepatitis Other hepatic disease Uremia Acromegaly Monoclonal gammopathies Drugs *alcohol*, anabolic steroids, corticosteroids, oral contraceptives (estrogens), isotretinoin (Accutane), β-blockers, thiazides, cyclosporins	Obesity Familial hypertriglyceridemia Lipoprotein lipase deficiency (especially heterozygotes) ?Apolipoprotein C-II deficiency (heterozygotes) Glycogen storage disease (Ia)	Achieve and maintain ideal body weight Exercise No ethanol Low saturated fat, low cholesterol, *low sugar*, high soluble fiber diet, with liberal fish intake Consider fish oil Niacin or gemfibrozil Consider adding lovastatin or pravastatin
Type I/V Fasting chylomicronemia Fasting triglycerides >400 mg/dl. Note: there is no clinically meaningful distinction between types I and V	Same as for type IV Systemic lupus erythematosus	Same as for type IV Lipoprotein lipase deficiency (especially homozygotes) Apolipoprotein C-II deficiency (homozygotes)	Same as type IV except very low fat diet (≤10% of total calories from fat) Fish oil often very effective

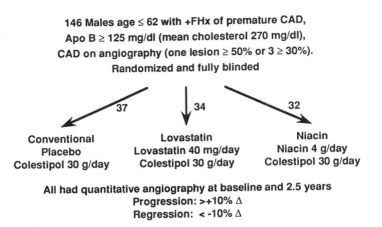

Figure 11   Design of the Familial Atherosclerosis Treatment Study (FATS). Adapted from Brown G, et al, Circulation 1989; 80(suppl II):II-264.

If one uses NCEP guidelines as definitions, a huge percentage of the United States population would be considered hypercholesterolemic. Fully 40–50% of U.S. men and women over age 30 have serum total cholesterol levels above 200 mg/dl. The proportion rises with age. If one applied the NCEP guidelines without regard to age, 2–10% of the population would be placed on antilipemic drugs, if it was assumed that diet reduced cholesterol 5–20% (100,101). Benefits for cholesterol lowering may diminish with age, although this is not at all clear at present (no intervention studies have been performed in the elderly). The physician must therefore weigh potential benefits and costs and be guided also by the patient's preferences. Many patients over 60 will be highly motivated because of recent onset of symptoms. The apparent reduction with age of relative risk for elevated serum cholesterol level may not be a universal phenomenon and there is no reason to avoid vigorous treatment in the otherwise healthy elderly patient who desires significant risk reduction or regression of coronary lesions. Intervention trials among the elderly are urgently needed, however, to assess the utility of an aggressive approach.

B. NCEP Guidelines for Management

Persons with serum total cholesterol <200 mg/dl should have repeat blood tests every 5 years. For the individual with a borderline high cholesterol (200–240 mg/dl), a low-saturated-fat, low-cholesterol diet is usually sufficient to reduce cholesterol below 200 mg/dl. For those with levels above 240 mg/dl, secondary causes of hyperlipidemia are sought and corrected. Diet is then applied vigorously for at least 6 months and the addition of drugs is considered when LDL cholesterol levels

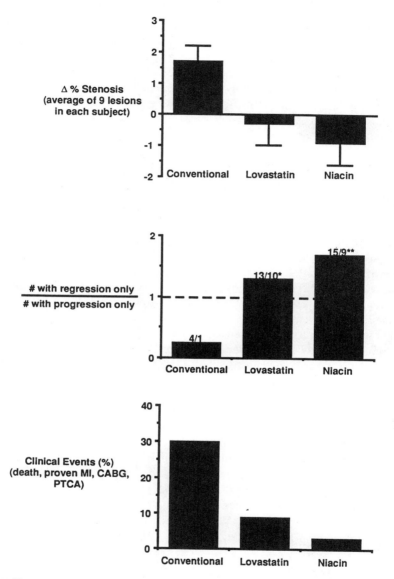

Figure 12   Principal results of the Familial Atherosclerosis Treatment Study (FATS). See Figure 11 for reference.

remain above 190 mg/dl. Lower action levels (LDL cholesterol > 160 mg/dl) for adding drugs are prompted by the presence of multiple risk factors including male sex, positive family history of CHD, severe obesity, hypertension, diabetes, cigarette smoking, and low HDL (<35 mg/dl). Cholestyramine, colestipol, and niacin are considered the agents of first choice, with niacin preferred when triglyceride levels are elevated. Blood should be drawn 4–6 weeks after use of a medication is started, and then every 3 months until lipids and other blood chemical values are stable. Thereafter, follow-up with blood analysis may be repeated every 6 months to 1 year.

The clinician must be aware that the NCEP guidelines, briefly outlined above, are meant only for normal persons and are primarily aimed at those ages 20–60. Protective ranges (total cholesterol well under 180 mg/dl and LDL under 100 mg/dl; Fig. 5) are more defensible goals for the patient with coronary artery disease in whom lesion regression is sought. In asymptomatic persons over age 75–80, serum lipid levels should probably be considered irrelevant except for the poor prognostic sign of a spontaneously falling serum cholesterol. A full lipid profile (with triglycerides, HDL cholesterol, and calculated LDL cholesterol) was not considered in NCEP guidelines to be necessary for persons in the borderline high risk range of total serum cholesterol values. However, most clinicians, especially in the light of increasing evidence of the importance of HDL cholesterol, would not base any treatment recommendations on a serum total cholesterol level alone. If high HDL levels cause moderate elevations in serum total cholesterol levels (most frequently seen in women), reassurance rather than treatment is indicated. Some types of hyperlipidemia require additional expertise to recognize and treat that are not emphasized in the NCEP schema. Much more vigorous treatments using drug combinations should be directed toward extremely high risk subjects, such as the patient with familial hypercholesterolemia. Moreover, the NCEP recommendations for drug treatment were made prior to completion of the Helsinki Heart Trial using gemfibrozil (Lopid), or the Family Atherosclerosis Treatment Study (FATS), which used combinations of colestipol with either niacin or lovastatin. Gemfibrozil (Lopid) and the HMG-CoA reductase inhibitors should now be included among the first-line agents.

C. Limitations and Use of Fredrickson Phenotypes

The classic Fredrickson hyperlipidemia phenotypes are useful clinical descriptions of hyperlipidemia. However, assigning a phenotype, except for type III, does not constitute a diagnosis. Phenotype definitions use cutoff values based on the 90th or 95th age and sex-specific percentile for plasma total or LDL cholesterol and plasma triglycerides and do not necessarily relate to cardiovascular risk. Furthermore, no mention was made in the original Fredrickson phenotype scheme of low HDL cholesterol. Low values of HDL cholesterol may occur in isolation or in the presence of hyperlipidemia, especially elevated triglycerides. Accordingly, the term "dyslipidemia" is more inclusive and relevant to prevention of CHD. Risks for CHD according to the most common Fredrickson phenotypes, as well as isolated low HDL, are shown in Figure 13 using data from the Framingham Offspring Study (102).

Perhaps the most practical use of Fredrickson phenotypes is to guide treatment. Thus, management of primary type IIa is similar, regardless of the cause. The same may be said for the other types. Definitions for the phenotypes, potential secondary and primary causes, and approaches to management are presented in Table 2. Note that without a specialized lipid laboratory to provide measured VLDL cholesterol levels (or at least gel or paper electrophoresis to detect a β-VLDL band) there is no way to differentiate type IIb from type III hyperlipidemia. A practical clue to type III hyperlipidemia is the finding of similarly elevated serum cholesterol and triglyceride levels, which change together with treatment. For example, a type III patient may be seen with a serum cholesterol level of 520 mg/dl and triglyceride values of 645 mg/dl. After weight loss and use of a careful low-fat diet, serum cholesterol levels might drop to 256 mg/dl and triglycerides to 245 mg/dl.

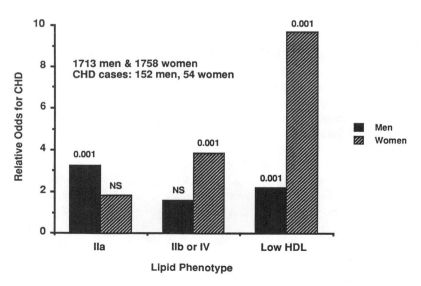

Figure 13 Isolated low HDL and premature coronary heart disease: The Framingham Offspring Study, 12 year follow-up. P-values for relative risks (when significantly greater than 1) are shown above bars. NS = non-significant. Data from Wilson PWF, Anderson KM, Arteriosclerosis 1989; 9:708a.

The original phenotyping scheme made a distinction between type I and type V hyperlipidemia, with type I defined by fasting chylomicronemia with normal VLDL levels and type V characterized by both fasting chylomicronemia and increased VLDL levels. However, there is no clinically meaningful distinction between these types since well-defined genetic syndromes (such as lipoprotein lipase deficiency) cause both types and there is no mechanistic reason to separate them. The vast majority of persons with triglyceride levels over 1,000 mg/dl have type V hyperlipidemia (unpublished observations).

D. Diagnosing Dyslipidemia by Cause

Diagnosis of dyslipidemia should be based on cause when possible. In broad terms, potential causes are primary (genetic or environmental) or secondary. Environmental causes include diets rich in saturated fat and cholesterol and low in soluble fiber, as well as excessive caloric intake resulting in obesity (with associated high triglycerides and low HDL). Diet (possibly together with genetically determined responsiveness or polygenic predisposition to higher serum cholesterol levels) is likely the most common cause of mild to modest hypercholesterolemia. For more severe dyslipidemias, and when associated with a strong family history of premature CHD, genetic causes predominate. Secondary causes of hyperlipidemia are much less common than primary dietary and genetic causes and occur most frequently in patients with hypertriglyceridemia. Diabetes occurred in 4–5%, and hypothyroidism in 5–21% of patients with hypertriglyceridemia (types IIb, IV, and V/I) in the Lipid Research Clinics Prevalence Study (103). There was no increase in the frequency of abnormal screening tests in type IIa. A useful rule of thumb is that if triglyceride levels are over 1000 mg/dl in a diabetic, a primary underlying cause is likely present even if the diabetes is in poor control. Other relatively common secondary causes of dyslipidemia include liver and renal disease, alcohol (especially type IV and V hyperlipidemias), use of birth control pills or estrogens (which raise triglyceride levels while they lower LDL and increase HDL cholesterol), progestins, isotretinoin (Accutane), corticosteroids, anabolic steroids, beta blockers without intrinsic sympathomimetic activity, and all diuretics other than indapamide (Lozol). A simple approach to excluding secondary hyperlipidemia is presented in Figure 14.

Diagnosis of genetic dyslipidemias is aided by recognition of a few important features. These are summarized in Table 3. Perhaps the most important message from this table is the fact that a reasonable diagnosis is often impossible without actual lipid measurements from most of the patient's first-degree relatives and sometimes other relatives as well. A thorough family history of coronary disease is critical to the diagnosis as well. Physicians who fail to obtain plasma lipid levels from family members when indicated are doing a disservice not only to their patients, who would be better served with an accurate diagnosis, but also to close

History:

Medical: pregnancy, stress (severe), diabetes, hypothyroidism, liver disease, renal disease, Cushing's syndrome, systemic lupus erythematosus, monoclonal gammopathies, acute intermittent porphyria, acromegaly

Current Medications: alcohol, oral contraceptives, thiazides, β-blockers, corticosteroids, anabolic steroids, isotretinoin (Accutane), cyclosporin

Laboratory:

Test:	Screen for:
Fasting glucose	Diabetes
Liver enzymes	Liver disease
Bilirubin	Liver disease
Albumin	Liver disease
Creatinine	Renal disease
BUN	Renal disease
Urinalysis	Diabetes, nephrotic syndrome
T4, TSH	Thyroid disorders

Note: Secondary causes are infrequent etiologic agents in dyslipidemia, especially without hypertriglyceridemia. In fact, except for type IIB and IV, there is no increase in the prevalence of abnormalities in the above laboratory tests in the LRC population of 1344 (Wallace et al. Circulation 1986;73 (suppl I):I62).

Figure 14 Excluding secondary causes of hyperlipidemia.

relatives and especially children who may be at extraordinarily high risk for premature coronary disease.

The most common cause of type IIa hyperlipidemia with serum total cholesterol levels between 240 and 350 mg/dl is probably polygenic predisposition, often aggravated by a poor diet. Mechanisms for such elevations probably include both increased production and, to a lesser extent, decreased removal of LDL cholesterol (104–106). When serum cholesterol levels rise above 350 mg/dl and triglyceride levels are normal, familial hypercholesterolemia (FH) becomes one of the most likely diagnoses. If such levels are found in children, FH is almost the only diagnosis. Indeed, the finding of a child with severe hypercholesterolemia practically ensures a diagnosis of FH. Screening family members reveals the extent of the problem.

E. Treating FH

In heterozygous FH, a genetic defect of one of the two LDL receptor genes causes a reduction of normal LDL receptor activity by one-half and a doubling of LDL cholesterol levels. Efforts to reduce LDL cholesterol levels are therefore aimed at

Table 3 Recognition of Common Genetic Dyslipidemias

Diagnosis	Lipid phenotypes	Mechanism	Clinical features	Family history
Familial hyper-cholesterolemia	Severe type IIa Total chol >300 LDL chol >220 Some IIb and III	LDL receptor defect → ↓ LDL fractional catabolic rate	Affects children. Tendinous xanthomas (not always present). Premature CVD	Dominant transmission of high LDL cholesterol. Multiple, striking, early MI cases
Familial combined hyperlipidemia	Types IIa, IIb, IV (and occasionally V) Less severe (90th percentile). Low HDL common	Typically, ↑ hepatic VLDL production. Also ↓ VLDL catabolic rate or both in some families.	Usually asymptomatic. Individuals switch between phenotypes (e.g. IV → IIa or IIb after weight loss)	Dominant transmission. At least 2 of 3 lipid phenotypes present among 1° relatives. Moderately early CHD
Polygenic hyper-cholesterolemia	Types IIa, (?)IIb Usually less severe than other forms	Variable. ↑ LDL synthesis or ↓ LDL fractional catabolic rate	Asymptomatic unless seen with premature CHD. Most common hyperlipidemia	Both parents have moderately high serum cholesterol. All sibs equally affected
Familial dysbeta-lipoproteinemia	Type III Over 95% of cases are apo E 2-2	Defective apo E binding to hepatic receptors → ↑ β-VLDL (chylomicron and VLDL remnants)	Highly variable severity. Total triglycerides and cholesterol similarly elevated (mg/dl). Tuberous xanthomas	Recessive transmission—thus usually negative family history of CHD. Very early CHD in affected may be seen

Hypoalphalipo-proteinemia (low HDL syndromes)	Low HDL levels—often without other lipid abnormalities	Multiple syndromes. Most common ones are poorly characterized. Both ↑ removal and ↓ production of HDL	Usually asymptomatic. Cataracts, large orange tonsils, other physical findings occur in some rare syndromes	Frequently positive for early CHD. Many cases are probably polygenic in origin
Familial hyper-triglyceridemia	Types IV, V/I Low HDL common	Mixed genetic causes. Apo CII deficiency probably similar to LPL deficiency. Both ↑ production and ↓ removal of VLDL	Usually asymptomatic. Acute pancreatitis and/or erruptive xanthomas may occur with severe hypertriglyceridemia	May or may not be associated with positive family history of CHD. Dominant transmission of less severe hypertriglyceridemia. Homozygotes more severely affected
Lipoprotein lipase (LPL) deficiency	Homozygotes (rare): types I/IV/V Heterozygotes: type IV, low HDL	↓ VLDL catabolic rate	Usually asymptomatic in heterozygotes. Homozygotes—eruptive xanthomas, pancreatitis	Highly age-dependent expression. Dominant transmission. Increased prevalence of high BP

stimulating the residual LDL receptor activity and reducing the production of LDL that contributes to the load that the receptors encounter.

The approach to treating FH provides a paradigm for patients with all other forms of type IIa and many with type IIb hyperlipidemia. With LDL cholesterol levels above 200–250 mg/dl, multiple drug regimens, along with careful diet intervention are almost always warranted. In our Preventive Cardiology Clinic we begin treatment with vigorous diet intervention, including formal, family group instruction from dietitians (107). If after 6 months (longer for children and young women, 3 months for persons with clinical CHD), plasma LDL cholesterol levels are not brought to target levels, a drug or combination of drugs is added. Drug treatment of FH has been thoroughly reviewed (108). Summary data from this review are presented below.

The drug regimen of choice for FH is an HMG-CoA reductase inhibitor combined with either cholestyramine or colestipol. The bile acid sequestrants alone at usual dosages (see Table 4) result in 20–35% reductions in LDL cholesterol in FH heterozygotes. Similar percentage reductions are seen in patients without FH, as illustrated by the LRC trial (Table 1). Lovastatin at 20 mg twice daily resulted in 27–39% reductions in several studies. The combination, however, of an HMG-CoA reductase inhibitor with a bile acid sequestrant results in 52–54% reductions. Similar decreases in LDL cholesterol occurred with lovastatin–niacin combinations. Reductions of 32–55% have been reported for combinations of a bile acid sequestrant and niacin in patients with FH. If a two-drug combination fails to reduce LDL cholesterol adequately, LDL cholesterol can usually be normalized, if not brought to protective levels (near 90 mg/dl), by combining a bile acid sequestrant, an HMG-CoA reductase inhibitor, and niacin. Indeed a mean 62% decrease in LDL cholesterol was reported using such a regimen. Gemfibrozil may be used cautiously as a substitute for niacin in combination regimens, but it tends to lower LDL cholesterol less effectively than niacin. Probucol may have a role in aiding tendinous xanthoma regression in FH patients (both heterozygotes and homozygotes) (109) but is otherwise not being used routinely until further clinical trials demonstrate efficacy in CHD prevention. Illustrations of vigorous diet and drug intervention in two male FH patients with histories of early CHD are presented in Figure 15.

In mild FH or in patients with moderate, isolated LDL cholesterol elevations with normal triglyceride levels (polygenic hypercholesterolemia or indeterminate cases), a single drug is often effective. The drug of choice in such cases is probably an HMG-CoA reductase inhibitor. In the past, a bile acid sequestrant was usually considered the drug of first choice in this setting. Indeed, a bile acid sequestrant is still probably preferable in children requiring LDL cholesterol reduction and is the only drug that can be used by pregnant women. Nevertheless, in the large group of patients for whom lipid intervention is most cost-effective (i.e., middle-aged men and older women as well as persons with clinical coronary disease), the HMG-CoA reductase inhibitors are probably a better choice for a single agent. Reasons for preferring HMG-CoA reductase inhibitors over bile acid sequestrants as single agents include greater efficacy, fewer side effects with greater ease of administration resulting in better patient compliance, and favorable cost-effectiveness (see below).

Laboratory follow-up of multidrug regimens should include a battery of tests including serum total cholesterol and liver function tests (such as a Chem 20) every 3 months. Some would include creatine kinase (CK) testing routinely in regimens that include lovastatin but unless this is part of an inexpensive panel, a more cost-effective approach might be to obtain CK levels only when general muscle pain presents as a problem. More frequent testing may be justifiable initially as suggested by NCEP guidelines. After tolerance is demonstrated and drug dosages are constant, less frequent laboratory testing may be appropriate. A full year or more is often required to arrive at a stable, well-tolerated, effective diet and drug program for an individual patient.

As with any intervention, treatment must be individualized. Children with heterozygous FH are treated vigorously with diet after age 2 and many authorities consider adding a bile acid sequestrant after age 8. Studies in younger children show no adverse effects of such treatment on growth or nutrient status (110,111). Efficacy of lovastatin or niacin in older children has been demonstrated (112) but no long-term safety evaluations of either lovastatin or niacin have been performed. Vigorous drug intervention usually begins after age 18–21 in men but may necessarily be postponed during childbearing years in female FH patients. Those with symptomatic CHD may benefit greatly from vigorous intervention and target total cholesterol levels should be in the range of 140–180 mg/dl. Finally, it would be difficult to justify vigorous drug intervention in the very elderly, even in the symptomatic FH patient. These age considerations, as well as drug costs, side effect profiles, and individual preferences must all be factored into decisions on an intervention program individualized for each patient.

Follow-up of severe hypercholesterolemia, as in FH, is lifelong and patients must be taught early in the course of treatment that relapse into old dietary habits or noncompliance with drug regimens will result in prompt return of serum lipids to untreated values. Instruction on the dynamic nature of lipoprotein metabolism and a clear understanding of factors that alter LDL levels facilitate the kind of long-term adherence required for effective treatment. A simple sketch emphasizing dynamic production and removal of lipoprotein particles is usually sufficient to remove false notions such as "If I stay on a good diet and take these drugs for a few months, then I will get the cholesterol out of my system and my high cholesterol will be cured." Understanding why their own cholesterol level is high and how each drug they take works greatly facilitates patients' long-term compliance.

Table 4 Drugs Used to Treat Hyperlipidemia

Drug	Usual dosage	Cost[a]	Mechanism and indications	Comments and precautions
Cholestyramine (Questran or Questran light)	2 scoops bid (1 scoop = 4 g). Increase gradually	$80	Binds intestinal bile acids, indirectly depleting the liver of cholesterol with upregulation of hepatic LDL receptors. Type IIa and some IIb. Often increases VLDL production—avoid in types IV and V/I. Increased efficacy in multiple drug combinations.	Concomitant psyllium helps mitigate constipation. Can raise serum triglycerides. Slight interference with fat soluble vitamin, folic acid, and iron absorption is rarely problematic. Decreases absorption of thiazides, digoxin, coumadin, tetracycline, phenobarbital, and thyroxin.
Cholestyramine (Cholybar)	1 bar = 1 scoop or 4 grams	$139	As above. An occasionally useful alternative to powders.	Potentially convenient alternative to powder but was the least preferred form of bile acid sequestrants among children.
Cholestipol (Cholestid)	2 scoops bid (1 scoop = 5 g)	$75	As above	Unflavored. Tends to be slightly more gritty than cholestyramine but preferences vary.
Niacin (nicotinic acid, not niacinamide)	1,000 mg bid. Increase gradually	$12–18	Mainly decreases VLDL synthesis with some increase in VLDL removal rate. Decreased hepatic cholesterol synthesis may contribute to cholesterol lowering effect. Types IIb, IV, V/I, and III.	Flushing is mediated by prostaglandins and is blocked by 1 aspirin an hour before taking. Flushing decreases with time on drug. Drug-free interval renews flushing. Time-release forms (even wax matrix) may be more heptatoxic than regular crystalline niacin.
Gemfibrozil (Lopid)	600 mg bid	$53	Increases lipoprotein lipase activity with increased VLDL and chylomicron removal rates. Apo AI synthetic rates increased. Types IIb, IV, V/I, and III.	Usually well tolerated. Resolution of high triglycerides may result in increased LDL cholesterol (increased fraction of VLDL converted to LDL). Reduced CHD risk mostly in men with initially low HDL.

Lovastatin (Mevacor)	20 mg qhs–bid	$55–110	Specific inhibitor of hepatic HMG-CoA reductase. Results in upregulation of hepatic LDL receptors. Types IIa, IIb alone or in combinations. (Occasionally III, IV or V/I—usually in combination with niacin.)	Usually well tolerated. Myositis and rhabdomyolysis are rare and mainly seen with niacin or gemfibrozil and especially cyclosporin combinations. Most effective in combinations but is an effective single agent. Can increase warfarin availability by displacing warfarin from albumin.
Pravastatin (Pravachol)	20 mg qhs	$50	Mechanism and indications same as lovastatin. Possibly less risk of rhabdomyolysis when used in combination therapy.	Usually well tolerated. Active uptake into liver. Hydrophilicity theoretically results in less penetration into peripheral tissues compared to lovastatin and simvastatin. No interaction with warfarin.
Simvastatin (Zocor)	10 mg qhs	$50	See Lovastatin	Very similar to Lovastatin, but somewhat more potent.
Probucol (Lorelco)	500 mg bid	$48	Mechanism of modest cholesterol-lowering unknown. Inhibits LDL oxidation. HDL_2 markedly decreased due to increased cholesterol ester transfer activity and, in part, decreased synthesis of apo AI. Evidence for enhanced reverse cholesterol transport. Adjunct in FH to aid tendinous xanthoma regression.	Usually well tolerated. May become more widely used if future human studies confirm antiatherosclerotic effects seen in animals. Decreases in HDL cholesterol are to be expected and may be as much as 50%.

aCost for 30 days treatment at usual dose (average wholesale price from Redbook Update, Medical Economics Company, New Jersey, December 1991).

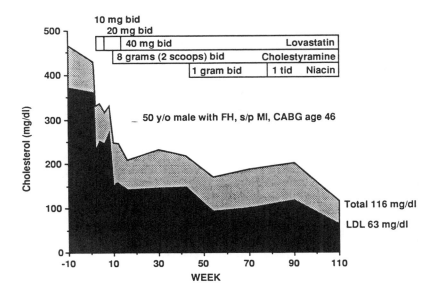

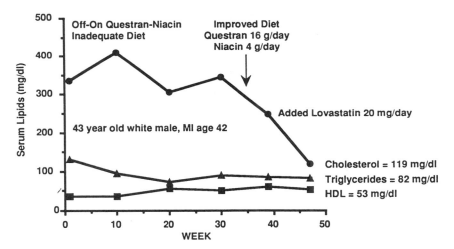

Figure 15 Pharmacologic treatment of familial hypercholesterolemia. In both these cases, niacin was reduced somewhat after the final points shown but total cholesterol has remained near 150 mg/dl in long term follow-up.

F. Familial Combined Hyperlipidemia and Mixed Hyperlipidemia

Familial combined hyperlipidemia (FCHL) is virtually impossible to diagnose without lipid values from multiple family members. Kinetic studies in individual subjects suggest excess production of VLDL apo B as the primary cause. However, the only family kinetic study showed that decreased removal rates of VLDL occurred in many family members as well as increased production (18). Given the potential mechanisms, efforts are directed first toward reducing VLDL production and second toward promoting VLDL and LDL removal. The same principles apply to most mixed lipid abnormalities.

While FCHL is often regarded as an easier condition to treat than FH, data regarding intervention in FCHL are very sparse. Guar gum significantly reduced serum cholesterol and triglycerides in FCHL patients (113) but no studies have been reported utilizing routine saturated fat and cholesterol restriction in patients with FCHL. Weight loss to near ideal and regular aerobic exercise are routinely recommended for any hyperlipidemia that includes elevated plasma triglyceride levels. Nevertheless, no data for efficacy of weight loss or exercise are available for FCHL. Weight loss, gemfibrozil, and fish oil effectively lower triglyceride levels in types IIb and IV (and V/I), but, at the same time, may result in increased serum LDL cholesterol in some individuals. This may be especially true for familial combined hyperlipidemia.

As in FH, goals of treatment of FCHL should include a reduction of LDL cholesterol to 130 mg/dl or lower for persons free of CHD and to under 100 mg/dl for those with CHD. At the same time, triglyceride levels should be maintained below 200–250 mg/dl and HDL cholesterol normalized to 35–45 mg/dl if initially low. These goals are, in some patients with FCHL, difficult to achieve without the use of drug combinations.

Niacin has been suggested as the drug of choice for patients with FCHL (and others with type IIb hyperlipidemia) (114). Unfortunately, no systematic studies of niacin in FCHL are available. Results for a single FCHL patient using niacin after failure of dietary therapy are shown in Figure 16.

Gemfibrozil (Lopid) at 600 mg twice daily may be an excellent alternative or initial choice for patients with FCHL and others with type IIb and IV or V/I who are reluctant to try niacin. One study noted a substantial reduction in plasma triglyceride levels in 9 type IIb FCHL patients treated with gemfibrozil alone (from 293 to 134 mg/dl), with a concomitant rise in HDL cholesterol from 38 to 48 mg/dl. The change in LDL cholesterol (from 229 to 221 mg/dl) was disappointing and not statistically significant, however. Only after addition of colestipol or lovastatin were there substantial reductions in LDL cholesterol in these patients (to 184 and 166 mg/dl, respectively). In eight type IV FCHL patients, comparable triglyceride and HDL changes occurred with gemfibrozil alone but LDL choles-

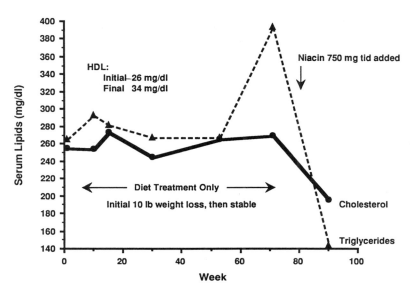

Figure 16 Treatment of 39-year-old male with hypertension and familial combined hyperlipidemia.

terol increased by 29% (from 146 mg/dl). Addition of colestipol to gemfibrozil lowered LDL cholesterol but raised triglycerides substantially in this group, while addition of lovastatin resulted in significant reduction in both triglycerides and LDL cholesterol (115). In a similar study, 13 patients with serum total cholesterol levels above 250 mg/dl and triglyceride levels above 250 mg/dl were given lovastatin, 40 mg twice daily. After 16 weeks, 9 subjects continued in the study with the addition of gemfibrozil 600 mg twice daily for another 8 weeks. Lovastatin alone resulted in 31% decrease in serum total cholesterol and a 34% drop in LDL cholesterol. A surprising finding was that triglyceride levels decreased from 485 to 336 mg/dl, a 31% decrease. HDL increased slightly but not significantly with lovastatin. Addition of gemfibrozil resulted in a marked additional decrease in triglycerides to 184 mg/dl but a small (statistically significant) 19% increase in LDL cholesterol levels (from 97 to 115 mg/dl). HDL levels increased significantly by 36% on the combination compared to placebo (116). In neither of these small studies were clinically significant adverse effects noted even with treatment using the drug combinations. Nevertheless, increased risk of myositis or rhabdomyolysis in patients using combinations of lovastatin with gemfibrozil or niacin probably preclude their routine use.

G. Type III Hyperlipidemia

Although rare in the general population (about 1:1,000–10,000, depending on the definition), type III hyperlipidemia may cause as many as 5% of early CHD cases (117). It is caused by the accumulation of abnormal VLDL and chylomicron remnant particles (collectively called β-VLDL) due to defective hepatic removal and remodeling process dependent on normal apolipoprotein E. Apo E isoforms include 2, 3, and 4. Inheriting two copies of the defective apo E2 isoform results in the propensity to type III, but another factor such as obesity or a gene causing excess production of VLDL seems to be required to result in frank type III hyperlipidemia. Definitive diagnosis requires a specialized lipid laboratory. Response to weight loss may be dramatic. In women, correcting estrogen deficiency can occasionally correct the hyperlipidemia. Response to drugs is usually marked, with 50–70% reductions in both total cholesterol and triglyceride levels when standard dosages of gemfibrozil or niacin are administered. Occasional unresponsive cases may require combined treatment with lovastatin and gemfibrozil or niacin if CHD risk is sufficiently high to warrant this aggressive treatment. Bile acid sequestrants are not used. Successful reduction of lipid levels in type III patients can result in gradual disappearance of tuberous xanthomas and improved blood flow in stenotic arteries (118).

H. Treating Severe Hypertriglyceridemia

Serum triglyceride levels above 250 mg/dl may be considered abnormal. Kinetic reasons for elevated levels include excess production of VLDL and decreased removal capacity, as in patients with homozygous or heterozygous lipoprotein lipase deficiency. In the clinical setting it is usually impossible to differentiate between these possibilities, but very low LDL cholesterol levels are a clue to diminished processing capacity for VLDL. HDL cholesterol is typically low and often will rise substantially when the triglyceride levels are reduced.

When initial serum triglyceride concentrations are in the range of 250–400 mg/dl, and sometimes for levels as high as 1,000 mg/dl, nonpharmacologic therapy may normalize levels. Weight loss and a regular, vigorous aerobic exercise program are important. In fact, weight loss may be the only effective treatment for some hypertriglyceridemic patients. Alcohol must be entirely eliminated in some individuals and low intakes should be encouraged for all patients with hypertriglyceridemia. A low-fat, high-fiber diet is helpful. Sugar must be avoided since some hypertriglyceridemic subjects experience marked increases in serum triglyceride levels on a diet rich in simple carbohydrates. Fish may be very helpful and even including modest amounts in the diet may aid in reducing serum triglycerides. For triglyceride levels under 1000 mg/dl, however, fish oil supplements are probably not warranted. Cholestyramine is avoided since it can increase

VLDL synthesis and result in markedly increased serum triglyceride values in some sensitive individuals (119). Gemfibrozil or niacin is probably warranted in patients whose triglyceride levels fail to drop below 400 mg/dl after the above measures are taken. Levels above 250 mg/dl may warrant drug therapy if accompanied by low HDL levels and/or the presence of clinical CHD.

For serum triglyceride levels higher than 1,000 mg/dl, and especially for levels above 2,000 mg/dl (the large majority of these patients will have fasting chylomicronemia and are thus type V/I), treatment is aimed at reducing the risk of pancreatitis, which is high in such individuals (120). Secondary causes of hyperlipidemia are more common with severe hypertriglyceridemia and should be carefully sought and treated vigorously. Alcohol is proscribed entirely. Fats, with the exception of fish oils, are most severely restricted to 10–15% of total calories or less. If warranted (as in a pregnant woman for whom drug therapy is contraindicated), hospitalization and elimination of dietary fat, together with oral or intravenous hydration and a modest supply of glucose, may dramatically reduce serum triglyceride levels and ward off an impending bout of acute pancreatitis.

In most patients, intervention as described above for less severe hypertriglyceridemia is usually effective. Fish oil supplements at a dosage of 3–5 capsules (1 g) 3 times daily (9–15 g oil/day), can be a remarkably effective addition to treatment of type V/I patients (121). Indeed, reductions in serum triglyceride levels of up to 81% have been reported for type V/I patients given large dosages of fish oil (122). Optimal regimens have not been defined for such patients and potentially effective combinations include an HMG-CoA reductase inhibitor with niacin or gemfibrozil, or possibly gemfibrozil with niacin. Again, benefits must be weighed carefully against risks when using lovastatin combined with gemfibrozil or niacin.

I. Isolated Low HDL Cholesterol

As shown in Figure 13, a low serum HDL level, even with normal serum LDL and triglycerides, confers a markedly increased risk of CHD. Management of low HDL remains primarily nonpharmacologic. Weight loss, vigorous regular exercise, and smoking cessation are the most effective nonpharmacologic means to raise HDL and can be recommended generally. Alcohol raises HDL in sedentary persons, but not necessarily in exercisers, and cannot be recommended for abstainers (123). Postmenopausal estrogen replacement in women will help raise HDL while androgenic steroids, often abused by athletes of either sex, can dramatically decrease HDL (124). Beyond these benign interventions, no data support attempts to raise HDL by pharmacologic means when other lipid values are normal (125). Furthermore, efforts to raise isolated low HDL cholesterol are often unsuccessful or minimally effective compared to treatment of hyperlipidemia. Nevertheless, there seems to be theoretical merit in minimizing LDL levels in patients with clinical CHD and low HDL, perhaps using an agent that can raise HDL as well, even if LDL levels are initially in the "normal" range. A clinical trial using such an approach is needed.

J. Further Clinical Considerations, Safety, Pharmacology, and Cost-Effectiveness of Lipid-Lowering Drugs and Combinations

1. Bile Acid Sequestrants

Cholestyramine or colestipol resins were traditionally considered the first-line agents for persons with hypercholesterolemia. They are safe drugs and the only agents that can currently be recommended for children and pregnant women. Clinically significant reductions in vitamin absorption are exceedingly rare (126). Nevertheless, annoying gastrointestinal side effects are common, as reported in the Lipid Research Clinic Coronary Primary Prevention Trial (see Table 5). Constipation can be severe if patients start immediately on a full dose. If one scoop is added each week up to a full dose of 2 scoops twice daily, constipation is often avoided. Higher dosages are associated with much more constipation. Psyllium (1 heaping teaspoon [about 3.5 g] 3 times daily) can reduce LDL cholesterol 9–20% as well as mitigate the constipation caused by the bile sequestrants (127,128). A handout with suggestions of different ways to use the resins (in juices, applesauce, etc.) may help improve compliance. Development of encapsulated forms of bile acid sequestrants is proceeding gradually and promises a more palatable means of administration (129,130). Bile acid sequestrants bind several other drugs in the intestine and care may be needed to adjust dosages or administration schedules

Table 5 Percent of Participants Reporting Moderate to Severe Gastrointestinal Side Effects in the First Year of Treatment in Cholestyramine (24 grams/day) and Placebo Groups of the Lipid Research Clinic Coronary Primary Prevention Trial

Side effect	Cholestyramine (N = 1,906)	Placebo (N = 1,900)	Chi-square[a]
Constipation	39	10	432
Gas	32	26	17
Belching or bloating	27	16	68
Heartburn	27	10	183
Nausea	16	8	58
Vomiting	6	5	ns
Abdominal pain	15	11	14
Diarrhea	10	11	ns
Any GI side effect	68	43	241

[a]Any chi-square value above 3.84 is statistically significant. ns = not significant.

properly. Drugs known to be bound to a clinically significant degree by the resins include digoxin (131), digitoxin (132), warfarin (133), propranolol, chlorothiazide (134), penicillin (135), tetracycline (136), phenobarbital, folic acid, iron salts, and thyroxine (137). Most lipid-lowering agents may be given together with the resins without significant effects on absorption.

Cholestyramine and colestipol effectively bind bile acid cations in exchange for chloride. Up to 10 g cholate can be bound by 24 g cholestyramine or 20 g colestipol in vitro (138). Actual binding of bile salts may be limited in vivo by free fatty acids, which also bind to these nonselective, anionic resins (139). Administration of bile acid binding resins increase fecal excretion of bile acids from about 100–500 mg/day to 1000–3000 mg/day (140). The increased excretion of bile acids depletes the hepatic pool and stimulates three compensatory mechanisms. First, the mass and total activity of the rate-limiting enzyme for bile acid synthesis, 7-α-hydroxylase, are increased in hepatocytes. Second, to compensate for increased conversion of cholesterol to bile acids, HMG-CoA reductase activity rises, accelerating de novo cholesterol synthesis of in the liver. Finally, the number of LDL receptors at the cell surface is increased, thereby promoting greater catabolism of LDL via the regulated LDL pathway. Although this mechanism has been amply demonstrated in animals, the relative contributions of the two metabolic pathways to replacing hepatic cholesterol vary widely between species. Indeed, some animals (such as rats) can compensate for cholesterol depletion entirely by increased synthesis of hepatic cholesterol without having to resort to upregulating the LDL pathway (141). Direct demonstration of the relative importance of these pathways in humans has only recently been achieved. Liver biopsies were obtained from normocholesterolemic patients with gallstones who were undergoing uncomplicated cholecystectomy. In 18 patients, cholestyramine (8 g twice daily) was given for 2–3 weeks before the surgery while 28 served as controls. Cholestyramine resulted in a 20% decrease in plasma total cholesterol. Compared to controls, cholestyramine stimulated a 6.2-fold increase in 7-α-hydroxylase activity, elevated HMG-CoA reductase activity by a factor of 5.4, and multiplied LDL receptor numbers by 2.8. Changes in these three pathways were closely correlated between individuals. An interesting finding was that compensatory mechanisms completely repleted hepatocyte cholesterol pools in these patients (142). In human kinetic studies by other investigators using radioisotopically labeled LDL, upregulation of the LDL pathway resulted in 70–100% increases in the fractional catabolic rate of LDL with no change in LDL synthesis. The increased fractional catabolic rate completely explained the reduction in LDL cholesterol (143,144). These studies illustrate the functional limitation of bile acid sequestrants in plasma LDL reduction due to the liver's substantial ability to compensate for cholesterol depletion by increased de novo cholesterol synthesis. Furthermore, the remarkable efficacy of bile acid sequestrant/HMG-CoA reductase inhibitor combinations is clearly explained by shifting the compensation for hepatic cholesterol depletion toward increased LDL degradation. Bile sequestrants (or presumably other agents that act only to increase LDL degradation via the LDL pathway) selectively deplete larger LDL, which appear to have greater affinity for LDL receptors compared to smaller LDL particles. The result is a relative enrichment of the remaining LDL particles with small, dense LDL. Since these particles are potentially more atherogenic than larger LDL, the reduction in CHD risk may be less than if the smaller LDL were removed as well (145). This effect may be exaggerated in patients who experience increases in plasma triglyceride levels associated with bile sequestrant therapy.

2. Niacin

Full-dosage (3000 mg/day in divided doses) niacin reduces serum triglyceride levels by 40–60% but has much smaller or negligible effects at dosages under 1500 mg/day. Niacin reduces LDL 15–20% when used as a single agent but is a very effective addition to various combined regimens. HDL is raised 26–31% on dosages as low as 500 mg twice daily (146,147). Low dosages may be especially advantageous in multiple drug regimens. Flushing is an expected and usually short-lived, although troublesome, side effect that wanes within a week or so of maintaining a constant dose. However, gastrointestinal (GI) and/or hepatic toxicity is a major problem limiting the usefulness of niacin for many patients. In the Coronary Drug Project, one of the most thorough evaluations of side effects ever conducted, fully 25% of the niacin group reported GI abnormalities (see Table 6). Only 12% had significant elevations of aspartate transferase (AST) (serum glutamic oxaloacetic transaminase [SGOT]). These results were obtained with regular crystalline niacin. Sustained-release forms may be more toxic. In 1 study of 71 hyperlipidemic subjects randomly assigned to receive either regular or sustained-release (Nicobid) niacin, flushing during the first month of treatment was more common with regular niacin. After 6 months, however, only 64% of a group taking a sustained-release form continued on treatment compared to over 90% taking regular niacin. Significantly more subjects taking sustained-released niacin experienced nausea (38% vs. 8%), vomiting (18% vs. 0%), diarrhea (45% vs. 22%), fatigue (24% vs. 3%), or impotence (22% vs. 3%). AST and alkaline phosphatase levels were slightly higher in the group receiving timed-release agent (148). Severe hepatic toxicity including fulminant hepatic failure with parenchymal necrosis may be seen with both forms of niacin (149) but has been reported within days of switching from crystalline to the sustained-release (not wax matrix) form (150). Even patients with no clinical or laboratory abnormalities while taking niacin apparently experience small histologic changes suggesting hepatotoxicity (151). Rechallenge with niacin has been particularly harmful in some patients after an initial untoward reaction and should probably be avoided. Nevertheless, a series of patients were presented who tolerated crystalline niacin after having experienced drug-induced hepatitis with the use of sustained-released niacin (152). Other

Table 6 Five-Year Incidence or Occurrence (%) of Adverse Effects Reported Significantly More Often for Niacin (3,000 mg daily) Compared with Placebo in The Coronary Drug Project. Data from The Coronary Drug Project Research Group, JAMA 1975; 231:360

Adverse effects	Niacin (N = 1,119)	Placebo (N = 2,789)	p value
Mortality in subgroups with:			
AV conduction defects	40.5	20.6	<0.01
Ventricular conduction defects	37.8	24.3	<0.01
Flushing	92.0	4.3	<0.00001
Pruritis	48.9	6.2	<0.00001
Urticaria	7.2	1.5	<0.0001
Excessive sweating	3.4	1.8	<0.01
Ichthyosis	3.1	0.8	<0.0001
Acanthosis nigricans	3.6	0.7	<0.0001
Hyperpigmentation	5.1	2.0	<0.0001
Other rash (by report)	19.8	5.9	<0.00001
Any skin abnormality (on exam)	26.3	15.8	<0.0001
Stomach pain	13.9	7.9	<0.0001
Nausea without vomiting	8.5	6.2	<0.01
Decreased appetite	4.1	1.5	<0.0001
Unexpected weight loss	2.7	0.9	<0.0001
Any diarrhea, nausea, vomiting, black stools, or stomach pain	21.4	14.3	<0.0001
Any GI abnormality	25.7	20.1	<0.0001
Acute gouty arthritis	6.4	4.3	<0.01
Prescription for gout medication	11.4	6.1	<0.0001
Rapid or irregular heart beat	3.7	2.6	<0.05
AST (SGOT) $\geqslant$70	11.9	8.4	<0.001
Alkaline phosphatase $\geqslant$16 (K-A units)	3.7	1.8	<0.001
Uric acid $\geqslant$10 mg/dl	13.0	4.0	<0.00001
Serum potassium <3.6 mmol/L	12.0	9.4	<0.05
Fasting glucose $\geqslant$120	23.8	15.9	<0.0001
1 hour glucose $\geqslant$240	18.9	12.9	<0.0001

important and well-recognized adverse effects from niacin include increased serum uric acid with occasional precipitation of acute gout, worsening of diabetes control, and activation of dormant peptic ulcer disease. Yet another toxic effect, although rare and reversible, is blurred vision due to cystoid macular edema (153,154). Niacin should probably not be given to patients with either atrioventricular or ventricular blocks since mortality in these subgroups was higher than with placebo in the Coronary Drug Project. Despite the apparently toxic nature of high-dosage niacin (3 g or more per day), niacin, however, remains the only lipid-lowering drug associated with long-term reduction in total mortality (155).

The mechanism of action of niacin must be considered unknown at the present time. There are conflicting theories and no convincing kinetic data. In early human kinetic studies, nicotinic acid reduced plasma LDL concentrations by reducing production rather than enhancing degradation of LDL (156). Effects on VLDL synthesis were not studied but have been assumed to be reduced by niacin. Only one kinetic study of niacin effects has been published subsequently. In a patient with type III hyperlipidemia, catabolism of VLDL and β-VLDL was accelerated after niacin therapy, suggesting possible effects on lipoprotein lipase, hepatic triglyceride lipase, or other removal mechanisms. The niacin therapy had resulted in a reduction of serum cholesterol levels from 1412 to 185 mg/dl, while triglyceride levels decreased from 2752 to 160 mg/dl in this severely affected but highly responsive type III patient. Removal mechanisms may have been saturated at such high levels. Higher apparent VLDL catabolic rates after niacin, may have been due simply to less saturated conversion of VLDL to LDL. VLDL synthetic rates were not reported (157). Niacin has been demonstrated to accelerate clearance rate of an intravenous fat load (158), but plasma lipoprotein lipase activity after heparin treatment did not change after niacin therapy (159).

Niacin effectively stimulates phosphodiesterase in adipose tissue (160), resulting in decreased cAMP levels (161) and reduced lipolysis (162). However, the antilipolytic effect of niacin lasts only 2–3 hr (about equal to niacin's plasma half-life) and is followed by a marked rebound and overshoot of plasma free fatty acid concentration (163). In fact, mean daily free fatty acid levels in patients treated with nicotinic acid were higher than before treatment despite a reduction in plasma cholesterol and triglyceride levels (164). Fatty acid flux was not measured in these studies. Other suggested mechanisms for niacin's hypolipemic activity include increased incorporation of fatty acids into adipose tissue (165) and reduction in hepatic cholesterol synthesis (166,167), possibly by inhibition of HMG-CoA reductase (168). Niacin apparently increases HDL (primarily HDL_3) by decreasing the fractional clearance of apo AI and AII (169). The reduction of LDL cholesterol with niacin was recently found to correlate strongly with elevations of serum liver enzymes, even though most of the enzyme levels remained in the normal or only slightly elevated range (170). Indeed, it is not unusual in clinical practice to observe profound reductions in serum cholesterol juxtaposed with more severe hepatic toxicity due to niacin.

3. *Gemfibrozil and Other Fibrates*

Gemfibrozil (Lopid) is one of the better tolerated lipid lowering drugs. It is almost always used at a dosage of 600 mg twice daily. It is useful in types IIb, III, IV, and

I/V, especially when HDL is low. In type V patients, triglyceride levels were reduced nearly 75% (from 1863 mg/dl) and HDL cholesterol values rose 27% while LDL cholesterol levels rose (as expected in type V patients) from 71 to 119 mg/dl (171). In normolipidemic subjects with low HDL cholesterol, gemfibrozil raised HDL only 9% while LDL cholesterol decreased slightly but nonsignificantly (172). Side effects that were reported by patients on gemfibrozil more frequently than for placebo include rash (2.1% vs. 0.8%) and gastrointestinal symptoms (1.6–6% vs. 0.6–4.8%) including nausea, vomiting, diarrhea, epigastric pain, and abdominal pain. In the Helsinki Heart Trial during the first year of treatment, 11.3% of the gemfibrozil-treated group reported moderate to severe gastrointestinal symptoms whereas 7.0% reported such symptoms in the placebo-treated group (p<0.001). Increased serum liver enzyme activities occur but are infrequent. Myositis and even rhabdomyolysis have been reported after treatment with other fibric acid derivatives, and rarely with gemfibrozil alone (173). The combination of gemfibrozil and lovastatin may cause myositis in as many as 5–8% of patients (174). The author has seen a middle-aged woman who had been treated with a combination of lovastatin and gemfibrozil and subsequently developed marked creatine phosphokinase (CPK) elevations with central muscle pain and weakness. These symptoms gradually resolved and CPK levels normalized when both lipid-lowering drugs were discontinued. When use of gemfibrozil was started several months later, however, the symptoms recurred and then resolved after use of the drug was stopped.

Gemfibrozil and other fibrates increase lipoprotein lipase activity (175). Gemfibrozil reduced plasma triglyceride levels from 379 to 185 mg/dl in 7 hypertriglyceridemic patients by reducing VLDL triglyceride production by 28% and increasing the fractional catabolic rate of VLDL triglyceride by 92% in 1 study. In the same study, clofibrate increased VLDL triglyceride fractional catabolic rate by 35% but did not affect the synthetic rate (176). Inability to inhibit VLDL triglyceride production effectively may help explain the poor response to clofibrate of some hypertriglyceridemic patients who were primarily overproducers of VLDL. In this same study, caloric restriction (to 100 kilocalories/day for 1 month) was an effective means of reducing VLDL triglyceride production in all subjects and resulted in greater reductions in plasma VLDL concentrations (177). Reduction of VLDL production by gemfibrozil may be explained by reduced peripheral lipolysis and decreased hepatic uptake of free fatty acids (178). HDL (primarily HDL_3) levels appear to be increased by gemfibrozil because of increased apo AI and AII production rather than decreased removal (179).

Newer fibrates, particularly bezafibrate (180,181), fenofibrate (182), and ciprofibrate (not yet available in the United States), appear to inhibit HMG-CoA reductase and have enhanced LDL-reducing activity by upregulating LDL receptors. Thus, bezafibrate was reported to reduce LDL cholesterol up to 35% in a small series of type IIa patients (including several with FH), while gemfibrozil was relatively ineffective in similar patients (183). Despite enhanced transport of LDL through the regulated LDL pathway, LDL cholesterol levels typically increase after treatment of patients with severe hypertriglyceridemia with fibrates because more VLDL particles escape direct catabolism before conversion to LDL (184) or because LDL catabolism via non-LDL receptor pathways is decreased (presumably due to changes in LDL composition) (185).

4. HMG-CoA Reductase Inhibitors

HMG-CoA reductase inhibitors are currently the most effective agents used singly for reducing LDL cholesterol. Lovastatin (Mevacor), pravastatin (Pravachol), and simvastatin (Zocor), are currently available in the United States. Other HMG-CoA reductase inhibitors such as fluvastatin will likely be available in the near future. The mechanism of action of these agents is relatively straightforward. HMG-CoA reductase is the rate-limiting step in cholesterol synthesis. By inhibiting this enzyme (primarily in the liver), hepatic cholesterol pools are depleted and LDL receptor expression increases (by about 180% as shown directly in patients undergoing cholecystectomy treated with pravastatin) (186). The cholesterol depletion results in marked induction of HMG-CoA reductase (increased enzyme quantities in hepatic microsomes, which remain inhibited as long as drug is present) and decreased bile saturation with cholesterol. Sudden withdrawal of lovastatin does not result in serum cholesterol overshoot, reflecting tight and rapid feedback control on cholesterol synthesis in the liver. Similar changes in human monocyte/macrophage cholesterol metabolism, including upregulation of LDL receptors, is seen with lovastatin administration (187) but not with pravastatin since it is water soluble and depends on a receptor-mediated mechanism for uptake into liver (188). Simvastatin administration resulted in upregulation of LDL receptors with increased fractional catabolic rates of LDL by 24% via the LDL receptor pathway and no change in removal rates through non-regulated pathways (189). No changes in LDL production rates were noted in this study.

All the HMG-CoA reductase inhibitors are generally very well tolerated. Reporting of side-effect profiles has been most extensive for lovastatin. Potential indications for use of HMG-CoA reductase inhibitors include heterozygous familial hypercholesterolemia, primary (polygenic) severe hypercholesterolemia, some high-risk subjects with moderate hypercholesterolemia, familial combined, or mixed hyperlipidemia, type III hyperlipidemia, diabetic dyslipidemia, hyperlipidemia of the nephrotic syndrome, and possibly isolated low HDL in patients with clinical CHD (190,191). Headache is the most commonly reported side effect of lovastatin (9.3% vs. 4.9% in placebo-treated patients in drug prescription literature). Constipation, dyspepsia, flatus, abdominal pains, and rash or pruritus occur in 4–6% of patients. These side effects were seen more often than in placebo-treated controls in drug prescription literature but not in other series. Insomnia in about 0.1% of patients taking lovastatin was also recently reported.

Concern was raised in the initial safety testing of lovastatin regarding a potential to cause cataracts. In fact, cataracts occurred in only one of the animal species tested (dogs) at enormous drug doses. Subsequent longer and more standardized follow-up in humans has failed to demonstrate any excess cataract formation beyond that expected with aging (192).

The EXCEL Study (193) was a randomized, double-blind, placebo-controlled study of 8245 patients with moderate hypercholesterolemia assigned to receive various dosages of lovastatin or placebo and evaluated for 48 weeks. Elevations of liver transaminase levels (3 times upper limit of normal) were found less frequently than in previous studies and were clearly dosage-related, with a 0.1% incidence in patients receiving 20 mg day of lovastatin, 0.9% for those taking 40 mg/day, and 1.5% for those taking 80 mg/day. Myositis, defined by muscle symptoms and CPK levels above 10 times the upper limit of normal, was rare in this study but apparently dosage related. There were no cases in those taking 20 mg/day, 1 case in over 3200 patients taking 40 mg/day (0.05%), and 4 among 1649 patients taking 80 mg/day (0.2%). Any CPK elevation (>10 times the upper limit of normal, with or without muscle symptoms) did not occur more frequently in those taking lovastatin than placebo. Prior studies, possibly using higher dosages, reported incidence rates for myalgia and/or muscle weakness with similar CPK elevations in 0.5–0.7% of subjects (194).

Rhabdomyolysis in patients taking lovastatin was originally reported to occur at high frequency in transplant patients who were concomitantly taking cyclosporin, probably due to several-fold increases in plasma lovastatin levels (195,196). These cases tended to be in patients receiving higher dosages of lovastatin. Erythromycin may also increase serum lovastatin levels, possibly by blocking liver metabolism, and lead to rhabdomyolysis (197). Nevertheless, motivated by findings in animals and humans that graft atherosclerosis is accelerated in the face of higher LDL levels, a Boston group safely maintained 11 cardiac transplant patients on lovastatin at dosages ≤60 mg/day for 1 year (198). They pointed out that several of the transplant patients in previous reports had been treated concomitantly with other drugs that can affect liver metabolism including gemfibrozil, niacin, erythromycin, and cimetidine. Furthermore, cyclosporin in combination with gemfibrozil or erythromycin had been noted to cause rhabdomyolysis in transplant patients. In a compiled series, 5% of 80 patients taking gemfibrozil and lovastatin developed myopathy—a rate at least 10 times higher than for patients taking lovastatin alone (199). Thus, despite the remarkable efficacy of lovastatin combinations, great caution must be exercised and benefits weighed against potentially serious adverse effects.

The water soluble agent pravastatin may theoretically be less likely to cause certain adverse effects compared to lovastatin or simvastatin, which are more lipid soluble. Rhabdomyolysis and myopathy have been less frequently reported among users of pravastatin in both controlled trials and usage surveillance when compared with lovastatin. Whether patient selection, concomitant drug therapy, or other factors may have accounted for part of this difference will need to be demonstrated in controlled clinical trials. Pravastatin is less protein bound than lovastatin and does not alter bleeding time or drug levels in patients taking warfarin. Lovastatin may result in prolonged bleeding time when added to a previously stable warfarin regimen and careful monitoring is necessary. As with other agents in this class, adverse clinical events occurred infrequently in pravastatin users compared with controls. Rash (4.0 vs. 1.1%) and influenza (2.4 vs. 0.7%) occurred significantly more frequently in the pravastatin group when all events were considered. When events attributed to the study drug were tabulated, only headache was seen more frequently in the pravastatin group (1.7%) compared to controls (0.2%). Increases in liver enzymes AST and ALT to 3 times the upper limit of normal were reported in 1.3% of patients on pravastatin in controlled trials. Pravastatin-induced hepatitis has been rarely reported. Nevertheless, addition of pravastatin to niacin did not result in an increase in the frequency of transaminase elevations in one small series. It is difficult to compare the incidence of these infrequent side effects in lovastatin and pravastatin studies because of differences in patient populations, control groups, and reporting methods. All the drugs in this class are generally well tolerated.

5. *Cost Effectiveness of Lipid-Lowering Agents*

Costs of the lipid lowering drugs in current use are provided in Table 4. From these costs and data from Table 1, a simple cost-effectiveness ratio can be determined for several drugs or combinations. Thus, (cost of drug per year)/(events prevented per year per 1000 persons treated/1000) gives the drug cost per event prevented. For cholestyramine, as reported for the most compliant group of the LRC trial, the cost per MI or CHD death prevented was $270,968 (assuming 20 g/day cholestyramine). For the most effective regimens in the highest-risk population (the FATS trial), costs were $14,944 and $31,938 per event prevented using colestipol combined with niacin or lovastatin, respectively. Thus, cost-effectiveness ratios can vary 20-fold simply due to differences in the background risk of patients being considered and the effectiveness of various drug regimens in preventing clinical endpoints. The cost of drug is actually only a portion (although a substantial one) of the total costs of hyperlipidemia treatment. More detailed cost effectiveness studies have been performed that include most other costs such as physician and dietitian visits for follow-up (200). In these analyses, the cost of treating hyperlipidemia with cholestyramine or lovastatin alone per additional year of life expectancy varied from $11,000 in a 40-year-old man with serum cholesterol over 300 mg/dl and at high risk (heavy smoker with hypertension and low HDL cholesterol) to about $1,400,000 in a 20-year-old man with total serum cholesterol level of 240 mg/dl at otherwise low risk of CHD. This analysis was based on risk data from the Framingham study and NCEP guidelines for follow-up. More extensive analyses will need to be performed using data from intervention trials before such data can be directly applied to the clinical setting. However, in terms of cost-effectiveness, middle-aged men at high risk for CHD who also have elevated serum cholesterol levels clearly stand to benefit most from lipid-lowering interventions.

Those for whom lipid-lowering intervention is most cost effective are persons with a history of clinical coronary artery disease. In a recent analysis, treatment with 20 mg/pr day of lovastatin of men aged 35–54 with a history of MI having cholesterol levels 250 mg/dl and above resulted in an actual dollar savings. That is, considering the costs of treating further acute events and the costs of treating serum lipid levels, the cost per year of life saved by treating lipids was actually negative (201). Treatment of other relatively high-risk groups who did not yet have cardiovascular disease (middle-aged men with moderate hypercholesterolemia) was also highly cost effective. These results are consistent with a recent meta-analysis of longitudinal studies that showed continued, strong prediction of subsequent acute events by lipid risk factors in patients after documented myocardial infarction (202). In the Lipid Research Clinics Follow-up Study among men with cardiovascular disease at baseline, 10 year mortality from cardiovascular disease was 5.9 times greater in men with LDL cholesterol levels above 160 mg/dl (4.13 mmol/L) compared to men with LDL below 130 mg/dl (3.35 mmol/L). HDL levels also continued to be highly predictive (relative risk 6.0 for men with HDL below 35 mg/dl vs. above 45 mg/dl) (203). Such analyses should be particularly motivating for cardiologists who see patients with coronary disease. Yet among patients with angiographically proven coronary artery disease and hypercholesterolemia studied between 1988 and 1989, only 35% or fewer were receiving either diet or drug therapy to lower their serum cholesterol levels (204). We hope that through further education or increased availability of specialized lipid treatment centers, this unfortunate undertreatment of patients who might benefit most will be corrected.

REFERENCES

1. Schucker B, Wittes JT, Cutler JA, et al. Change in physician perspective on cholesterol and heart disease. Results from two national surveys. JAMA 1987; 258:3521–6.

2. Clarke CB. Physician attitudes toward elevated lipid levels: an international perspective. In: Grundy SM, Bearn AG, eds. The role of cholesterol in atherosclerosis: new therapeutic opportunities. Philadelphia: Hanley & Belfus, 1988: 213–32.

3. Hopkins PN. Unpublished observations.

4. Nash DT. Hypercholesterolemia during hospitalization. The case for closer surveillance. Postgrad Med 1986; 79:303–10.

5. Landzberg JS, Heim CR. Physician recognition and treatment of hypercholesterolemia. Arch Intern Med 1989; 149:933–5.

6. Amsterdam EA, Walker N, Arons D, Baker L. Disparity in physician approach to hyperlipidemia and hypercholesterolemia. Arteriosclerosis 1990; 10:836a.

7. Steinberg D. The cholesterol controversy is over. Why did it take so long? Circulation 1989; 80:1070–8.

8. Moore TJ. The cholesterol myth. Atlantic Monthly, September 1989:37–70.

9. Leaf A. Management of hypercholesterolemia. Are preventive interventions advisable? N Engl J Med 1989; 321:680–4.

10. Fries JF, Green LW, Levine S. Health promotion and the compression of morbidity. Lancet 1989; 1:481–3.

11. Weinstein ND. Reducing unrealistic optimism about illness susceptibility. Health Psychol 1983; 2:11–20.

12. Weinstein ND. Why it won't happen to me: perception of risk factors and susceptibility. Health Psychol 1984; 3:431–57.

13. Pierce DK, Connor SL, Sexton G, Calvin L, Connor WE, Matarazzo JD. Knowledge of and attitudes toward coronary heart disease and nutrition in Oregon families. Prev Med 1984; 13:390–5.

14. Snyder DR, Ingram RE. Company motivates and miserable: the impact of consensus information on help seeking for psychological problems. J Pers Soc Psychol 1983; 45:1118–27.

15. Taylor WC, Pass TM, Shepard DS, Komaroff AL. Cholesterol reduction and life expectancy. A model incorporating multiple risk factors. Ann Intern Med 1987; 106:605–14.

16. Hill AB. Principles of medical statistics, 9th ed. New York: Oxford University Press, 1971:309–23.

17. Spitzer WO. The scientific admissibility of evidence on the effectiveness of preventive interventions. In: Goldbloom RB, Lawrence RS, eds. Preventing disease. Beyond the rhetoric. New York: Springer-Verlag, 1990:1–4.

18. Hopkins PN, Williams RR. Human genetics and coronary heart disease: a public health perspective. Annu Rev Nutr 1989; 9:303–45.

19. Clarkson TB, Prichard RW, Bullock BC, et al. Pathogenesis of atherosclerosis: some advances from using animal models. Exp Mol Pathol 1976; 24:264–86.

20. Constantinides P. Experimental atherosclerosis. New York: Elsevier, 1965.

21. Leary T. The genesis of atherosclerosis. Arch Pathol Lab Med 1941; 32:507–55.

22. Kritchevsky D, Davidson LM, Shapiro IL, et al. Lipid metabolism and experimental atherosclerosis in baboons: influence of cholesterol-free, semisynthetic diets. Am J Clin Nutr 1974; 27:29–50.

23. Ross AC, Minick CR, Zilversmit DB. Equal atherosclerosis in rabbits fed cholesterol-free, low fat diet or cholesterol-supplemented diet. Atherosclerosis 1978; 29:301–15.

24. Wissler R, Vesselinovitch D. The effects of feeding various dietary fats on the development and regression of hypercholesterolemia and atherosclerosis. Adv Exp Med Biol 1975; 60:65–76.

25. Minick CR. Immunologic arterial injury in atherogenesis. Ann NY Acad Sci 1976; 275:210–27.

26. Prescott MF, McBride CH, Cooley J, Hasler-Rapacz J, Attie A, Rapacz J. Develop

ment of complex atherosclerotic plaques in pigs bearing mutant alleles for apo-lipoprotein B. Circulation 1989; 80(Suppl II):II–64.

27. Wissler RW. Current status of regression studies. Atherosclerosis Rev 1978; 3:213–29.
28. St. Clair RN. Atherosclerosis regression in animal models: current concepts of cellular and biochemical mechanisms. Prog Cardiovasc Dis 1983; 26:109–32.
29. Kim DN, Schmee J, Ho H-T, Thomas WA. The "turning off" of excessive cell replicative activity in advanced atherosclerotic lesions of swine by a regression diet. Atherosclerosis 1988; 71:131–42.
30. Working Group on Arteriosclerosis of the National Heart, Lung, and Blood Institute. Prevention. Report of the Working Group on Arteriosclerosis of the National Heart, Lung, and Blood Institute, Vol 2. Bethesda, MD: US Department of Health and Human Services, Public Health Service, National Institutes of Health, NIH Publication No 81-2035, September 1981; 261–422.
31. Hopkins PN, Williams RR. Identification and relative weight of cardiovascular risk factors. Clin Cardiol 1986; 4:3–31.
32. Welch CC, Proudfit WL, Sheldon WC. Coronary arteriographic findings in 1,000 women under age 50. Am J Cardiol 1975; 35:211–5.
33. Cohn PF, Gabbay SI, Weglicki WB. Serum lipid levels in angiographically defined coronary artery disease. Ann Intern Med 1976; 84:241–5.
34. Welch CC, Proudfit WL, Sones FM, et al. Cinecoronary arteriography in young men. Circulation 1970; 42:647–52.
35. Gordon T, Garcia-Pamieri MR, Kagan A, et al. Differences in coronary heart disease in Framingham, Honolulu and Puerto Rico. J Chron Dis 1974; 27:329–44.
36. Williams RR, Hasstedt SJ, Wilson DE, Ash KO, Yanowitz FF, Reiber GE, Kuida H. Evidence that men with familial hypercholesterolemia can avoid early coronary death. An analysis of 77 gene carriers in four Utah pedigrees. JAMA 1986; 255:219–224.
37. Schettler G, Nussel E, Buchholz L. Epidemiological research in Western Europe. Atherosclerosis Rev 1978; 3:201–11.
38. Nicholson J, Gartside PS, Siegel M, Spencer W, Steiner PM, Glueck CJ. Lipid and lipoprotein distributions in octo- and nona-genarians. Metabolism 1979; 28:51–60.
39. Postiglione A, Corese C, Fischetti A, et al. Plasma lipids and geriatric assessment in a very aged population in South Italy. Atherosclerosis 1989; 80:63–8.
40. Stokes J. Dyslipidemia as a risk factor cardiovascular disease and untimely death: the Framingham Study. Atherosclerosis Rev 1988; 18:49–57.
41. Butler WJ, Ostrander LD, Carman WJ, et al. Mortality from coronary heart disease in the Tecumseh Study. Long-term effect of diabetes mellitus, glucose tolerance and other risk factors. Am J Epidemiol 1985; 121:541–7.
42. Stamler J, Wentworth D, Neaton JD, for the MRFIT Cooperative Research Group. Is the relationship between serum cholesterol and risk of death from coronary heart disease continuous and graded? Findings on the 356,222 primary screenees of the Multiple Risk Factor Intervention Trial (MRFIT). JAMA 1986; 256:2823–8.
43. Gordon T, Castelli WP, Hjortland MC, Kannel WB, Dawber TR. Predicting coronary heart disease in middle-aged and older persons. The Framingham Study. JAMA 1977; 238:497–9.

44. Benfante R, Reed D. Is elevated serum cholesterol level a risk factor for coronary heart disease in the elderly? JAMA 1990; 263:393–6.

45. Zimetbaum P, Frishman W, Ooi WL, Derman M, Aronson M, Eder H. Relationship between plasma lipids and the incidence of cardiovascular events in the old old: The Bronx Longitudinal Aging Study (Abstract).

46. Blankenhorn DH, Aoaupovic P, Wickham E, Chin HP, Azen SP. Prediction of angiographic change in native human coronary arteries and aortocoronary bypass grafts. Lipid and nonlipid factors. Circulation 1990; 81:470–6.

47. Campeau L, Enjalbert M, Lesperance J, et al. The relation of risk factors to the development of atherosclerosis in saphenous-vein bypass grafts and the progression of disease in the native circulation. A study 10 years after aortocoronary bypass surgery. N Engl J Med 1984; 311:1329–32.

48. Anderson KM, Castelli WP, Levy D. Cholesterol and mortality. 30 years of follow-up from the Framingham Study. JAMA 1987; 257:2176–80.

49. Williams RR, Sorlie PD, Feinleib M, et al. Cancer incidence by levels of cholesterol. JAMA 1981; 245:247–52.

50. International Collaborative Group. Circulating cholesterol level and risk of death from cancer in men aged 40 to 69 years: experience of an international collaborative group. JAMA 1982; 248:2853–9.

51. Sherwin RW, Wentworth DN, Cutler JA, et al. Serum cholesterol and the risk from cancer in men. JAMA 1987; 257:943–8.

52. Schatzkin A, Hoover RN, Taylor PR, et al. Serum cholesterol and cancer in the NHANES I Epidemiologic Follow-up Study. Lancet 1987; 2:298–302.

53. Cowan LD, O'Connell DL, Criqui MH, Barrett-Connor E, Bush TL, Wallace RB. Cancer mortality and lipid and lipoprotein levels. The Lipid Research Clinics Program Mortality Follow-up Study. Am J Epidemiol 1990; 131:468–82.

54. Winawer SJ, Flehinger BJ, Buchalter J, Herbert E, Shike M. Declining serum cholesterol levels prior to diagnosis of colon cancer. A time-trend, case-control study. JAMA 1990; 263:2083–5.

55. Isles CG, Hole DJ, Gillis CR, Hawthrone VM, Lever AF. Plasma cholesterol, coronary heart disease, and cancer in the Rengrew and Paisley survey. Br Med J 1989; 298:920–4.

56. Forette B, Tortrat D, Wolmark Y. Cholesterol as risk factor for mortality in elderly women. Lancet 1989; 1:868–70.

57. Henriksson P, Eriksson M, Ericsson S, et al. Hypocholesterolaemia and increased elimination of low-density lipoproteins in metastatic cancer of the prostrate. Lancet 1989; 2:1178–80.

58. Anonymous. Severe acquired hypocholesterolemia: two case reports. Nutr Rev 1989; 47:202–7.

59. Heiss G, Johnson NJ, Reiland S, Davis CE, Tyroler HA. The epidemiology of plasma high-density lipoprotein cholesterol levels. The Lipid Research Clinics Program Prevalence Study Summary. Circulation 1980; 62(suppl IV):IV-116–36.

60. Gordon DJ, Rifkind BM. High-density lipoprotein—the clinical implications of recent studies. N Engl J Med 1989; 321:1311–6.

61. Castelli WP. Epidemiology of coronary heart disease: the Framingham Study. Am J Med 1984; 76(suppl 2A):4–12.

62. Castelli WP, Wilson PWF, Levy D, Anderson K. Serum lipids and risk of coronary artery disease. Atherosclerosis Rev 1990; 21:7–19.

63. Superko HR, Bachorik PS, Wood PD, High-density lipoprotein cholesterol measurements. A help or hindrance in practical clinical medicine. JAMA 1986; 256:2714–7.

64. Grundy SM, Goodman DWS, Rifkind BM, Cleeman JI. The place of HDL in cholesterol management. A perspective from the National Cholesterol Education Program. Arch Intern Med 1989; 149:505–10.

65. Miller GJ, Miller NE. Dietary fat, HDL cholesterol, and coronary disease: one interpretation (letter). Lancet 1982; 1270–1.

66. Austin MA. Plasma triglyceride as a risk factor for coronary heart disease. The epidemiologic evidence and beyond. Am J Epidemiol 1989; 129:249–59.

67. Castelli WP. The triglyceride issue: a view from Framingham. Am Heart J 1986; 112: 432–7.

68. Wilson PWF, Anderson KM. Isolated hypoalphalipoproteinemia and premature heart disease: the Framingham offspring. Arteriosclerosis 1989; 9:708a.

69. Williams RR, Hopkins PN, Hunt SC, et al. Population-based frequency of dyslipidemia syndromes in coronary-prone families in Utah. Arch Intern Med 1990; 150: 582–8.

70. Brunzell JD, Schrott HG, Motulsky AG, et al. Myocardial infarction in the familial forms of hypertriglyceridemia. Metabolism 1976; 25:313–20.

71. Vega GL, Beltz WF, Grundy SM. Low density lipoprotein metabolism in hypertriglyceridemic and normolipidemic patients with coronary heart disease. J Lipid Res 1985; 26:115–26.

72. Schwenke DC, Carew TE. Initiation of atherosclerotic lesions in cholesterol-fed rabbits. II. Selective retention of LDL vs. selective increases in LDL permeability in susceptible sites of arteries. Arteriosclerosis 1989; 9:908–18.

73. Florentin RA, Nam KT, Thomas WA. Increased 3.H-thymidine incorporation into endothelial cells of swine fed cholesterol for 3 days. Exp Mol Pathol 1969; 10:250–5.

74. Steinberg D, Parthasarathy S, Carew TE, Khoo JC, Witztum JL. Beyond cholesterol. Modifications of low density lipoprotein that increase its atherogenicity. N Engl J Med 1989; 320:915–24.

75. Berliner JA, Territo M, Almada L, Carter A, Shafonskyh E, Fogelman AM. Monocyte chemotactic factor produced by large vessel endothelial cells in vitro. Arteriosclerosis 1986; 6:254–8.

76. Goldstein JL, Brown MS. Lipoprotein metabolism in the macrophage: implications for cholesterol deposition in atherosclerosis. Annu Rev Biochem 1983; 52:223–61.

77. Ross R. The pathogenesis of atherosclerosis—an update. N Engl J Med 1986; 314: 488–500.

78. Small DM. Progression and regression of atherosclerotic lesions. Insights from lipid physical biochemistry. Arteriosclerosis 1988; 8:103–29.

79. Smith EB, Slater RS. Relationship between low density lipoprotein in aortic intima and serum lipid levels. Lancet 1972; 1:463–9.

80. Niehaus CE, Nicoll A, Wootton R, et al. Influence of lipid concentrations and age on transfer of plasma lipoprotein into human arterial intima. Lancet 1977; 2:469–71.
81. Carvalho ACA, Colman RW, Lees RS. Platelet function in hyperlipoproteinemia. N Engl J Med 1974; 290:434–8.
82. Hassall DG, Forrest LA, Bruckdorfer R, et al. Influence of plasma lipoproteins on platelet aggregation in a normal male population. Arteriosclerosis 1983; 3:332–8.
83. Davi G, Averna M, Novo S, et al. Effects of synvinolin on platelet aggregation and thromboxane B2 synthesis in type IIa hypercholesterolemic patients. Atherosclerosis 1989; 79:79–83.
84. Simpson HCR, Mann JI, Meade TW, Chakrabarti R, Stirling Y, Woolf L. Hypertriglyceridemia and hypercoagulability. Lancet 1983; 1:786–90.
85. Hamsten A, Wiman B, de Faire U, Blomback M. Increased plasma levels of a rapid inhibitor of tissue plasminogen activator in young survivors of myocardial infarction. N Engl J Med 1985; 313:1557–63.
86. Crutchley DJ, McPhee, Terris MF, Canossa-Terris MA. Levels of three hemostatic factors in relation to serum lipids. Monocyte procoagulant activity, tissue plasminogen activator, and type-1 plasminogen activator inhibitor. Arteriosclerosis 1989; 9;934–9.
87. Sundell IB, Nilsson TK, Hallmans G, Hellsten G, Dahlen GH. Interrelationships between plasma levels of plasminogen activator inhibitor, tissue plasminogen activator, lipoprotein(a), and established cardiovascular risk factors in a North Swedish population. Atherosclerosis 1989; 80:9–16.
88. Elkeles RS, Chakrabarti R, Vickers M, Stirling Y, Meade TW. Effect of treatment of hyperlipidaemia on haemostatic variables. Br Med J 1980; 281:973–4.
89. Khanna PK, Seth HN, Balasubramanian V, Hoon RS. Effect of submaximal exercise on fibrinolytic activity in ischaemic heart disease. Br Heart J 1975; 37:1273–6.
90. Niort G, Bulgarelli A, Cassader M, Pagano G. Effect of short-term treatment with bezafibrate on plasma fibrinogen, fibrinopeptide A, platelet activation and blood filterability in atherosclerotic hyperfibrinogenemic patients. Atherosclerosis 1988; 71:113–9.
91. Tall AR. Plasma high density lipoproteins. Metabolism and relationship to atherogenesis. J Clin Invest 1990; 86:379–84.
92. Hjermann I, VelveByre K, Holme I, Leren P. Effect of diet and smoking intervention on the incidence of coronary heart disease. Report from the Oslo Study Group of a randomized trial in healthy men. Lancet 1981; 2:1304–10.
93. Holme I, Hjermann I, Helgeland A, Leren P. The Oslo Study: diet and antismoking advice. Additional results from a 5-year primary preventive trial in middle-aged men. Prev Med 1985; 14:279–92.
94. Ornish D, Brown SE, Scherwitz LW, et al. Can lifestyle changes reverse coronary heart disease? The Lifestyle Heart Trial. Lancet 1990; 336:129–33.
95. Manninen V, Elo MO, Frick MH, et al. Lipid alterations and decline in the incidence of coronary heart disease in the Helsinki Heart Study. JAMA 1988; 260:641–51.
96. Manninen V, Koskinen P, Manttari M, Huttunen JK, Canter D, Frick HM. Predictive value for coronary heart disease of baseline high-density and low-density

lipoprotein cholesterol among Fredrickson type IIa subjects in the Helsinki Heart Study. Am J Cardiol 1990; 66:24–7A.

97. Kane JP, Malloy MJ, Ports TA, Phillips NR, Diehl JC, Havel RJ. Regression of coronary atherosclerosis during treatment of familial hypercholesterolemia with combined drug regimens. JAMA 1990; 264:3007–12.

98. Wysowski DK, Gross TP. Deaths due to accidents and violence in two recent trials of cholesterol-lowering drugs. Arch Intern Med 1990; 150:2169–72.

99. The Expert Panel. Report of the National Cholesterol Education Program Expert Panel on detection, evaluation, and treatment of high blood cholesterol in adults. Arch Intern Med 1988; 148:36–69.

100. Wilson PWF, Christiansen JC, Anderson KM, Kannel WB. Impact of national guidelines for cholesterol risk factor screening. The Framingham offspring study. JAMA 1989; 262:41–4.

101. Sempos C, Fulwood R, Haines C, et al. The prevalence of high blood cholesterol levels among adults in the United States. JAMA 1989; 262:45–52.

102. Wilson PWF, Anderson KM. Isolated hypoalphalipoproteinemia and premature heart disease: the Framingham offspring study (abstract). Arteriosclerosis 1989; 9:708a.

103. Wallace RB, Pomrehn P, Heiss G, Chambless LE, Johnson N, Patten R, Lippel K, Rifkind BM. Alterations in clinical chemistry levels associated with the dyslipoproteinemias. The Lipid Research Clinics Program Prevalence Study. Circulation 1986; 73(suppl I):I-62–I-69.

104. Kesaniemi YA, Grundy SM. Significance of low density lipoprotein production in the regulation of plasma cholesterol level in man. J Clin Invest 1982; 70:13–22.

105. Turner PR, Konarska R, Revill J, et al. Metabolic study of variation in plasma cholesterol level in normal men. Lancet 1984; 2:663–5.

106. Grundy SM, Vega GL, Bilheimer DW. Kinetic mechanisms determining variability in low density lipoprotein levels and rise with age. Arteriosclerosis 1985; 5:623–30.

107. McMurry MP, Hopkins PN, Gould R, et al. Family-oriented nutrition intervention for a lipid clinic population. J Am Diet Assoc 1991; 91:57–65.

108. Illingworth DR, Bacon S. Treatment of heterozygous familial hypercholesterolemia with lipid-lowering drugs. Arteriosclerosis 1989; 9(suppl I):I-121–34.

109. Yamamoto A, Hara, H, Takaichi S, Wakasugi J-I, Tomikawa M. Effect of probucol on macrophages, leading to regression of xanthomas and atheromatous vascular lesions. Am J Cardiol 1988; 62:31–6B.

110. Glueck CJ, Tsang RC, Mellies MJ. Long-term (2 to 6 year) therapy of familial hypercholesterolemia and hypertriglyceridemia in childhood. In: Lauer RM, Shekelle RB, eds. Childhood prevention of atherosclerosis and hypertension. New York: Raven Press, 1980:155–66.

111. Glueck CJ, Mellies, MJ, Dine M, Perry T, Laskarzewski P. Safety and efficacy of long-term diet and diet plus bile acid-binding resin cholesterol-lowering therapy in 73 children heterozygous for familial hypercholesterolemia. Pediatrics 1986; 78: 338–48.

112. Stein EA. Treatment of familial hypercholesterolemia with drugs in children. Arteriosclerosis 1989; 9(suppl I):I-145–51.

113. Bosello O, Cominacini L, Zocca I, et al. Effects of guar gum on plasma lipoproteins

and apolipoproteins C-II and C-III in patients affected by familial combined hyperlipoproteinemia. Am J Clin Nutr 1984; 40:1165–74.

114. Grundy SM, Chait A, Brunzell JD. Familial combined hyperlipidemia workshop. Arteriosclerosis 1987; 7:203–7.

115. East C, Bilheimer DW, Grundy SM. Combination drug therapy for familial combined hyperlipidemia. Ann Intern Med 1988; 109:25–32.

116. Vega GL, Grundy SM. Management of primary mixed hyperlipidemia with lovastatin. Arch Intern Med 1990; 150:1313–9.

117. Williams RR, Hopkins PN, Hunt SC, et al. Population-based frequency of dyslipidemia syndromes in coronary-prone families in Utah. Arch Intern Med 1990; 150: 582–8.

118. Mahley RW, Rall SC. Type III hyperlipoproteinemia (dysbetalipoproteinemia): the role of apolipoprotein E in normal and abnormal lipoprotein metabolism. In: Scriver CR, Beaudet AL, Sly WS, Valle D, eds. The metabolic basis of inherited disease. New York: McGraw-Hill, 1989:1195–213.

119. Beil U, Krouse JR, Enarsson K, Grundy SM. Effects on interruption of the enterohepatic circulation of bile acids on the transport of very low density lipoprotein triglycerides. Metabolism 1982; 31:438–44.

120. Brunzell JD. Familial lipoprotein lipase deficiency and other causes of the chylomicronemia syndrome. In: Scriver CR, Beaudet AL, Sly WS, Valle D, eds. The metabolic basis of inherited disease, 6th ed. New York: McGraw-Hill, 1989; 1165–80.

121. Harris WS, Rothrock DW, Fanning et al. Fish oils in hypertriglyceridemia: a dose–response study. Am J Clin Nutr 1990; 51:399–406.

122. Phillipson BE, Rothrock DN, Connor WE, Harris WS, Illingworth DR. Reduction of plasma lipids, lipoproteins and apoproteins by dietary fish oils in patients with hypertriglyceridemia. N Engl J Med 1985; 312:1210–6.

123. Wilson PWF. High-density lipoprotein, low-density lipoprotein and coronary artery disease. Am J Cardiol 1990 66:7A–10A.

124. Riccardi G. Hormones, diabetes mellitus and lipoprotein metabolism. Cur Opin Lipidol 1990; 1:237–43.

125. Grundy SM, Goodman DWS, Rifkind BM, Cleeman JI. The place of HDL in cholesterol management. A perspective from the National Cholesterol Education Program. Arch Intern Med 1989; 149:505–10.

126. Glueck CJ. Therapy of familial and acquired hyperlipoproteinemia in children and adolescents. Prev Med 1983; 12:835–47.

127. Anderson JW, Zettwoch N, Feldman T, Tietyen-Clark J, Oeltgen P, Bishop CW. Cholesterol-lowering effects of psyllium hydrophilic mucilloid for hypercholesterolemic men. Arch Intern Med 1988; 148:292–6.

128. Levin EG, Miller VT, Muesing RA, Stoy DB, Balm TK, LaRosa JC. Comparison of psyllium hydrophilic mucilloid and cellulose as adjuncts to a prudent diet in the treatment of mild to moderate hypercholesterolemia. Arch Intern Med 1990; 150: 1822–7.

129. Zavoral JH, Kwiterovich PO, Marquis NR, Hutton GD, Kafonek SD. Comparative efficacy of cholestyramine tablets and powder. Arteriosclerosis 1990; 10:801a.

130. Superko HR, Haskell WL, Cianciola C. LDLC reduction, colestipol granules versus new tablet. Arteriosclerosis 1989; 9:766a.

131. Hall WH, Shappell SD, Doherty JE. Effect of cholestyramine on digoxin absorption and excretion in man. Am J Cardiol 1977; 39;213–6.

132. Caldwell JH, Bush CA, Greenberg NJ. Interruption of the enterohepatic circulation of digitoxin by cholestyramine. II. Effect on metabolic disposition of tritium-labeled digitoxin and cardiac systolic intervals in man. J Clin Invest 1971; 50:2638–44.

133. Hanigan JJ. Colestid-warfarin drug interaction study: a comparison of plasma warfarin concentrations following oral administration of 10 mg of sodium warfarin both with and without an anionic exchange resin (colestipol HCL or choles-tyramine). The Upjohn Co., Domestic Pharmaceutical Medical Affairs, Colestid Study, Clinical Services No. 032. 1975.

134. Kauffman RE, Azarnoff DL. Effect of colestipol on gastrointestinal absorption of chlorothizid in man. Clin Pharmacol Ther 1973; 14:886–90.

135. Brown RD. The effect of Colestid and Questran on penicillin G serum levels after concomitant administration of Colestid (colestipol hydrochloride, Upjohn) and Pentids (penicillin G potassium tablets, Squibb) or Questran (cholestyramine, Mead Johnson) and Pentids. The Upjohn Co., Domestic Pharmaceutical Medical Affairs, Colestid Study, Clinical Services No. 033. 1977.

136. Brown RK. The effect of concomitant administration of colestipol hydrochloride or cholestyramine and tetracycline hydrochloride on the bioavailability of orally administered tetracycline hydrochloride. The Upjohn Co., Domestic Pharmaceutical Medical Affairs, Colestid Study, Clinical Services No. 031. 1975.

137. Northcutt RC, Stiel JN, Hollifield JW, et al. The influence of cholestyramine on thyroxine absorption. JAMA 1969; 208:1857–61.

138. Johns WH, Bates TR. J Pharm Sci 1969; 58:179–83.

139. Johns WH, Bates TR. J Pharm Sci 1970; 59:329–33.

140. Grundy SM. Arch Intern Med 1972; 130:638–48.

141. Spady DK, Turley SD, Dietschy JM. Rates of low density lipoprotein uptake and cholesterol synthesis are regulated independently in the liver. J Lipid Res 1985; 26:465–72.

142. Reihner E, Angelin B, Rudling M, Ewerth S, Bjorkhem I, Einarsson K. Regulation of hepatic cholesterol metabolism in humans: stimulatory effects of cholestyramine on HMG-CoA reductase activity and low density lipoprotein receptor expression in gallstone patients. J Lipid Res 1990; 31:2219–26.

143. Shepherd J, Packard CJ, Bicker S, Lawrie TDV, Morgan HG. Cholestyramine promotes receptor-mediated low-density-lipoprotein catabolism. N Engl J Med 1980; 302:1219–22.

144. Thompson GR, Soutar AK, Spengel FA, Jadhav A, Gavigan SJ, Myant NB. Defects of receptor-mediated low density lipoprotein catabolism in homozygous familial hypercholesterolemia and hypothyroidism in vivo. Proc Natl Acad Sci USA 1981; 78:2591–5.

145. Young SG, Witztum JL, Carew TE, Krauss RW, Lindgren FT. Colestipol-induced changes in LDL composition and metabolism. II. Studies in humans. J Lipid Res 1989; 30:225–38.

146. Alderman JD, Pasternack RC, Sacks FM, Smith HS, Monrad ES, Grossman W. Effect of a modified, well-tolerated niacin regimen on serum total cholesterol, high density lipoprotein cholesterol and the cholesterol to high density lipoprotein ratio. Am J Cardiol 1989; 64:725–9.

147. Luria MH. Effect of low-dose niacin on high-density lipoprotein cholesterol and total cholesterol/high density lipoprotein cholesterol ratio. Arch Intern Med 1988; 148:2493–5.

148. Knopp RH, Ginsberg J, Albers JJ, et al. Contrasting effects of unmodified and time-release forms of niacin on lipoproteins in hyperlipidemic subjects: clues to mechanism of action of niacin. Metabolism 1985; 34:642–50.

149. Clementz GL, Holmes AW. Nicotinic acid-induced fulminant hepatic failure. J Clin Gastroenterol 1987; 9:582–4.

150. Mullin GE, Greenson JK, Mitchell MC. Fulminant hepatic failure after ingestion of sustained-release nicotinic acid. Ann Intern Med 1989; 111:253–5.

151. Baggenstoss AG, Christensen NA, Berge KG, Baldus WP, Spiekerman RE, Ellefson RD. Fine structural changes in the liver in hypercholesterolemic patients receiving long-term nicotinic acid therapy. Mayo Clin Proc 1967; 42:385–99.

152. Henkin Y, Johnson KC, Segrest JP. Rechallenge with crystalline niacin after drug-induced hepatitis from sustained-release niacin. JAMA 1990; 264:241–3.

153. Gass JDM. Nicotinic acid maculopathy. Am J Ophthalmol 1973; 76:500–10.

154. Millay RH, Klein ML, Illingworth DR. Niacin maculopathy. Ophthalmology 1988; 95:930–6.

155. Canner PL, Berge KG, Wenger NK, et al. Fifteen year mortality in Coronary Drug Project patients: long-term benefit with niacin. J Am Coll Cardiol 1986; 8:1245–55.

156. Levy RI, Langer T. Hypolipidemic drugs and lipoprotein metabolism. Adv Exp Med Biol 1972; 26:155–63.

157. Kushwaha RS, Haffner SM, Foster DM, Hazzard WR. Compositional and metabolic heterogeneity of alpha 2- and beta-very-low-density lipoproteins in subjects with broad beta disease and endogenous hypertriglyceridemia. Metabolism 1985; 34:1029–38.

158. Froberg SO, Boberg J, Carlson LA, Eriksson M. Effect of nicotinic acid on the diurnal variation of plasma levels of glucose, free fatty acids, triglycerides and cholesterol and of urinary excretion of catecholamines. In: Gey KF, Carlson LA, eds. Metabolic effects of nicotinic acid and its derivatives. Bern: Hans Huber, 1971:167–81.

159. Nikkila EA. Effect of nicotinic acid on adipose tissue lipoprotein lipase and removal rate of plasma triglycerides. In: Gey KF, Carlson LA, eds. Metabolic effects of nicotinic acid and its derivatives. Bern: Hans Huber, 1971:487–95.

160. Krishna G, Weiss B, Davies JI, et al. Mechanism of nicotinic acid inhibition of hormone-induced lipolysis. Fed Proc 1966; 25:719.

161. Butcher RS, Baird CE, Sutherland EW. Effects of lipolytic and antilipolytic substances on adenosine 3′, 5′-monophosphate levels in isolated fat cells. J Biol Chem 1968; 243:1705–12.

162. Carlson LA, Oro L, Ostman J. Effect of nicotinic acid on plasma lipids in patients with hyperlipoproteinemia during the first week of treatment. J Atherosclerosis Res 1968; 18:667–77.

163. Pereira JN. The plasma free fatty acid rebound induced by nicotinic acid. J Lipid Res 1967; 8:239–44.

164. Carlstrom S, Laurell S. The effect of nicotinic acid on the diurnal variation of the free fatty acids of plasma. Acta Med Scand 1968; 184:121–3.

165. Carlson LA, Eriksson I, Walldius G. A case of massive hypertriglyceridaemia and impaired fatty acid incorporation into adipose tissue glycerides (FIAT), both corrected by nicotinic acid. Acta Med Scand 1973; 194:363–9.

166. Parsons BW. Reduction in hepatic synthesis of cholesterol from C14-acetate in hypercholesterolemic patients by nicotinic acid. Circulation 1961; 24:1099–100.

167. Kudchokar BJ, Sodhi HS, Horlick L, Mason DT. Clin Pharmacol Ther 1978; 24: 354–73.

168. Gamble W, Wright LD. Effect of nicotinic acid and related compounds on incorporation of mevalonic acid into cholesterol. Proc Soc Exp Biol Med 1971; 107:161–2.

169. Packard CJ, Stewart JM, Third JLHC, Morgan HG, Lawrie TDV, Shepherd J. Effects of nicotinic acid therapy on high density lipoprotein metabolism in type II and type IV hyperlipoproteinemia. Biochim Biophys Acta 1980; 618:53–62.

170. Keenan JM, Fontaine PL, Wenz JB, Myers S, Huang Z, Ripsin CM. Niacin revisited. A randomized, controlled trial of wax-matrix sustained-release niacin in hypercholesterolemia. Arch Intern Med 1991; 151:1424–32.

171. Leaf DA, Connor WE, Illingworth EF, Bacon SP, Sexton G. The hypolipidemic effects of gemfibrozil in type V hyperlipidemia. A double-blind, crossover study. JAMA 1989; 262:3154–60.

172. Vega GL, Grundy SM. Comparison of lovastatin and gemfibrozil in normolipidemic patients with hypoalphalipoproteinemia. JAMA 1989; 262:3148–53.

173. Magarian GJ, Lucas LM. Gemfibrozil-induced myopathy. Arch Intern Med 1991; 151:1873–4.

174. Pierce LR, Wysowski DK, Gross TP. Myopathy and rhabdomyolysis associated with lovastatin-gemfibrozil combination therapy. JAMA 1990; 264:71–5.

175. Wolfe BM, Kane JP, Havel RJ, Brewster H. Mechanisms of the hypolipemic and hyperketonemic effects of clofibrate in postabsorptive man. J Clin Invest 1973; 52: 2146–59.

176. Kesaniemi YA, Grundy SM. Influence of gemfibrozil and clofibrate on metabolism of cholesterol and plasma triglycerides in man. JAMA 1984; 251:2241–6.

177. Kesaniemi YA, Beltz WF, Grundy SM. Comparison of clofibrate and caloric restriction on kinetics of very low density lipoprotein triglycerides. Arteriosclerosis 1985; 5:153–61.

178. Kissebah AH, Adams PA, Wynn V. Lipokinetic studies with gemfibrozil (CI-719). Proc Roy Soc Med 1976; 69(suppl 2): 98–100.

179. Saku K, Gartside PS, Hynd BA, Kashyap ML. Mechanism of action of gemfibrozil on lipoprotein metabolism. J Clin Invest 1985; 75:1702–12.

180. Berndt J, Gaumert R, Still J. Atherosclerosis 1978; 30:147–52.

181. Stewart JM, Packard CJ, Lorimer AR, Boag DE, Shephard J. Effects of Bezafibrate on receptor mediated and receptor independent low density lipoprotein catabolism in type II hyperlipoproteinemic subjects. Atherosclerosis 1982; 44:355–65.

182. Schneider A, Stange EF, Ditschuneit HH, Ditschuneit H. Atherosclerosis 1985; 56: 2257–62.
183. Nakandakare E, Garcia RC, Rocha JC, Sperotto G, Oliveira HCF, Quintao ECR. Effects of simvastatin, bezafibrate and gemfibrozil on the quantity and composition of plasma lipoproteins. Atherosclerosis 1990; 85:211–7.
184. Packard CJ, Munro A, Lorimer AR, Gotto AM, Shepherd J. The metabolism of apolipoprotein B in large triglyceride-rich very low density lipoprotein of normal and hypertriglyceridemic subjects. J Clin Invest 1984; 74:2178–92.
185. Shepherd J, Caslake MJ, Lorimer AR, Vallance BD, Packard CJ. Fenofibrate reduces low density lipoprotein catabolism in hypertriglyceridemic subjects. Arteriosclerosis 1985; 5:162–8.
186. Reihner E, Rudling M, Stahlberg D, Berglund L, Ewerth S, Bjorkhem I, Einarsson K, Angelin B. Influence of pravastatin, a specific inhibitor of HMG-CoA reductase, on hepatic metabolism of cholesterol. N Engl J Med 1990; 323:224–8.
187. Raveh D, Israeli A, Arnon R, Eisenberg S. Effects of lovastatin therapy on LDL receptor activity in circulating monocytes and on structure and composition of plasma lipoproteins. Atherosclerosis 1990; 82:19–26.
188. Kempen HJM, Vermeer M, de Wit E, Havekes LM. Vastatins inhibit cholesterol ester accumulation in human monocyte-derived macrophages. Arterio Thromb 1991; 11:146–53.
189. Malmendier CL, Lontie J-F, Delcroix C, Magot T. Effect of simvastatin on receptor-dependent low density lipoprotein catabolism in normocholesterolemic human volunteers. Atherosclerosis 1989; 80:101–9.
190. Grundy SM, Vega GL, Garg A. Use of 3-hydroxy-3-methylglutaryl conenzyme A reductase inhibitors in various forms of dyslipidemia. Am J Cardiol 1990; 66:31–8B.
191. Illingworth DR, Bacon SP, Larsen KK. Long-term experience with HMG-CoA reductase inhibitors in the therapy of hypercholesterolemia. Atherosclerosis Rev 1988; 18:161–87.
192. Mantell G, Burke MT, Staggers J. Extended clinical safety profile of lovastatin. Am J Cardiol 1990; 66:11B–15B.
193. Bradford RH, Shear CL, Chremos AN, et al. Expanded clinical evaluation of lovastatin (EXCEL) Study results. Arch Intern Med 1991; 151:43–9.
194. Pierce LR, Wysowski DK, Gross TP. Myopathy and rhabdomyolysis associated with lovastatin–gemfibrozil combination therapy. JAMA 1990; 264:71–5.
195. Norman DJ, Illingworth DR, Munson J, Hosenpud J. Myolysis and acute renal failure in a heart-transplant recipient receiving lovastatin. N Engl J Med 1988; 318: 46–7.
196. East C, Alivizatos PA, Grundy SM, Jones PH, Farmer JA. Rhabdomyolysis in patients receiving lovastatin after cardiac transplantation. N Engl J Med 1988; 318: 47–8.
197. Spach DH, Bauwens JE, Clark CD, Burke WG. Rhabdomyolysis associated with lovastatin and erythromycin use. West J Med 1991; 154:213–5.
198. Kuo PC, Kirshenbaum JM, Gordon J, et al. Lovastatin therapy for hypercholesterolemia in cardiac transplant recipients. Am J Cardiol 1989; 64:631–5.

199. Tobert JA. Reply (letter). N Engl J Med 1988; 318:48.

200. Taylor WC, Pass TM, Shepard DS, Komaroff AL. Cost effectiveness of cholesterol reduction for the primary prevention of coronary heart disease in men. In: Goldbloom RB, Lawrence RS, eds. Preventing disease. Beyond the rhetoric. New York: Springer-Verlag, 1990:437–41.

201. Goldman L, Weinstein MC, Goldman PA, Williams LW. Cost-effectiveness of HMG-CoA reductase inhibition for primary and secondary prevention of coronary heart disease. JAMA 1991; 265:1145–51.

202. Rossouw JE, Lewis B, Rifkind BM. The value of lowering cholesterol after myocardial infarction. N Engl J Med 1990; 323:1112–9.

203. Pekkanen J, Linn S, Heiss G, Suchindran CM, Leon A, Rifkind BM, Tyroler HA. Ten-year mortality from cardiovascular disease in relation to cholesterol level among men with and without preexisting cardiovascular disease. N Engl J Med 1990; 322: 1700–7.

204. Cohen MV, Byrne M-J, Levine B, Gutowski T, Adelson R. Low rate of treatment of hypercholesterolemia by cardiologists in patients with suspected and proven coronary artery disease. Circulation 1991; 83:1294–1304.

205. Committee on Principal Investigators, WHO Clofibrate Trial. A cooperative trial in the primary prevention of ischaemic heart disease using clofibrate. Br Heart J 1978; 40:1069–1118.

206. Lipid Research Clinics Program. The Lipid Research Clinics Coronary Primary Prevention Trial results. I. Reduction in incidence of coronary heart disease. JAMA 1984; 251:351–64.

207. Gordon DJ. Personal communication, 1990.

208. Frick MH, Elo O, Haapa K, et al. Helsinki Heart Study: primary-prevention trial with gemfibrozil in middle-aged men with dyslipidemia. N Engl J Med 1987; 317: 1237–45.

209. Group of Physicians of the Newcastle Upon Tyne Region. Trial of clofibrate in the treatment of ischaemic heart disease. Br Med J 1971; 4:767–75.

210. Research Committee of the Scottish Society of Physicians. Ischaemic heart disease: a secondary prevention trial using clofibrate. Br Med J 1971; 4:775–84.

211. Coronary Drug project Research Group. The Coronary Drug Project: findings leading to further modifications of its protocol with respect to dextrothyroxine. JAMA 1972; 220:996–1009.

212. Coronary Drug Project Research Group. Clofibrate and niacin in coronary heart disease. JAMA 1975; 231:360–81.

213. Brensike JF, Levy RI, Kelsey SF, et al. Effects of therapy with cholestyramine on progression of coronary arteriosclerosis: results of the NHLBI Type II Coronary Intervention Study. Circulation 1984; 69:313–24.

214. Blankenhorn DH, Nessim SA, Johnson RL, Sanmarco ME, Azen SP, Cashin-Hemphill L. Beneficial effects of combined colestipol–niacin therapy on coronary atherosclerosis and coronary venous bypass grafts. JAMA 1987; 257:3233–40.

215. Carlson LA, Rosenhamer G. Reduction of mortality in the Stockholm Ischaemic Heart Disease Secondary Prevention Study by combined treatment with clofibrate and nicotinic acid. Acta Med Scand 1988; 223:405–18.

216. Brown BG, Lin JT, Schaefer SM, Kaplan CA, Dodge HT, Albers JJ. Niacin or lovastatin, combined with colestipol, regress coronary atherosclerosis and prevent clinical events in men with elevated apolipoprotein B. Circulation 1989; 80(suppl II):266.

217. Buchwald H, Varco RL, Matts JP, et al. Effect of partial ileal bypass surgery on mortality and morbidity from coronary heart disease in patients with hypercholesterolemia. N Engl J Med 1990; 323; 946–55.

218. Dorr AE, Gundersen K, Schneider JC, Spencer TW, Martin WB. Colestipol hydrochloride in hypercholesterolemic patients—effect on serum cholesterol and mortality. J Chron Dis 1978; 31:5–14.

219. Lipid Research Clinics Program. The Lipid Research Clinics Coronary Primary Prevention Trial results. II. The relationship of reduction in incidence of coronary heart disease to cholesterol lowering. JAMA 1984; 251:365–74.

9

Control of Hypertension in Prevention of Coronary Heart Disease

NEMAT O. BORHANI
University of Nevada School of Medicine, Reno, Nevada
University of California School of Medicine, Davis, California
University of Tennessee, Memphis, Tennessee

I. NATURE OF THE PROBLEM

A. Introduction

Diseases of the heart remain the leading cause of death in the United States, accounting for approximately 32% of all deaths (1). More than two-thirds of deaths attributed to diseases of the heart are caused by clinical consequences of atherosclerosis, such as acute myocardial infarction.

The pathogenesis of atherosclerosis includes two distinct, but interconnected, mechanisms. One is predominantly an abnormality in lipid metabolism, and the other a subtle injury to the surface of endothelium (2). The mechanism by which abnormal lipids, especially high levels of low-density lipoprotein (LDL) cholesterol, enhance the formation of atherosclerosis, and block the lumen of arteries, is well established (2–5). The role of chronic and subtle injury to the surface of endothelium, as a cause of atherosclerosis, is perhaps less appreciated.

Chronic and uncontrolled hypertension causes minute injuries on the surface of endothelium, which lead to changes in endothelial permeability and function, smooth muscle cell proliferation, accumulation of vascular connective tissues, and eventually the formation of atheroma. This process, demonstrated convincingly by research at the cellular level, makes hypertension a strong risk factor for atherosclerosis, as has been reported consistently by numerous clinical and epidemiologic studies (6,7). Judicious treatment of hypertension, on the other hand, is effective in reducing the level of blood pressure in hypertensive patients (8–12). It is, therefore, reasonable to consider the control of hypertension as an effective means of primary prevention of atherosclerosis and clinical manifestation of diseases associated with it.

B. Epidemiology of Hypertension: Prevalence

Blood pressure is a biological quantitative variable, that is, the level of blood pressure in the general population forms a continuous distribution. Therefore, any definition of hypertension based on a dichotomy of this frequency distribution (above or below a certain level) is arbitrary. Nevertheless, it is customary in practice to use a cut off of 140–160 mmHg for systolic blood pressure and 90–95 mmHg for diastolic blood pressure as the levels above which we define hypertension. Because of the arbitrary nature of this definition, estimates of the prevalence of hypertension in a population depend upon the cut point used. For example, in the Hypertension Detection and Follow-up Program (HDFP), which screened 158,906 persons aged 30–69 years in their homes, the prevalence of hypertension was 25.3% when the cut off point for diastolic blood pressure was chosen at 90 mmHg; it was 14.5% when the cut off point was set at 95 mmHg (13,14). In addition to the choice of the cut off point, a realistic picture of the prevalence of hypertension in a community depends upon the number of hypertensive persons who may be taking antihypertensive medication at the time of screening. Thus, the actual prevalence of hypertension would include not only those individuals whose blood pressures are above the chosen cut off point but also those whose blood pressure are below the cut off point, but who are taking antihypertensive medication at the time of the survey (13).

Another important point in estimating the prevalence of hypertension is the inherent problem of blood pressure variability. For example, in the HDFP the observed changes in diastolic blood pressure between the first screening (conducted at home) and the second screening (conducted a week later in the HDFP clinics) were dramatic. Among those with a diastolic blood pressure (DBP) in the range of 95–104 mmHg at the first screen, 39% of blacks and 46% of whites had a diastolic blood pressure below 90 mmHg at the second screen, notwithstanding the possible impact a clinic visit may have on blood pressure level, the so-called "white coat syndrome." Even in the next highest stratum (i.e., DBP 105–114 mmHg), 20% of the blacks and 22% of the whites had a diastolic blood pressure below 90 mmHg at the second screen (13,14).

Prevalence of hypertension in the community varies markedly by sex and by race. The higher prevalence of hypertension in black Americans, however, is a well-documented epidemiologic feature of hypertension in the United States. For example, in the HDFP the prevalence of hypertension (i.e., DBP $\geq$ 95 mmHg) was

28.1% in black men and 13.1% in white men. Among women the prevalence was 23.1% in blacks and 8.4% in whites. Black to white ratio in the prevalence of hypertension was 2.1 for men and 2.7 for women (13). This ratio increased dramatically in the highest stratum of hypertension (i.e., DBP ≥ 115 mmHg), in which it was 5.4 for men and 7.1 for women. prevalence of hypertension is slightly higher in men than in women. However, when the number of the individuals who may have a "normal" blood pressure at the time of screening but are on antihypertensive medication is added to the number of individuals with high blood pressure (i.e., "actual" hypertension), there seems to be no difference between men and women, even though the difference between blacks and whites persists. In the HDFP the prevalence of "actual" hypertension (i.e., those with DBP ≥ 95 mmHg, and those with DBP < 95 mmHg but on antihypertensive medication) was 36% in black men and 37% in black women; it was 19% in white men and 18% in white women (13). This phenomenon may be due to the fact that more women than men, in both races, choose to seek medical care and receive antihypertensive medication.

In addition to sex and race, other sociodemographic and cultural factors seem to influence the prevalence of hypertension. For example, the prevalence of hypertension is inversely associated with the level of education, both in blacks and in whites (15,16). The greater the number of school years completed, the lower the prevalence of hypertension. It should be emphasized, however, that at least two factors could confound this relationship. Adults with lower educational achievements are likely to be older, hence having a higher DBP. Also, since body weight is positively associated with hypertension and age, it could confound the univariate relationship between education and blood pressure. However, in the HDFP when age was taken into account, the inverse relationship between hypertension and education was not totally eliminated. Indeed, the largest relative difference in prevalence of hypertension between educational classes was found in the younger age groups. This difference was more striking in blacks than in whites. Among the youngest blacks (30–39 years of age), those with a college education had a prevalence rate of 13.7%, compared to a rate of 26.6% among those with less than 10 years of formal education (15). It should be pointed out, however, that education alone, as an index of social and economic status, does not by itself explain the observed difference in the prevalence of hypertension between blacks and whites in the United States.

II. HYPERTENSION–CORONARY HEART DISEASE CONNECTION

A. Hypertension as a Risk for Morbidity and Premature Mortality

Elevated blood pressure, when left uncontrolled, leads to clinical manifestations of end-organ damage, or atherosclerosis, or both. Congestive heart failure, renal insufficiency, stroke, and coronary heart disease are only a few catastrophic consequences of uncontrolled hypertension (6–8). Both systolic and diastolic blood pressure exert independent risk on morbidity and premature mortality. Even at very low levels of diastolic blood pressure (e.g., DBP 80–84 mmHg) a small increase in systolic blood pressure (SBP) is associated positively with a correspondingly high incidence of morbidity and premature mortality.

To the extent that endothelial injury plays a role in the pathogenesis of atherosclerosis, it is useful to review the role of hypertension as a risk factor in this context. Hypertension causes major changes in the arterial wall. Some of these changes are thought to be associated with a remodeling of the artery so that it could withstand the increase in the intravascular pressure caused by hypertension (16). Other changes are due to the response to endothelial injury, which predisposes the artery to formation of atherosclerosis with its known catastrophic consequences. It seems that the culprit in the whole process of atherosclerosis is the injury to the surface of endothelium. Uncontrolled elevation of blood pressure over a long period of time causes subtle injury to the surface of endothelium. This injury causes platelet aggregation and platelet adherence at the site of injury. Release of platelet-derived growth factor (PDGF) establishes a vicious cycle by inducing vasoconstriction (17), and by stimulating the migration of smooth muscle cells (SMC) into the intima, and causing SMC hypertrophy and polyploidy (18,19). The injury to the endothelium also increases permeability to lipid molecules and leads to the infiltration of LDL cholesterol into arterial wall. Entrapment of LDL molecule in the intima, its modification (perhaps by oxidation), and increased uptake of such modified LDL molecules by macrophages will lead to the formation of foam cells and fatty streaks, hence the formation of atherosclerosis. The process of atherosclerosis is discussed in more detail in Chapter 2.

Although the relative risk of premature mortality increases proportionally with a corresponding increment in the level of blood pressure, the magnitude of hypertension as a risk factor in the community can be appreciated best when one considers the attributable risk, which depicts the excess number of deaths in the community due to hypertension. Data from the follow-up study of more than 360,000 men aged 35–57 years who participated in the original screening for the Multiple Risk Factor Intervention Trial (MRFIT) indicate that although an increase of 5 mmHg in diastolic blood pressure at baseline was associated with a concomitant increase of 21% in relative risk of coronary heart disease mortality in the subsequent 6 years, the excess coronary heart disease death due to hypertension, as a percentage of all coronary heart disease death in this population, was more than 35% in 6 years (6). The largest excess death due to hypertension was observed in the youngest age group in this cohort (6). The attributable risk of hypertension in a given population is highest in the lowest stratum of hypertension (e.g., DBP 90–104 mmHg). The reason for this phenomenon is the high percentage of individuals in a given community who are likely to be in this stratum of hypertension. Among the HDFP screenees who were identified as hypertensive, 75% were in this stratum (13). It has been estimated that if the medical profession could successfully treat all patients with a diastolic blood pressure of 100 mmHg and above, which is a very unlikely assumption, there would still remain a 43% level of excess deaths due to hypertension among those in the lowest stratum. Thus, it is important to consider the attributable risk of hypertension when one thinks of hypertension as a community health problem.

In considering hypertension as a risk factor, two additional points should be emphasized; both have significant clinical implications. One is the synergism between blood pressure and other risk factors, such as cigarette smoking, hyperlipidemia, and glucose intolerance. Although there is an independent risk associated with the level of blood pressure, the strength of this association is increased dramatically in the presence of other risk factors. For example, a systolic blood pressure of 180 mmHg in a 55-year-old man carries with it a known risk for clinical manifestation of coronary heart disease, such as acute myocardial infarction, which is higher than when the systolic blood pressure is around 130 or 140 mmHg. However, this relative risk increases manyfold when other risk factors such as hyperlipidemia and glucose intolerance are added to the equation. The second point is that uncontrolled hypertension, even in its lowest stratum (e.g., DBP 90–104 mmHg), creates its own vicious cycle, increasing the danger of progression toward target organ damage, such as left ventricular hypertrophy, hence increasing the risk of premature mortality. This phenomenon has significant clinical implications; it brings to focus the fact that deleterious effects of hypertension begin early at the onset of the disease, necessitating early detection and treatment to halt the progression of the process. For this reason recent clinical trials on the efficacy of treatment have focused on the effect of antihypertensive treatment, not as much on the reduction in morbidity and mortality but on halting the progression of atherosclerosis itself (20).

B. The Efficacy of Treatment

1. Total Mortality

Results of the Veterans Administration Cooperative Group Study on the efficacy of antihypertensive agents (known as the VA Study) have shown clearly that hypertensive patients who were treated with antihypertensive drugs experienced a lower incidence of morbid events than a comparable group of patients treated with placebo (21–23). Other large-scale clinical trials conducted since then in the United States and elsewhere have confirmed the benefit of drug treatment of hypertension. These clinical trials include the Hypertension Detection and Follow Up Program (HDFP), the Medical Research Council Trial of the UK (MRC), the Australian Therapeutic Trial in Mild Hypertension (the Australian Study), and others (8–13,24–31). Among these, the HDFP was one of the largest clinical trial;

it was a population-based study in which participants were randomly selected from a defined base population in 14 U.S. communities. Thus, a brief discussion of the design and the results of this clinical trial will be presented as an example (10,13–15,23–30).

The HDFP was a community-based, randomized clinical trial, conducted under a stringent standardized protocol in 14 U.S. communities. The study population included men and women 30–69 years old with average home screening blood pressures (average of three readings) of 95 mmHg and above. Each HDFP clinical center defined a base population (e.g., a city, or a county) from which the hypertensive patients would be identified. In 1 of the 14 centers a large industrial complex was identified as the base population. In each base population a census was conducted that included a complete enumeration. Thus, fairly extensive baseline demographic and other relevant information was gathered on a total of 442,056 enumerated individuals in 14 U.S. communities. Using a probability sample, a total of 159,468 men and women in the age group 30–69 years were then identified as the HDFP base population. These individuals were screened at their home (first screening), which included a comprehensive determination of health status and a health care interview. A series of 3 blood pressure measurements were taken at 5 min intervals, using a standard mercury sphygmomanometer and appropriately sized cuff placed on the right arm with the participant in a seated position and at rest for 5 min. Systolic blood pressure was defined as the first and diastolic pressure as the fifth Korotkoff sounds. If the average of the 3 separate readings of diastolic blood pressure was 95 mmHg or above, the participant was invited to come to the HDFP clinic within 1 week for a second screening.

At the second screening in the clinic, the participant's blood pressure was measured four times, using both a standard mercury sphygmomanometer, and a Selman-Hawksley random-zero sphygmomanometer. If the average of the second and fourth diastolic blood pressure readings was 90 mmHg or higher, the subject was invited to participate in the trial and was randomized into either a stepped care or referred care group.

Of the 159,468 individuals screened at home, 22,650 had a DBP 95 mmHg or above and were invited to the HDFP clinics for the second screening. Of these 17,187 individuals completed the second screen, and 11,237 had a DBP higher than 90 mmHg. Of these, 10,940 met all the entry criteria for the study and were randomized into stepped care (SC = 5485) and referred care (RC = 5455) groups and were evaluated for 5 years. The result of this random assignment was not revealed to the clinic staff until all baseline data (including medical history, complete physical, laboratory, x-ray, and electrocardiographic [ECG] examinations) had been collected at the third screening visit. The RC group was referred to the primary source of care each participant had identified, and the SC group was treated in the HDFP clinic using a standardized regimen of stepwise drug treatment. This consisted of a defined dosage increment, and/or addition of a specified drug until blood pressure control was achieved. Participants who entered the trial with a DBP of 100 mmHg and above were assigned a goal blood pressure of 90 mmHg. For those with DBP of 90–99 mmHg, the goal blood pressure was a 10 mmHg reduction in their DBP. Those who were already receiving antihypertensive drug treatment at baseline were assigned a DBP goal of 90 mmHg. The details of the HDFP drug treatment protocol are summarized in Table 1.

Certain salient features of the HDFP findings have direct implications for clinical practice, especially when the objective is the prevention of atherosclerosis by early identification and treatment of hypertension. For example, blood pressure distribution in the HDFP population, as in the U.S. population as a whole, was related to race (i.e., blacks had higher blood pressure, and more severe hypertension than whites). Also, the history of being on antihypertensive medication at baseline was almost always associated with the presence of end-organ damage (e.g., left ventricular hypertrophy), or other disease states, such as diabetes mellitus. The history of being on antihypertensive drugs was also associated with high levels of serum uric acid, and was more common in older patients and in women. Cigarette smoking was related to lean body weight; this relationship was more common in whites than in blacks. Thus, it is useful to review briefly the results of the HDFP, taking into account the possible confounding effect of these variables and their observed association with the efficacy of treatment.

a. Cigarette Smoking. Five-year mortality in HDFP was consistently higher in smokers than in nonsmokers, but in each age, sex, and race group the SC participants, in both smoker and nonsmoker groups, showed a lower mortality than the RC group (Table 2). The SC–RC difference in mortality was consistent by chi-square test for smokers and nonsmokers and was highly significant ($p = 0.008$), after adjustment for baseline smoking status.

Table 1 Stepped Care Drug Treatment Protocol in HDFP

Step	Drug(s)	Dosage (mg/day)	Duration (wks)
1	Chlorthalidone[a]	25–100	12
2	Add reserpine or methyldopa	0.1–0.25	12
		500–2,000	
3	Add hydralazine	30–200	16
4	Add guanethidine	10–200	—
5	Add or substitute additional agents as needed	—	—

[a]Spironolactone (24–100 mg/day) or triamterine (50–300 mg/day) was used in addition or alternatively when clinically indicated.
Source: Ref. 10.

Table 2 Age-, Sex-, and Race-Adjusted 5 Year Mortality Rate
Per 1000 According to Smoking Status at Baseline in HDFP

Smoking Status	Mortality rate per 1,000	
	Stepped care group	Referred care group
All participants		
Smokers	87.4	102.9
Nonsmokers	48.8	58.2
DBP 90–104 mmHg		
Smokers	80.4	96.3
Nonsmokers	41.1	54.3

Source: Ref. 31.

b. *Serum Cholesterol.* Five-year mortality in HDFP was lower in the SC group than in the RC group irrespective of the level of serum cholesterol. The beneficial effect of step care treatment was similar in those with baseline serum cholesterol below 250 mg/dl and in those with serum cholesterol above that level (Table 3). As was the case for smokers and nonsmokers, the SC–RC difference in mortality was consistent by chi-square test for those with serum cholesterol level below 250 mg/dl and these above, and was highly significant ($p = 0.009$).

c. *Fasting Plasma Glucose.* In view of recent reports of glucose metabolism abnormalities in hypertensive patients (a subject discussed in further detail below), the HDFP findings in this regard are of particular interest. For all HDFP participants, those with fasting plasma glucose levels below 140 mg/dl had a lower mortality in the SC group than in the RC. This was not the case for those with

Table 3 Age-, Sex-, and Race-Adjusted 5 Year Mortality Rate Per 1,000 According to Level of Serum Cholesterol at Baseline in HDFP

Serum cholesterol (mg/dl)	Mortality rate per 1,000	
	Stepped care group	Referred care group
All participants		
Less than 250	61.6	75.3
250 and above	68.1	77.6
DBP 90–104 mmHg		
Less than 250	56.5	72.1
250 and above	53.2	77.3

Source: Ref. 31.

Table 4 Age-, Sex-, and Race-Adjusted 5 Year Mortality Rate Per 1,000 According to Level of Fasting Plasma Glucose at Baseline in HDFP

Fasting plasma glucose (mg/dl)	Mortality rate per 1,000	
	Stepped care group	Referred care group
All participants		
Less than 140	58.2	70.3
140 and above	112.0	108.5
DBP 90–104 mmHg		
Less than 140	51.8	67.8
140 and above	74.9	104.1

Source: Ref. 31.

fasting plasma glucose levels above 140 mg/dl, even though the difference between the two was small (112.0 vs. 108.5). The chi-square test failed to show a significant nonhomogeneity of response to drug treatment for those with fasting plasma glucose levels above 140 mg/dl compared to those below that level. However, when adjusted for baseline level of fasting plasma glucose, the chi-square test for the SC–RC difference in mortality was highly significant ($p = 0.01$) (Table 4).

Among all randomized HDFP participants (10,940), 772 reported previously diagnosed diabetes mellitus at baseline (7.1%). The SC mortality rate was lower than the RC in both groups with and without history of diabetes. However, the percentage reduction in 5 year mortality in the SC was much lower in those with a history of diabetes than in those without (4.9% vs. 16.5%) (Table 5). Furthermore,

Table 5 Age-, Sex-, and Race-Adjusted 5 Year Mortality Rate Per 1,000 According to History of Diabetes at Baseline in HDFP

History of diabetes	Mortality rate per 1,000	
	Stepped care group	Referred care group
All participants		
Negative	61.2	73.3
Positive	103.3	108.6
DBP 90–104 mmHg		
Negative	56.3	71.2
Positive	58.0	78.9

Source: Ref. 31.

the 5 year mortality rate was much higher in both the SC and RC groups among those with a history of diabetes than in those without.

In multivariate analyses of the HDFP data, using both the multiple linear and logistic regression models, which included factors associated with increased mortality (e.g., hyperlipidemia or cigarette smoking), although these factors were related to 5 year mortality, the drug treatment of hypertension showed a significant favorable impact on mortality, which was independent of all of the other 18 variables included in the model.

2. Coronary Heart Disease Mortality

Although the HDFP results show a reduction in coronary heart disease (CHD) mortality among the SC group compared with the RC group, not all clinical trials have confirmed this finding. This inconsistency in the results of clinical trials on the efficacy of antihypertensive drug treatment has caused a controversy about the effect of treating hypertension as a means for preventing coronary heart disease. Further, whereas the observed reduction in total mortality, or stroke mortality, among drug-treated groups in these clinical trials is consistent with the predicted expectation based on the extrapolation from the findings of the observational population studies, this is not the case for CHD. For example, findings of longitudinal observational studies, such as the Framingham Study, would predict that an average reduction of 5–6 mmHg in DBP should be associated with at least a 30–40% reduction in stroke mortality in 5 years. Indeed, pooled data from all clinical trials show that exactly a reduction of this magnitude has been observed (i.e., 40–42% reduction in 5 years). For CHD mortality, however, this does not seem to be the case. Whereas the extrapolation from the findings of observational studies would indicate that a 5–6 mmHg reduction in DBP should yield at least a 25–28% reduction in CHD mortality, the pooled results of all clinical trials show an average reduction in CHD mortality of 8–14% (9); the HDFP results showed a reduction of only 15% in 5 years. The observed reduction in CHD mortality, even in clinical trials that have reported a favorable outcome, falls short of the expectation.

One possible explanation for this shortfall could be that it is perhaps due to chance. In other words, the observed less than expected reduction in CHD mortality in these clinical trials has been purely a random event. This is a plausible explanation and is usually referred to as a type II error: the probability of not observing a positive result when in reality the positive result had occurred. Another possible explanation could be that none of these clinical trials, with an average follow-up period of 5 years, evaluated their patients long enough to observe the "real" result. In other words, as has been suggested, about one-half of the expected reduction in CHD mortality had occurred "rapidly" in the course of these clinical trials, and that the trials were terminated presumably before the other half could be observed (9).

A third explanation could be that the metabolic adverse effects of treatment itself, or perhaps some chronic disease processes, had blunted the effect of drug therapy. For this reason some of the salient points about the HDFP were discussed in detail earlier in this chapter. Foremost among these metabolic reasons for the observed shortfall in CHD mortality is the relationship between hypertension and glucose metabolism, and the role of some of the antihypertensive drugs on glucose and lipid metabolism.

C. Hypertension and Glucose Metabolism

As noted above, the presence of diabetes mellitus, or an abnormal fasting plasma glucose level, carried not only a high risk of mortality in the HDFP but it also blunted the efficacy of antihypertensive treatment. Findings from the epidemiologic observational studies (e.g., Framingham Study) indicate that the presence of hyperglycemia, or abnormal glucose tolerance, has a synergistic effect on the impact of other CHD risk factors, such as high blood pressure or elevated plasma cholesterol levels. The addition of glucose intolerance to hypertension causes a pronounced impact on the risk of CHD that is more than just the sum of the two independent risk factors. Furthermore, patients with hypertension do suffer from an abnormality in glucose metabolism, and most of them are insulin-resistant, that is, the tissue (cells) are unable to respond normally to insulin-stimulated glucose uptake. In other words, hypertension by itself is an insulin-resistant state, and insulin resistance contributes to impaired glucose tolerance, abnormal lipid levels, atherosclerosis, and increased CHD risk (31–33).

Some of the drugs used to treat hypertension accentuate this inherent metabolic abnormality. For example, treatment of hypertension with thiazides, or a combination of thiazides and some of the beta blockers, shifts the plasma glucose and the insulin curves upwards, after a glucose load. This upward shift is more pronounced than the upward shift in the curve observed in hypertensive patients not receiving treatment (31,32). For these reasons a new concept has evolved considering hypertension as a risk factor for atherosclerosis. The concept identifies hypertension as an insulin-resistant state, which causes hyperinsulinemia, hyperglycemia, impaired glucose tolerance, hypertriglyceridemia, and perhaps decreased high-density lipoprotein (HDL) cholesterol levels. These abnormal risk factors accelerate the formation of atherosclerosis.

D. Metabolic Side Effects of Treatment

Some of the drugs commonly used in the treatment of hypertension cause metabolic side effects in certain patients. For example, thiazides, in addition to their effect on glucose metabolism, have been shown to cause an abnormal lipid profile in some patients (34–39). A 5% increase in the level of total serum cholesterol in 1 year after thiazide therapy, and a 10% increase in LDL cholesterol, have been reported (34,35). Therefore, it is important to consider these problems before choosing antihypertensive drugs for a given patient.

III. DETECTION, EVALUATION, AND TREATMENT IN CLINICAL PRACTICE

A. Detection and Evaluation

Based on early discussion, it should be clear that detection of hypertension in practice must depend not only on the level of systolic and diastolic blood pressure but also on the entire clinical profile of the patient. The most logical guideline to follow must be that a systolic blood pressure of 160 mmHg or a diastolic blood pressure of 100 mmHg in a 50-year-old white male patient would present quite a different clinical picture if this patient does not smoke cigarettes, does not have abnormal glucose tolerance, or ECG abnormality, compared to a patient in the same age sex and race who has one or perhaps all of these risk factors.

Thus, the first foremost step in evaluating patients for diagnosis and treatment is a comprehensive clinical work-up. This implies that physicians and community health workers must avoid the temptation of putting people on treatment based only on the results of blood pressure screening. Those with sustained elevation of blood pressure must be referred to a source of medical care for clinical evaluation. The guidelines of the Joint National Committee on Detection, Evaluation, and Treatment of High Blood Pressure with regards to measurement of blood pressure, confirmation and follow up should be followed (40) (see Table 6). Clinical evaluation should include a comprehensive medical and personal history, a physical examination, including an evaluation of the cardiovascular system, and a minimum of laboratory tests, including the following:

1. Urinalysis
2. Routine blood work
3. Analysis of blood chemistry, which must include lipids, fasting glucose, insulin, electrolytes, and other routine tests
4. A 12-lead resting ECG

The determination of glucose tolerance is considered, by some, essential in the clinical work-up of a hypertensive patient. If this is done, measurement of plasma insulin level, both fasting and after glucose load, must be part of the test. The determination of insulin level in conjunction with glucose level is important to detect the presence of insulin resistance, which, if present, would dictate an entirely different and highly specific therapeutic regimen. Patients with hypertension ". . . as a group are insulin resistant . . .," and ". . . lowering of blood pressure does not necessarily lead to an improvement in these metabolic abnormalities" (33). Thus, a careful determination of the patient's lipid profile espe-

Table 6 Classification of Blood Pressure and Recommended Follow-Up[a]

Range (mmHg)	Classification of diastolic blood pressure	Recommended follow-up
<85	"Normal"	Recheck within 2 years
85–89	High normal	Recheck within 1 year
90–104	Mild hypertension	Confirm treat
105–114	Moderate hypertension	Evaluate and treat promptly
>114	Severe hypertension	Evaluate and treat promptly

Classification of systolic blood pressure when diastolic blood pressure is below 90 mmHg

<140	Normal	Recheck within 2 years
140–159	Borderline systolic hypertension	Confirm within 2 months
160–200	Isolated systolic hypertension	Confirm and treat
>200	Severe systolic hypertension	Evaluate and treat promptly

[a]Adapted from The 1988 Report of The Joint National Committee on Detection, Evaluation, and Treatment of High Blood Pressure.
Source: Refs. 40, 50.

cially the levels of triglycerides and HDL cholesterol, and glucose and insulin metabolism must be given serious consideration in the evaluation of patient with hypertension before the therapeutic regimen is decided upon.

B. Nonpharmacologic Therapy

The goal of treatment should be to prevent morbidity and mortality associated with hypertension. The objective should be twofold. One, "to achieve and maintain arterial blood pressure below 140/90 mmHg, if possible" (40), and the other, to avoid interfering with patients' quality of life and minimize the undesirable side effects. The 1988 Report of the Joint Nation Committee on Detection, Evaluation, and Treatment of High Blood Pressure points out that, based on available scientific evidence, nonpharmacologic modes of therapy, such as weight reduction, restriction of alcohol and sodium, avoidance of tobacco,and participating in regular physical exercise, should be used ". . . both as definitive intervention and as an adjunct to pharmacologic therapy . . ." (40). Indeed, in the individualized therapy for hypertension, the Joint Committee Report lists nonpharmacologic modes of therapy as step one in the therapeutic regimen (40). It is important to consider, however, that adherence to nonpharmacologic modes of therapy may not be uniform among all patients with hypertension. Furthermore, some patients may not respond as might be expected. For this reason, it is incumbent upon the practicing physician to monitor carefully the patient's response to a nonpharmacologic therapeutic regimen. These patients must be educated as to the benefits and limitations of nonpharmacologic modes of therapy, and they should be evaluated at regular intervals. If a patient's blood pressure does not respond to the regimen within 5–6 months, the appropriate antihypertensive drug therapy must be added to the regimen. One must avoid giving these patients a false sense of security that might persuade them to ignore the necessity of visiting their physicians at regular intervals, or even slip away from practicing the changes in lifestyle they had been encouraged to follow.

It is instructive to review briefly the findings of a recently completed clinical trial on hypertension prevention by changes in lifestyle. The study, known as the Hypertension Prevention Trial (HPT), was a multicenter study with a large sample size. Participants were instructed and counseled to make changes in their dietary habits such as restriction in sodium intake or weight reduction programs. They were evaluated for 3 years to study the effects of weight loss and sodium restriction on blood pressure (41). An important aspect of HPT on the use of nonpharmacologic modes of therapy was a determination of the reasons for dietary failures and problems reported by participants (42). The HPT results indicated that men perceived their problems in adherence to a dietary regimen to be more controllable than did women (42). These findings are in concert with previous reports in the literature that prior to entry into a weight loss program, men express more confidence in their ability to lose weight than women, but they report more difficulty than women in dealing with temptation to eat, or not to follow the prescribed regimen (43). Thus, practicing physicians who choose to begin the treatment of hypertension with nonpharmacologic regimen need to become aware of complicated psychological issues involved in changing a person's behavior and lifestyle. The nonpharmacologic therapeutic regimen must be planned in specific terms for each patient, taking into consideration age, sex, race, socioeconomic status, and other personal characteristics. These programs must be administered by highly trained professional staff and patients must be counseled and evaluated under strict supervision of these professional staff (e.g., a qualified nutritionist, exercise physiologist, or psychologist).

C. Pharmacologic Treatment

Selection of antihypertensive drugs need to be based, as a minimum, upon the following criteria:

1. Efficacy: The chosen drug must have demonstrated a proven efficacy in reducing the level of blood pressure within the desirable range.
2. Safety: The drug must be safe to administer and proven to have a minimum adverse effect on the patient. In other words, practicing physicians should be knowledgeable of the drug's adverse side effects, and be confident that the drug they choose has a minimum risk to the patient.
3. Coronary heart disease risk factors: The chosen drug should be at least

neutral or, if possible, beneficial toward other coronary heart disease risk factors, especially plasma lipid levels and glucose metabolism.

4. Patient acceptance: The drug must be acceptable to the patient, especially in terms of the drug's effect on quality of life. For example, if a patient perceives that the drug might cause impotence, it is the physician's responsibility to listen to the patient's complaint and correct the situation, even if in the opinion of the physician the presenting complaint is "perceived" and not "real." Otherwise, the patient may not follow the therapeutic regimen.

D. The "Ideal" Treatment

The "ideal" antihypertensive drug of the 1990s is expected to have the following characteristics:

1. The drug should reduce blood pressure effectively, safely, and with no serious side effect.
2. The drug should not worsen the lipid profile.
3. The drug should not adversely affect glucose or insulin metabolism or result in electrolyte imbalance.
4. The drug should not induce weight gain and should not interfere with physical exercise.

These are but some of the few, albeit important, characteristics of the "ideal" antihypertensive drugs. With prudence, physicians could select the drug of choice for a given patient, and evaluate the patient regularly to monitor not only blood pressure response to drug therapy but also the metabolic side effects of the drug. In addition to the careful selection of a drug that will suit a patient's particular clinical and metabolic profile, an important consideration is the dosage of the drug. It is important to begin the pharmacologic therapy with the smallest recommended dosage of the chosen drug and evaluate the patient to monitor the response. If the patient does not respond as expected, the dosage of the drug could be increased gradually to reach the maximum effective dosage. Or, if necessary, additional drugs, in small dosages, could be added to the regimen to achieve a satisfactory result. The Joint National Committee recommends a "step-down" procedure as well. This means that depending on the patient's response the dosage of the drug, or combination thereof, could be, and should be, reduced if the desired blood pressure goal could be maintained with smaller dosages or fewer drugs. This practice reduces the probability of adverse side effects and will increase compliance.

Drug treatment of hypertension should consider both short-term goals (i.e., reduction of blood pressure) and long-term implications (i.e., adverse effect on other coronary heart disease risk factors). Furthermore, selection of initial therapy should be individualized according to the patient's clinical profile. For example, for some patients the use of an entirely different class of diuretics from thiazide diuretics may be the choice. Some of the newly introduced diuretics such as indapamide may be an ideal choice for initial therapy. In others an angiotensin-converting-enzyme (ACE) inhibitor, beta blocker, calcium channel blocker, or one of the new alpha blockers may be the drug of choice. Whatever drug or class of drugs is chosen as monotherapy, the dosage should be kept low to avoid adverse side effects. If monotherapy is ineffective in low dosages of the chosen drug, a second drug with a different mechanism of action should be added, or substituted, as necessary. In all cases of drug therapy, physicians should consider potential drug interactions and protect the patient's quality of life.

IV. CONTROVERSIES AND UNRESOLVED ISSUES

On the need to detect and treat hypertension early, there is no controversy today. There is, however, some debate in the scientific community at the present time regarding the issues discussed below.

A. Ambulatory Blood Pressure Measurement

There is considerable debate about the utility of ambulatory blood pressure monitoring (44). On the one hand, it has been demonstrated that blood pressure measurements among hypertensive patients visiting physicians offices are, on the average, higher than the readings obtained by automated ambulatory recording. Thus, it is argued that many patients are unnecessarily diagnosed as having hypertension, and put on drug treatment, when they may not need it (45). On the other hand, there are practical and financial problems associated with the routine use of ambulatory blood pressure devices in clinical practice. These techniques are cumbersome and expensive to use. It is not clear at this time whether the third party payees or government health agencies would pay for the cost involved.

B. Role of Plasma Renin

Proponents of measuring plasma renin activity argue that patients with hypertension could be classified into low-, normal-, or high-renin groups (46). It is argued that the choice of appropriate antihypertensive drug should depend on the renin profile of the patient. That is, patients with low renin activity would respond best to certain drugs, while patients with high renin activity would respond best to other classes of drugs. Also, it has been reported that hypertension as a risk factor for coronary heart disease is a lesser evil in patients with low renin activity than in those with high renin (47,48). Although these hypotheses have scientific validity in the context of the renin-angiotensin system, there is no universally accepted consensus to mandate a common therapeutic strategy at this time. We hope that a consensus will emerge in the near future based on the results of larger longitudinal studies, controlled clinical trials, or both.

C. Isolated Systolic Hypertension

Although isolated systolic hypertension (ISH), defined as systolic blood pressure above 160 mmHg in the presence of diastolic pressures below 90 mmHg, is a recognized risk factor for morbidity and premature mortality, especially among the elderly, the need for pharmacologic therapy or the efficacy of treatment was not known until very recently. A multicenter randomized clinical trial has been underway in the United States to test the efficacy and safety of drug treatment of ISH in the elderly (49). This multicenter clinical trial, known as the systolic hypertension in the elderly program (SHEP) was completed early in 1991.

Final results of the systolic hypertension in SHEP have been recently published (50). The main objective of this multicenter clinical trial was to determine the efficacy of drug treatment in reducing the incidence of stroke in patients with ISH. A total of 4,736 patients, 60 years of age and older, with confirmed ISH (systolic blood pressure $\geq$ 160 mmHg and diastolic blood pressure < 90 mmHg), were randomized into two groups: one receiving active antihypertensive drug treatment and the other placebo. The average systolic blood pressure at baseline was 170 mmHg (50). The active drug treatment group received a step-care drug treatment regimen, beginning with chlorthalidone 12.5 mg a day; this was increased to 25 mg a day if necessary. The step 2 drug was atenolol 25 mg a day, which was increased to 50 mg a day if necessary. The placebo group received matching placebo in each step. The study was a double-blind, placebo-controlled clinical trial. Neither the patient nor clinic physicians knew the nature of the drug being administered.

After 5 years of follow-up, the average systolic blood pressure in the placebo-treated group was 155 mmHg. For the group receiving active drug treatment, it was 143 mmHg. The average diastolic blood pressure was 72 and 68 mmHg, respectively, in the placebo- and actively treated groups (50). There was a concomitant reduction in the 5 year incidence of stroke among the patients randomized to receive the active drug treatment. The 5 year incidence of stroke was 5.2: 100 patients in the actively treated group and 8.2: 100 patients in the placebo-treated group, a reduction of 36% (p = 0.0003). The absolute benefit in favor of active drug treatment was estimated at 5 years as 30 events: 1000 patients (50). These impressive results were observed despite the fact that during the course of the trial 35% of patients who were randomized into the placebo-treated group were prescribed (by their source of medical care) and took known antihypertensive drugs, hence diluting the true difference that would have been observed between actively treated and placebo groups.

Thus, the final results of SHEP demonstrate conclusively that treatment of ISH in individuals over the age of 60 years is beneficial (50,51). Therefore, there should be no "controversy" on this issue. The positive SHEP results were achieved with a minimum effective dosage of antihypertensive drugs in a stepped care regimen associated with only an infrequent excess of adverse effects, and no evidence of increase in dementia or depression (50).

V. CONCLUSION

The problems in methodology, or the adverse side effects of some antihypertensive drugs, may explain the shortfall in the observed reduction in CHD mortality reported thus far by clinical trials on the efficacy of antihypertensive drug treatment. The lessons we have learned from the findings of observational epidemiologic studies and these clinical trials should be considered in aggregate, in light of the consistent observations reported from clinical and laboratory studies on the role of hypertension in the pathogenesis of atherosclerosis.

1. Hypertension is a strong risk factor for atherosclerosis in general, and for clinical manifestation of CHD in particular.
2. Hypertension should be detected early and treated effectively.
3. Drug treatment for hypertension must be administered in the context of recognizing the abnormal hemodynamic and metabolic features of the disease.
4. Hypertension seems to be an insulin-resistant state, with abnormal glucose tolerance in the face of elevated levels of plasma insulin.
5. Hypertension drug treatment must protect the patient against aggravating other CHD risk factors, and must be an adjunct to lifestyle changes, such as weight reduction, increased physical activity, smoking cessation, and reduced intake of alcohol.
6. Isolated systolic hypertension (ISH) is a recognized risk factor for morbidity and premature mortality, especially in individuals above the age of 60 years. There is now conclusive evidence that treatment of ISH in the elderly is beneficial in reducing the incidence of stroke and other cardiovascular complications of ISH.

REFERENCES

1. Health United States 1989. U.S. Department of Health and Human Services, National Center for Health Statistics Pub. No. 90-1232, 1989.
2. Steinberg D. Lipoproteins and atherosclerosis. A look back and a look ahead. Atherosclerosis 1983; 3:283–301.
3. Goldstein JL, Brown MS. The low density lipoprotein pathway and its relation to atherosclerosis. Ann Biochem 1977; 46:897–930.

4. Steinberg D. Lipoproteins and pathogenesis of atherosclerosis. Circulation 1987; 76: 508–14.

5. Brown MS, Goldstein JL. How LDL receptors influence cholesterol and atherosclerosis. Sci Am 1984; 251:58–66.

6. Stamler J, Newton JD, Wenworth DN. Blood pressure and risk of fatal coronary heart disease. Hypertension 1989; 13 (Suppl I):2–12.

7. McMahon S, Peto R, Cutler J, Collins R, Sorlie P, Newton J, Abbott R, Godwin J, Dyar A, Stamler J. Blood pressure, stroke and coronary heart disease, part I: prolonged differences in blood pressure: prospective observational studies corrected for the regression dilution bias. Lancet 1990; 335:765–74.

8. Borhani, NO. Primary prevention of coronary heart disease in practice. JAMA 1985; 254:257–62.

9. Collins R, Peto R, McMahon S, Hebert P, Fiebach NH, Eberlein KA, Godwin J, Qizilbash N, Taylor J, Hennekens CH. Blood pressure, stroke, and coronary heart disease part II. Short-term reductions in blood pressure, overview of randomized drug trials in their epidemiological context. Lancet 1990; 335:827–38.

10. Hypertension Detection and Follow Up Program (HDFP) Cooperative Group. Five-year finding of the HDFP; I. Reduction in mortality in persons with high blood pressure, including mild hypertension. JAMA 1979; 242:2562–71.

11. Australian National Blood Management Committee. The Australian therapeutic trial in hypertension. Lancet 1980; 1:1261–7.

12. Medical Research Council Working Party. MRC trial of treatment of mild hypertension, principal results. Br Med J 1985; 291:97–104.

13. The HDFP Cooperative Group. Blood pressure studies in 14 communities, a two stage screen for hypertension. JAMA 1977; 237:2385–91.

14. Wassertheil-Smoller S, Apostolidis A, Miller M, Oberman A, Tham T, on Behalf of the HDFP Cooperative Group. Recent status of detection, treatment and control of hypertension in the community. J Commun Health 1979; 5:82–93.

15. The HDFP Cooperative Group. Race, education and prevalence of hypertension. Am J Epidemiol 1977; 106:351–61.

16. Tyroler H. Socioeconomic status in the epidemiology and treatment of hypertension. Hypertension 1989; 13 (Suppl. I):94–7.

17. Chobanian AY. The 1989 Corcoran lecture: adaptive and maladaptive responses of the arterial wall to hypertension. Hypertension 1990; 15:666–74.

18. Berk BC, Alexander RN, Brock TA, Gimbrone MA, Webb RC. Vasoconstriction, a new biological activity of platelet derived growth factor. Science 1986; 232:87–90.

19. Owens GK, Geisterfer AT, Yang YW, Komoriya A. Transforming growth factor-B–induced growth inhibition and cellular hypertrophy in cultured vascular smooth muscle cells. J Cell Biol 1988; 107:771–80.

20. Borhani NO, Brugger SB, Byington RP, on behalf of the U.S. MIDAS research group. Multicenter study with isradipine and diuretics against atherosclerosis. J Cardiovasc Pharmacol 1990; 15 (Suppl. I):23–9.

21. Veterans Administration Cooperative Study Group on Antihypertensive Agents. Effects of treatment on morbidity in hypertension; I. Results in patients with diastolic blood pressures 115–129 mmHg. JAMA 1967; 202:116–22.

22. Veterans Administration Cooperative Study Group on Antihypertensive Agents. Effects of treatment on morbidity in hypertension; II. Results in patients with diastolic blood pressures ranging 90 through 114 mmHg. JAMA 1970; 213:1143–52.

23. Veterans Administration Cooperative Study Group on Antihypertensive Agents. Effects of treatment on morbidity in hypertension; III. Influence of age, diastolic pressure, and prior cardiovascular disease; further analysis of side effects. Circulation 1972; 45:991–1004.

24. Hypertension Detection and Follow Up Program Cooperative Group. Five year findings of the HDFP; II. Mortality by race, sex and age. JAMA 1979; 242:2572–7.

25. Hypertension Detection and Follow Up Program Cooperative Group. Five year findings of the HDFP; III. Reduction in stroke incidence among persons with high blood pressure. JAMA 1982; 247:633–8.

26. Hypertension Detection and Follow Up Cooperative Group. The effect of treatment on mortality in "mild" hypertension. N Engl J Med 1982; 307:976–80.

27. Hypertension Detection and Follow Up Cooperative Group. Effect of stepped care treatment on the incidence of myocardial infarction and angina pectoris. Hypertension 1984; 6 (Suppl. I):198–206.

28. Hypertension Detection and Follow Up Cooperative Group. Five-year findings of the HDFP, mortality by race-sex and blood pressure level, a further analysis. J Commun Health 1984; 9:314–27.

29. Hypertension Detection and Follow Up Cooperative Group. The effect of antihypertensive drug treatment on Mortality in the presence of resting electrocardiographic abnormalities at baseline. Circulation 1984; 70:996–1003.

30. Hypertension Detection and Follow Up Cooperative Group. Five-year finding of the HDFP, prevention and reversal of left ventricular hypertrophy with antihypertensive drug therapy. Hypertension 1985; 7:105–12.

31. Hypertension Detection and Follow Up Cooperative Group. Mortality finding for stepped care and referred care participants in the HDFP stratified by other risk factors. Prev Med 1985; 14:312–335.

32. Ferrannini E, Buzzigoli G, Bonadonna R. Insulin resistance in essential hypertension. N Engl J Med 1987; 317:350–357.

33. Swislocki A, Hoffman B, Reaven GM. Insulin resistance, glucose intolerance and hyperinsulinemia in patients with hypertension. Am J Hypertension 1989; 2:419–23.

34. Modan M, Halkin H, Almong S. Hyperinsulinemia, a link between hypertension, obesity and glucose intolerance. J Clin Invest 1985; 75:809–17.

35. Wilhelmsen L, Berglund G, Elmfeldt D, Fitzsimons T, Holzgreve H, Hosie J, Horukvist PE, Pennert K, Tuomiletho J, Wedel H, on behalf of the Heart Attack Primary Prevention in Hypertension Trial Research Group. Beta blockers versus diuretics in hypertensive men; main results from the happy trial. J Hypertension 1987; 5:561–72.

36. Pollare T, Lithell H, Berne C. A comparison of the effect of hydrochlorothiazide and captopril on glucose and lipid metabolism in patients with hypertension. N Engl J Med 1989; 321:868–73.

37. Grimm RH, Hunninghake DB. Lipids and hypertension, implications of new guidelines for cholesterol management for treatment of hypertension. Am J Med 1986; 80 (Suppl. 2A):56–63.

38. Lardinois CK, Newman SL. The effect of antihypertensive agents on serum lipids and lipoproteins. Arch Intern Med 1988; 148:1280–8.
39. Wiedman P, Uehlinger DE, Gerber A. Antihypertensive treatment and serum lipoproteins. J Hypertension 1985; 3:297–306.
40. The 1988 Joint National Committee Report on Detection, Evaluation and Treatment of High Blood Pressure. Arch Intern Med 1988; 148:1023–38.
41. Meinert CL, Borhani NO, Langford HG, for the Hypertension Prevention Trial Research Group. Design, methods and rationale in the HPT. Control Clin Trial 1989; 10 (Suppl. III):1–29.
42. Jeffery RW, French SA, Schmid TL. Attributions for dietary failures: problems reported by participants in the hypertension prevention trial (HPT). Health psychol 1990; 9:315–29.
43. Foster JL, Jeffery RW. Gender differences related to weight history, eating patterns, efficacy expectations, self-esteem, and weight loss among participants in a weight reduction program. Addict Behav 1986; 11:141–7.
44. Cox J, O'Malley K, Atkins N, and O'Brien E. A comparison of the 24-hour blood pressure profile in normotensive and hypertensive subjects. J Hypertension 1991; 9 (Suppl. I):3–6.
45. Pickering TG, James GD, Boddie C, Harshfield GA, Blank S, Laragh JH. How common is white coat hypertension? JAMA 1988; 259:255–8.
46. Laragh JH. The renin-angiotensin-aldosterone system for blood pressure regulation and for subdividing patients to reveal and analyze different forms of hypertension. In: Laragh JH, Buhler FR, Seldin DW, eds. Frontiers in hypertension Research, New York: Springer-Verlag 1981; 183–94.
47. Brunner HR, Laragh JH, Baer L, et al. Essential hypertension: renin and aldosterone, heart attack and stroke. N Engl J Med 1972; 286:441–4.
48. Laragh JH, Sealy JE. The renin-angiotensin-aldosterone system in hypertensive disorders: a key to two forms of arteriolar vasoconstriction and a possible clue to risk of vascular injury (heart attack and stroke) and prognosis. In: Laragh JH, Brunner HR, eds. Hypertension, pathophysiology, diagnosis, and management. New York: Raven Press, 1990; 1329–48.
49. Borhani NO, Applegate WB, Cutler JA, Davis BR, Furberg CD, Lakatose Page L, Perry HM, Smith WM, Probstfield JL. Systolic hypertension in the elderly program (SHEP) design and rationale. Hypertension 1991; 17 (Suppl. II):1–15.
50. SHEP Cooperative Research Group. Prevention of stroke by antihypertensive drug treatment in older persons with isolated systolic hypertension—final results of the systolic hypertension in the elderly program (SHEP). JAMA 1991; 265:3255–64.
51. Winker MA, Murphy MB. Isolated systolic hypertension in the elderly (editorial). JAMA 1991; 265:3301–2.

Smoking and Coronary Heart Disease

JOHN H. HOLBROOK and FRANCES M. GOUGH
University of Utah School of Medicine
Salt Lake City, Utah

I. INTRODUCTION

Cigarette smoking is an addictive behavior that has become a major scourge of the twentieth century. In industrialized nations, cigarette smoking is the major cause of premature death and disease. The annual toll in the United States for tobacco-caused premature death is an estimated 390,000 lives; thus, cigarette smoking accounts for more than one out of every six deaths in the United States (1).

Because Third World countries have been targeted by multinational tobacco companies as prospective growth areas for tobacco use, developing nations face the same tobacco-caused epidemic currently seen in the Western world. Each year, worldwide, an estimated 2.5 million premature deaths occur, and ultimately as many as 200 million children under the age of 20 years may die because of the use of tobacco products (2).

II. SMOKING BEHAVIOR

Significant changes are occurring in smoking behavior in the United States (3). Between 1965 and 1987 the prevalence of smoking among men decreased from 50.2 to 31.2%; among women during the same period of time the prevalence of smoking decreased from 31.9 to 26.5%. The overall prevalence for adult U.S. smokers in 1987 was 28.8% (Table 1) (3). Annual per capita cigarette consumption

Table 1 Percentage of Adults Who
Smoke Cigarettes According to Sex
and Age, United States, 1987

Age (yrs)	Men	Women	Total
18–24	28.1	26.1	27.1
25–44	35.6	30.8	33.2
45–64	33.5	28.6	30.9
65–74	20.2	18.0	19.0
≥75	11.3	7.5	8.9
Total	31.2	26.5	28.8

Source: Ref. 3.

by adults in the United States decreased from 4345 cigarettes in 1963 to 3196 in
1987. This represents a 26% decrease. In the United States in 1985 there were an
estimated 56 million smokers and 43 million former smokers. Thus, approximately 44% of living American adults, who had ever smoked cigarettes, had quit
smoking. However, among blacks, blue-collar workers, and less-educated individuals, the smoking prevalence remains higher than in the overall population. The
decline in smoking prevalence among U.S. women has been slower than among
men, and since 1977 the prevalence of teenage smoking among girls has exceeded
that among boys. More than 75% of smokers began smoking as teenagers (4).

III. PRINCIPAL ADVERSE EFFECTS

Tobacco smoke contains more than 4000 compounds including those that are
carcinogenic, toxic, mutagenic, and pharmacologically active. A typical cigarette
smoker, who puffs more than 70,000 times a year, repetitively exposes multiple
organ systems to toxic substances. Understanding the diverse biological effects of
tobacco smoke and the cigarette's remarkably efficient substance delivery system
provides a framework for studying the numerous harmful effects of smoking (5).

Cigarette smokers' overall mortality is greater than that of nonsmokers because
they are at increased risk of dying from five of the six leading causes of death in the
United States including coronary heart disease (CHD), cancer, cerebrovascular
disease, chronic obstructive pulmonary disease, and pneumonia/influenza (6).
The principal adverse effects of cigarette smoking are summarized in Table 2 (1).

IV. TOBACCO ADDICTION

Cigarette smoking was once viewed as a "habit." In 1980 "tobacco dependence"
was introduced as a diagnostic category in the *Diagnostic and Statistical Manual*

Table 2 Summary of the Principal Effects of Cigarette Smoking

---

Mortality and morbidity
Overall mortality increased
Overall morbidity increased
Cardiovascular
A major cause of coronary heart disease
A cause of cerebrovascular disease
Increased mortality from atherosclerotic aortic aneurysm
A major cause of atherosclerotic peripheral vascular disease
Cancer
The major cause of lung cancer
The major cause of laryngeal cancer
A major cause of oral cancer
A contributory factor for bladder cancer
A contributory factor for pancreatic cancer
A contributory factor for renal cancer
An association with gastric cancer
An association with cervical cancer
Pulmonary
The major cause of chronic bronchitis
The major cause of emphysema
Gastrointestinal
A probable cause of peptic ulcer disease
Pregnancy
A cause of intrauterine growth retardation
A probable cause of unsuccessful pregnancies
Other effects
An addictive behavior
A cause of disease, including lung cancer, in healthy nonsmokers
Adverse occupational interactions that increase the risk of cancer
Adverse interactions with alcohol that increase the risk of cancer
Adverse drug reactions
An association with nonmalignant oral disease

Source: Adapted from Ref. 1.

of Mental Disorders (*DSM-III*) published by the American Psychiatric Association (7). The revised third edition of this manual (*DSM-III-R*) published in 1987 changed this diagnostic category to "nicotine dependence" (8). The landmark 1988 Report of the Surgeon General, "Nicotine Addiction," listed criteria for establishing tobacco use as addicting (Table 3) (9). The report concluded that: 1. Cigarettes and other forms of tobacco are addicting. 2. Nicotine is the drug in

Table 3 Criteria for Establishing Tobacco Use as Addicting

1. User's behavior is largely controlled by psychoactive substance.
2. Compulsive substance use despite damage to the individual.
3. Pharmacologic activity of substance is sufficiently rewarding to maintain self-administration.
4. Tolerance results from continued use of substance.
5. Physical dependence on the substance can occur; a withdrawal syndrome usually accompanies substance abstinence.
6. With cessation of substance use, tendency to relapse is strong.

Source: Adapted from Ref. 9.

tobacco that causes addiction. 3. The pharmacologic and behavioral processes that determine tobacco addiction are similar to those that determine addiction to drugs such as heroin and cocaine. The 1989 Report of the Surgeon General also commented that smoking is "an addiction influenced by a wide range of interacting factors including pharmacologic effects of nicotine; conditioning of those effects to numerous activities, emotions, and settings; socioeconomic factors; personal factors such as coping resources; and social influence factors" (1). An understanding of this addictive behavior may help health professionals to have realistic treatment goals and may help smokers to understand the course leading to smoking cessation.

V. CIGARETTE SMOKING AND CORONARY HEART DISEASE

A. Causal Evidence

When Hammond and Horn first reported in 1958 on the relationship between smoking and death rates in a study involving 187,783 men, cigarette smokers had a 68% higher death rate than nonsmokers, and CHD accounted for 52% of the excess deaths (10). At that time it was not clear that a causal relationship existed between cigarette smoking and CHD. In the intervening 32 years a wealth of epidemiologic, pathologic, experimental, and clinical data have established cigarette smoking as a major cause of CHD (11). In 1985 in the United States cigarette smoking was estimated to account for the following percentages of deaths due to CHD: 45% in men less than 65 years old, 41% in women less than 65 years old, 21% in men 65 years of age and older, and 12% in women 65 years of age and older (1).

1. Epidemiology

Large prospective epidemiologic studies have been carried out in North America, northern Europe, and Japan using CHD mortality as an endpoint (Table 4) (11). In

Table 4 Coronary Heart Disease Mortality Ratios, Major Prospective Studies

Population/study	Size	No. of CHD deaths	Mortality ratio Nonsmoker	Mortality ratio Cigarette smoker
U.S. veterans	290,000 males	34,874	1.00	1.58
ACS 9-State study	188,000 males	5,297	1.00	1.70
Japanese in 29 health	122,000 males	3,351	1.00	1.71
districts	143,000 females	2,653	1.00	1.78
ACS 25-State study	358,000 males	10,771	1.00	1.90–2.55
	483,000 females	4,048	1.00	•
Canadian veterans	78,000 males	3,405	1.00	1.60
British physicians	34,000 males	3,191	1.00	1.62
	6,195 females	179	1.00	•
Swedish study	27,000 males	916	1.00	1.70
	28,000 females	457	1.00	1.30
California males in 9 occupations	68,000 males	1,718	1.00	1.60
Swiss physicians	3,749 males	280	1.00	1.33–2.18

Source: Ref. 11.

the largest studies, which included over 20 million person-years of observation, smokers experienced a 70% greater CHD-related death rate than nonsmokers. Heavy cigarette smokers have CHD-related death rates 200–300% greater than nonsmokers. Cigarette smokers also experience a 200–400% greater incidence of CHD and risk for sudden death than nonsmokers.

Early studies documented lower CHD death rates for women than men; however, in more recent studies in women whose smoking patterns were similar to those of men, increased CHD risks were reported for women that were comparable to those of men (11). Cigarette smoking produces a greater relative CHD risk in younger smokers (those under the age of 50 years) than in those 50 years of age and older (12). The actual number of CHD deaths due to smoking is greater in older populations because of the rapid rise in CHD mortality with increasing age in both smokers and nonsmokers.

As exposure to cigarette smoke increases, CHD mortality increases (11). This dose–response relationship has been documented for the number of cigarettes smoked per day, the depth of inhalation, the age at which smoking began, and the number of years of smoking. There is no evidence that smoking cigarettes with reduced yields of tar and nicotine reduces CHD risk (13).

Cigarette smoking is a major risk factor for CHD that is independent of other major CHD risk factors such as hypertension and hypercholesterolemia. When other major CHD risk factors are present, in addition to smoking, a multiplicative increase in CHD risk results. The net effect is that the presence of two risk factors may produce a fourfold increase in CHD risk, and the presence of three risk factors may produce an eightfold increase in CHD risk (Fig. 1) (1,92).

Some CHD risk factor interactions have been studied. Cigarette smoking decreases the high-density lipoprotein (HDL)/low-density lipoprotein (LDL) cholesterol ratio (14). Smokers who are hypertensive are more likely to develop malignant hypertension and to die from hypertensive complications than hypertensive patients who are nonsmokers (12). Smokers whose families are at high risk for CHD, such as those with familial hypercholesterolemia, may be especially vulnerable to the harmful effects of smoking (15). Diabetic smokers also have a greatly increased risk for CHD mortality (1). Women who smoke and use oral contraceptives concurrently have a markedly increased risk for CHD (12).

2. *Pathologic*

Both prospective studies with autopsy follow-up and autopsy studies with retrospective smoking data have shown that cigarette smoking contributes to the development of atherosclerosis. This effect is most marked for aortic atherosclerosis, but it is also demonstrable for coronary atherosclerosis (11). Auerbach et al. (16) found more severe coronary atherosclerosis in cigarette smokers than

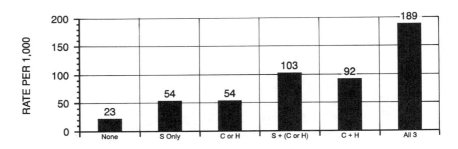

MAJOR RISK FACTOR COMBINATIONS

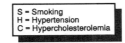

S = Smoking
H = Hypertension
C = Hypercholesterolemia

Figure 1   Ten-year incidence of first major coronary heart disease (CHD) event in men aged 30–39 years at entry, based on major risk factor combinations at entry. C, hypercholesterolemia, defined as >250 mg/dl; H, hypertension, defined as diastolic BP >90 mm Hg; S, any current use of cigarettes at entry. All rates were age-adjusted by 10-year age groups to the U.S. white male population (from Refs. 1,61).

nonsmokers and also noted a dose-response relationship. Former smokers' levels of atherosclerosis were intermediate between smokers and nonsmokers. Strong et al. performed a careful analysis of coronary atherosclerosis with a special emphasis on evaluation of lesions, collection of smoking information, and problems of autopsy selection (17). They reported that coronary atherosclerosis was more extensive in heavy smokers than in nonsmokers.

Angiographic studies have confirmed that coronary atherosclerosis is increased in smokers compared to nonsmokers (18,19). Autopsy studies have also shown increased intimal thickening of intramyocardial arteries and arterioles in smokers compared to nonsmokers; such lesions may contribute to a cardiomyopathy that is associated with smoking (12,20).

Endothelial injury is thought to be an important factor leading to the development of atherosclerosis. Experimental studies have shown that cigarette smoke exerts a toxic endothelial effect. Davis et al. reported that cigarette smoking produced an acute endothelial desquamating effect in male patients with CHD (21). Asmussen and Kjeldsen noted degenerative endothelial changes in the umbilical arteries of mothers who smoked; this endothelial damage was not observed in the umbilical arteries of nonsmoking mothers (22).

3. *Experimental and Clinical*

The pathogenesis of CHD is multifactorial, complex, and incompletely understood. Cigarette smoking contributes to both the chronic atherosclerotic process and acute ischemic, occlusive, and arrhythmic coronary events (11).

There are several possible mechanisms through which smoking contributes to the development of atherosclerosis (23). Toxic tobacco smoke constituents such as nicotine and carbon monoxide or other constituents, such as an antigenic glycoprotein, may cause repetitive endothelial injury. Lipid infiltration of the arterial intima is a major feature of atherosclerosis; cigarette smoking decreases the HDL/LDL cholesterol ratio and this may promote lipid deposition in the intima. Another characteristic of atherosclerosis is intimal smooth muscle proliferation. Cigarette smoking is associated with increased adherence of platelets to arterial endothelium. Adherent platelets may release mediators that promote proliferation and migration of smooth muscle into the arterial intima (11,24). Other atherosclerosis-promoting mechanisms have been proposed such as smoking-induced abnormalities in the synthesis of thromboxane A_2 and prostacyclin in apparently healthy individuals (25). Such an effect may lead to platelet and intimal dysfunction.

In normal individuals inhalation of cigarette smoke produces several nicotine-mediated, acute cardiovascular responses such as increases in blood pressure, heart rate, cardiac output, and coronary blood flow. With repetitive nicotine dosing by the smoker, a cyclic hyperadrenergic state results. In smokers with significant coronary artery stenosis, coronary blood flow may not increase or may decrease, despite the increase in myocardial oxygen demand; the resulting imbalance between oxygen supply and demand may precipitate a clinical coronary event (26,32).

Other smoking-mediated mechanisms impair delivery of oxygen to the myocardium, an effect that may be clinically important in those with CHD. For example, cigarette smokers are chronically exposed to low levels of carbon monoxide. The resulting elevation of carboxyhemoglobin causes cellular hypoxia by reducing the total amount of oxygen carried by red cells and by shifting the oxyhemoglobin dissociation curve to the left, which in turn reduces the amount of oxygen released at the cellular level. Allred et al. showed in men with CHD that low level carboxyhemoglobin elevations, found commonly in smokers, exacerbated myocardial ischemia during graded exercise (27).

Thrombosis plays a key role in most cases of acute myocardial infarction. Cigarette smokers demonstrate increased platelet adhesiveness, aggregation, and activation (24). In several cross-sectional studies increased fibrinogen levels have been found in smokers compared to nonsmokers (24). These elevated fibrinogen levels have, in turn, been associated with an increased CHD risk, independent of other CHD risk factors. With smoking cessation, fibrinogen levels return to the levels observed in nonsmokers. Thus, cigarette smoking may mediate some of its acute adverse effects through contributing to a hypercoagulable state.

Spasm of the coronary arteries is an important cause of myocardial ischemia and infarction. Cigarette smoking exerts well-documented vasoconstrictive effects on the coronary circulation (26,32). Smokers are much more likely than nonsmokers to experience vasospastic angina pectoris (28). Some of this effect may be mediated by acute increases in platelet and plasma vasopressin that occur with smoking (24).

Cardiac arrhythmias may precipitate an acute myocardial infarction and may constitute one of the major complications of acute myocardial infarction. Studies in animals have documented that cigarette smoking decreases the ventricular fibrillation threshold (29). Sudden death, which is usually due to a lethal arrhythmia, accounts for more than 50% of all coronary deaths; cigarette smokers have a 200–400% greater chance than nonsmokers of experiencing sudden death (11).

CHD presents as one of several clinical syndromes including angina pectoris, variant angina pectoris, nonfatal acute myocardial infarction, fatal acute myocardial infarction, silent myocardial ischemia, and sudden death. Smoking exerts a deleterious effect on these various manifestations of CHD. Patients with stable angina pectoris, who smoke, have a worse prognosis than those who do not smoke (30). Barry et al. recently demonstrated, with continuous ambulatory monitoring of patients with stable angina pectoris, that smokers had ischemic episodes that were 3 times more frequent and 12 times more sustained than nonsmokers (31). Most of these ischemic events were silent. Variant angina pectoris is more commonly seen in smokers than in nonsmokers (28). Patients who have had an acute myocardial infarction and continue to smoke are more likely to experience a recurrent acute myocardial infarction and sudden death than those who quit smoking (33).

B. Smoking Cessation and CHD Risk Reduction

Epidemiologic studies in apparently healthy men and women have consistently shown a decrease in CHD risk with smoking cessation. Case–control, cohort, and interventional studies have yielded the same result: smoking cessation is beneficial and reduces CHD risk (24). Studies in patients with diagnosed CHD have likewise shown that smoking cessation reduces the likelihood of additional morbidity and mortality from CHD. The reduction in CHD risk is independent of baseline differences between continuing smokers and those who quit smoking (34).

1. Studies of Apparently Healthy Smokers

The results of case–control studies are summarized in Table 5 (24). Current smokers had a CHD risk that was, on average, three times greater than that of nonsmokers. Former smoker CHD risk declined over time and was often the same as that of nonsmokers within 3 years of quitting. These studies are notable because they documented the benefits of smoking cessation for men less than 55 years of age and for women less than 50 years of age.

The results of very large cohort studies are summarized in Table 6 (11). In each of these studies smoking cessation resulted in a reduction in CHD risk. Smokers with a greater lifetime exposure to cigarettes had some residual CHD risk that was proportional to their total smoke exposure. Preliminary data from a new American Cancer Society cohort study with more than 1.2 million participants were recently published (1). This study documented that the benefits of cessation may be delayed in those who quit because of symptomatic illness and that some residual CHD risk may persist in former smokers for several years (24). A recent large cohort study of 119,404 female nurses is important because it demonstrated the benefits of smoking cessation in women (35). More recently published cohort studies on CHD and smoking cessation were summarized in the 1990 Report of the Surgeon General (24). These studies corroborate and amplify those described previously.

Intervention trials have extended the knowledge base on CHD and risk factor modification. In these studies investigators attempted to modify coronary risk factors in individual patients or groups and to follow the CHD experience of the intervention group compared to the control group. Such studies pose challenging problems in design and analysis, such as assessing the independent effect of smoking cessation. The results of the major intervention trials are summarized in Table 7 (24). In the Multiple Risk Factor Intervention Trial mortality rates for CHD were 10.6% lower for men who received special intervention than in men who received usual care (36). Those who quit smoking had more than a 40% reduction in CHD mortality compared to continuing smokers. The Whitehall intervention

Table 5 Case–Control Studies of CHD Risk among Former Smokers

Reference	Population	Number of cases	Number of controls	Source of controls	Number of cases among former smokers	Relative risk as compared with never smokers[a]	
						Former smokers	Current smokers
Willett et al. (1981)	Nurses Health Study: women aged 30–55	263	5,260	Nested in cohort	29	Overall 1.0 (0.7–1.6) Quit 1–4 yr 1.5 (0.7–3.1) Quit 5–9 yr 1.5 (0.8–3.0) Quit ≥10 yr 0.6 (0.3–1.3)	3.0 (2.3–4.0)
Rosenberg, Kaufman, Helmrich, Shapiro (1985)	Eastern US men aged <55	1,873	2,775	Hospital-based	348	1.1 (0.9–1.4)	2.9 (2.4–3.4)
Rosenberg, Kaufman, Helmrich, Miller et al. (1985)	Eastern US women aged <50	555	1,864	Hospital-based	35	1.0 (0.7–1.6)	1.4–7.0 depending on cig/day
LaVecchia et al. (1987)	Italian women aged <55	168	251	Hospital-based	3	0.8 (0.2–3.8)	3.6–13.1 depending on cig/day
Rosenberg, Palmer, Shapiro (1990)	Eastern US women aged <65	910	2,375	Hospital-based	149	Overall 1.2 (1.0–1.7) Quit <24 mo 2.6 (1.8–3.8) Quit 24–35 mo 1.3 Quit ≥36 mo 0.8–1.1	3.6 (3.0–4.4)

[a]95% confidence interval shown in parentheses when available.
Source: Ref. 24.

Table 6 Cessation of Smoking and Coronary Heart Disease Mortality Ratios, Prospective Studies

Study	Continuing smoker		Exsmoker	
U.S. veterans	1.58		1.16	
Swedish males	1.70		1.50	
females	1.30		1.50	
American Cancer Society 25-state males	1–19[a]	20+	1–19	20+
	1.87	2.05	1.26	1.62
Canadian veterans	1.60		1.46	
British physicians males	1.62		1.29	
Japanese males in 29 health districts	1.71		1.34	

[a]Number of cigarettes smoked daily.
Source: Ref. 11.

trial was unique because it was the only study designed to assess the effect of smoking cessation, alone, on CHD mortality (24). There was a 19% reduction in CHD mortality in the intervention group compared to the normal care group.

2. Studies of Patients with Coronary Heart Disease

Studies of smoking cessation in patients with diagnosed CHD usually deal with survivors of an acute myocardial infarction, but they may also include those who were smokers at the time angina pectoris was diagnosed and those who smoked at the time CHD was diagnosed by angiography. Twenty studies have been published in which the CHD experience of persistent smokers was compared with that of those who quit smoking (24). Mulcahy summarized the results of several of these investigations and concluded that those who quit smoking experience about one-half the risk experienced by continuing smokers for a recurrent myocardial infarction or CHD death (37).

3. Implications

The studies reviewed in this section document the efficacy of smoking cessation for primary and secondary prevention of CHD. Within 1 year after stopping smoking, an approximately 50% reduction in CHD risk occurs; thereafter, a more gradual decline in CHD risk occurs over several years (24). This pattern of CHD risk reduction is consistent with the pathophysiological mechanisms described in a prior section: smoking contributes to acute coronary events and to the chronic atherosclerotic process.

VI. SMOKING CESSATION STRATEGIES IN CLINICAL PRACTICE

A behavioral revolution has occurred in the United States. Millions of cigarette smokers have quit smoking, and the ranks of former smokers are increasing by 1.3

Table 7 Intervention Trials of Smoking Cessation and CHD Risk

Reference[a]	Population	Intervention	Outcome
Hughes et al. (1981); MRFIT Research Group (1982, 1986); Grimm (1986)	MRFIT: 12,866 healthy US men aged 35–57 at high CHD risk	Diet, reduction in weight, hypertension, and smoking	CHD deaths
Ockene et al. (1990)	MRFIT: 7,663 participant smokers at entry	Diet, reduction in weight, hypertension, and smoking	CHD deaths
	MRFIT: 6,943 participant smokers at entry	Diet, reduction in weight, hypertension, and smoking	CHD deaths
Hjermann et al. (1981)	Oslo study: 1,232 healthy Oslo men aged 40–49 at high CHD risk	Diet and smoking	Fatal and nonfatal MI
Kornitzer et al. (1983)	19,409 male Belgian factory workers, aged 40–59	Antismoking, hypertension control	Fatal and nonfatal MI
Rose, Tunstall-Pedoe, Heller (1983)	12 pairs of factories in UK. 18,210 men aged 40–59	Diet, antismoking, hypertension control	Nonfatal MI and CHD deaths
Rose et al. (1982)	1,445 healthy British civil servants all smoking at high CHD risk	Antismoking advice	CHD deaths
Wilhelmsen et al. (1986)	10,004 random Göteborg men aged 45–55	Antihypertensive, dietary, antismoking advice	Major CHD

[a]These references are from the original report and are not cited in this chapter.
Source: Ref. 24.

million persons each year. Smoking is no longer considered "normal" or, in many settings, socially acceptable. Of all adults who smoked during the year 1985–1986, 70% had made one or more serious quit attempts during their lifetime, and one-third stopped smoking for at least 1 day during that year (1). Unfortunately, only about 8% of those who try to quit are successful each year (38).

Table 7 Continued

Cases among former smokers	Overall effect of intervention	Effect of smoking cessation (nonrandomized)
15	7% decline in intervention group	44% reduction compared with persistent smokers
33	—	Quitters had 42% reduction (16–60%) comparing quitters at first annual exam to smokers at that time
12	—	Quitters had 65% reduction (37–80%) comparing 3-yr persistent quitters with persistent smokers
16	47% decline in intervention group	Smoking cessation accounted for about 25% of the difference between the groups
169	24.5% reduction in intervention group	No specific analysis conducted for effect of smoking cessation
403	4% net reduction in prevalence of current smoking, virtually no difference in outcome between the two groups	No specific analysis of ex-smokers
49	19% reduction in intervention group	19% CHD reduction in group offered antismoking advice, not statistically significant
NR	No difference	Intervention achieved only small differences between the groups for smoking and other risk factors

A. Cessation and the Patient

Peer pressure and other psychosocial forces in the teenage years usually lead to initiation of cigarette smoking. Smoking is often maintained because of tobacco addiction: smokers continue to smoke to avoid the psychological and physiological withdrawal associated with cessation. The influence of personal, social, and economic factors also contributes to continuation of smoking. The most important influence motivating smokers to consider quitting is personal concern about the adverse health effects of tobacco products. Social concerns and influences may also play an important motivational role in quitting, such as wanting to set a good example for children, receiving pressure from family and friends to quit, and sensing public disapproval of smoking. The cost of cigarettes is an important reason to quit for only about 10% of both current and former U.S. cigarette smokers (39). According to the U.S. 1986 Adult Use of Tobacco Survey, about 90% of quitters used individual methods to stop smoking. Quitting "cold turkey" was by far the most effective method, accounting for 82% of successful quitters (38,40). Product-assisted methods, such as using nicotine-containing chewing gum, and formal cessation programs accounted for 5% and 2% of the quitters, respectively (39). Those who quit "cold turkey" were more likely to remain nonsmokers than those who were involved in cessation programs. This observation is not based on a clinical trial in which smokers were randomly assigned to unassisted or assisted cessation programs. Rather, it may mean that those who enter structured cessation programs are not able to stop smoking on their own. Formal cessation programs appear to serve a small population of smokers, including heavy smokers, who are at highest risk for the harmful effects of smoking (38). Smokers who were advised by physicians to stop smoking were nearly twice as likely to attempt to quit, compared to those who received no advice. Among successful quitters 66% succeeded after one or two attempts, 20% succeeded after three or four attempts, and 12% succeeded after five or six attempts (38).

B. Cessation and the Physician

Physicians have unique opportunities to promote smoking cessation. Approximately 70% of the nation's 54 million smokers visit a physician at least once a year, with the average smoker making 4.3 physician visits per year (41,43). Physicians have contact with patients when they are experiencing symptomatic disease; in this setting patients may be most responsive to a smoking cessation message. Patients view physicians' advice to stop smoking as important in making the decision to quit, and physicians rank smoking cessation as a very important health-promoting behavior (41).

Although physicians are in a key position to promote smoking cessation, many are not advising their patients to quit. For example, in a recent survey of Michigan adults, Anda et al. found that only 44% of respondents reported having ever been told to quit smoking by a physician (41). Surveys indicate that about half of physicians report advising their patient to stop smoking (42). Those most likely to receive smoking cessation advice included those with smoking-related disease, those who had smoked for longer periods, and those who had made three prior attempts to quit.

There are several deterrents to greater physician involvement in smoking cessation efforts. Most practicing physicians have not received formal training in counseling about smoking cessation, and few physicians feel confident about their skills or about the success of their counseling efforts (43). Other barriers include the lack of third-party reimbursement for counseling, concern that some patients may be alienated by counseling efforts, and the view held by some physicians that counseling is a low-priority item in the busy practice of medicine.

C. Scientific Data Base

Schwartz reviewed 416 smoking cessation trials performed in North America (44). The intervention methods included the following: self-help, educational, group therapy, medication, nicotine chewing gum, hypnosis, acupuncture, physician advice or counseling, aversive conditioning, self-monitoring, and multicomponent cessation programs. Because of problems in study design and methodology, useful comparisons between interventions could not be made. Most interventions produced 1 year quit rates that varied between 10 and 40%. The variation in cessation rates appeared to be due more to differences in the selection of smokers in the cessation trials than to significant differences in the treatment methods (1). Physician intervention, involving more than counseling, produced a median cessation rate of 23% at 1 year. When physician intervention was restricted solely to cardiac patients, the median cessation rate at 1 year was 43%, one of the highest of any cessation method reviewed (1).

Kottke et al. used meta-analysis to evaluate 39 controlled smoking cessation trials in clinical practice (45). The studied cessation techniques involved various combinations of counseling, distribution of self-help materials, prescription of nicotine gum, and other interventions such as hypnosis. The smoking cessation rates of unselected patients averaged 8.4% higher for intervention groups than for controls at 6 months and remained 5.8% higher at 12 months. The authors concluded that reinforcement of the smoking cessation message produced the successful outcomes. Thus they emphasize giving a clear nonsmoking message in a repetitive, consistent fashion that employs a variety of "delivery systems" such as personalized advice, printed self-help materials, the mass media, and smoke-free environments.

Nicotine gum has been studied in several randomized controlled trials of smoking cessation (4). When used alone it has not been effective. When used correctly and in combination with physician counseling, it enhances long-term smoking cessation rates by about one-third. It may be especially helpful for those who are very nicotine dependent (4). Other drugs such as clonidine may prove to be useful, but data are not adequate to allow firm recommendations on their use at this time.

Brief, effective smoking cessation messages can be provided by physicians during routine office visits. In a recent study of such a physician intervention, Cummings et al. found physician counseling to be at least as cost-effective as many other accepted medical practices such as treating mild hypertension and hypercholesterolemia (46).

The cessation stage model of Prochaska and Diclemente suggests that smoking cessation involves more than the decision to quit (1,44). According to this model stopping smoking involves four steps occurring over time: precontemplation, contemplation, cessation, and maintenance. In the precontemplation phase smokers ignore or are indifferent to cessation messages. During the contemplation phase, smokers consider quitting and evaluate smoking cessation data. In the cessation stage smokers have not smoked for less than 6 months. The maintenance phase involves long-term abstinence from smoking. The implications of this model include tailoring physician messages to a specific stage, such as helping the "precontemplator" to consider stopping smoking.

D. Physician Education

1. *Knowledge Base*

In order to assist smokers effectively to quit smoking, physicians should possess a fundamental knowledge of smoking cessation. This data base includes knowledge of the potential impact that physicians may exert on smoking cessation, the health effects of smoking and of smoking cessation, the obstacles to quitting, and factors associated with successful smoking cessation.

Physicians should view cigarette smoking as a clinical opportunity to help the patient achieve better health and as a chronic medical problem that requires skillful treatment and follow-up. Management of this problem is at least as cost-effective as that of treating other CHD risk factors such as mild hypertension and hypercholesterolemia. Even with just brief physician counseling, sustained 5% cessation rates can be expected. In an individual practice this may not appear significant; however, when such a success rate is projected to the entire U.S. smoking population, approximately 2.1 million additional smokers would quit each year (39). As already noted, cardiac patients are especially responsive to smoking cessation messages. Sixty-three percent smoking cessation rates have been reported in patients hospitalized with an acute myocardial infarction (43). Patients at high risk for CHD may also be especially responsive to smoking cessation messages; in such individuals 1 year cessation rates of 50% have been observed (43).

Although patients are aware of the health risks of smoking, they often do not understand the relative significance of smoking as the most important cause of preventable death in the United States. Understanding how smoking contributes to the pathophysiology of CHD (see above) and how quitting smoking exerts a salutary impact on this process can be of value to patients considering quitting. For example, it is useful to point out to those in the contemplative or cessation stages that the risk of CHD decreases by approximately 50% within 1 year after quitting.

Because nicotine addiction is the major obstacle to quitting, physicians should be acquainted with the nicotine withdrawal syndrome and be prepared to help the patient cope with it. Features of the syndrome include: 1. craving for nicotine; 2. irritability, frustration, or anger; 3. anxiety; 4. difficulty concentrating; 5. restlessness; 6. decreased heart rate; 7. increased appetite or weight gain (9). Withdrawal may be detected within 2 hr of quitting, may peak within 24 hr of quitting, and usually decreases in intensity over a period of several days to a few weeks. Those experiencing the withdrawal syndrome can be reassured that it is not life-threatening, that intense cravings usually last only a few minutes, and that simple activities such as taking a walk can distract the quitter until the intense craving passes. Smokers should also appreciate that many former smokers failed at least once before they succeeded. Thus, continuing smokers should be encouraged to learn from their previous attempts to quit and to work toward another quit date.

Orleans has outlined factors associated with successful smoking cessation, including motivational factors, effective quitting skills, social supports, psychological assets, and smoking habit factors (48). Understanding and assessing these factors in an individual patient may allow the physician to develop a more effective, personalized cessation strategy.

2. Specific Skills

Physicians should possess specific skills in order to assist patients effectively to quit smoking. The requisite skills include the ability to assess individual patient needs, to teach about the risks of smoking and the benefits of cessation, to counsel about quitting, to prescribe nicotine gum correctly, and to manage smoking effectively as a chronic medical problem.

Physician assessment skills include the ability to take a detailed smoking history and to determine if the patient is interested in quitting smoking. If the patient is not interested, the physician should be ready and able to help motivate the smoker to move from the precontemplative to the contemplative stage.

If the patient is interested in quitting, the physician should be able to assess the patient's medical status and to explain in a personally relevant fashion the risks of continuing to smoke and the benefits of quitting. The physician should also be able to allay concerns of smokers about quitting, such as fear of weight gain. Common patient concerns and possible physician responses are presented in Table 8 (49).

Counseling skills include the ability to provide a repetitive and clear recommendation to stop smoking, to encourage the patient to set a quit date, and to follow up with the patient to help prevent or deal with relapse.

The physician should understand the proper use, contraindications, and side effects of nicotine gum. The gum should not be used as an aid to tapering smoking and should only be used when the patient has stopped smoking. The gum should

Table 8 Responses to Patients' Common Questions and Concerns

1. Won't I gain weight if I stop smoking?
   Not every person who stops smoking gains weight.
   Average weight gains are small for people who do gain (5–10 lbs).
   The risks to health from smoking are far greater than the risks to health from a small weight gain.
   Don't diet now: there will be time after you are an established nonsmoker.
   Exercise is an effective technique to cope with withdrawal and to avoid weight gain.
   Avoid high-calorie snacks. Vegetables (such as carrot sticks) and fruits are good snacks.
2. I smoke only low-tar/low nicotine cigarettes, so I don't need to stop.
   There is no such thing as a safe cigarette.
   Many smokers inhale more often or more deeply to compensate for low nicotine levels in these cigarettes.
3. Is it better to stop "cold turkey" or over a long period of time?
   There is no "best way."
   Most successful former smokers quit "cold turkey."
4. What about insomnia?
   Many smokers report having problems sleeping after they stop smoking. If these symptoms are related to nicotine dependence, they should disappear within 2–3 weeks.
5. Why do I cough more now that I've stopped?
   About 20% of former smokers report an increase in coughing after they stop smoking. This is a temporay response thought to be caused by an increase in the lung's ability to remove phlegm, so it actually represents recovery of the lung's defense mechanisms.
6. Now that I've stopped, can I smoke a cigarette occasionally?
   No. Nicotine addiction seems to be retriggered quickly in most former smokers. Don't risk geting hooked again.
7. What should I do when I get an urge to smoke?
   Some people relieve cravings by chewing gum, sucking on a cinnamon stick, or eating a carrot stick.
   Cravings for cigarettes are a normal part of withdrawal.
   Most cravings last for only a few minutes and then subside.
   Cravings become rare after a few weeks.
   Use nicotine gum, if prescribed.
8. When I don't smoke, I feel restless, and I can't concentrate.
   These are normal symptoms of nicotine withdrawal.
   These symptoms are most acute in the first 3 days after stopping.
   These symptoms will disappear after a few weeks.
9. What other withdrawal symptoms will I have?
   Some smokers have few or no withdrawal symptoms.
   Other common symptoms include anxiety, irritability, mild headache, and gastrointestinal symptoms such as constipation.
   Few smokers experience all these symptoms.
   Like other symptoms, they are only temporary.

Table 8 Continued

10. I'd like to use the nicotine gum you recommend, but I'm afraid I'll become addicted to it. A small percentage of people do use nicotine gum for longer than the recommended 3–6 months. Most people are able to reduce the amount of nicotine gum they use gradually, without discomfort until they stop completely.

Source: Adapted from Ref. 49.

be chewed slowly and allowed to rest against the oral mucosa through which it is absorbed. When using the gum, the patient should not eat or drink. Most patients should use the gum for at least 3 months. The gum is contraindicated in women who are pregnant or nursing and in those who have had a recent myocardial infarction or serious arrhythmia. Patients with dentures and those who cannot chew should not receive the gum.

Follow-up skills include the ability to encourage the former smoker to remain a nonsmoker and to provide guidance to avoid relapse. The former smoker should throw away all cigarettes and smoking equipment, avoid situations formerly associated with smoking, develop coping mechanisms other than smoking, and establish networks of supportive friends and relatives.

If relapse occurs, the physician should attempt to help the patient learn from the experience and set another quit date. Relapse should not be viewed as a failure; rather, it is a step on the road to cessation (50). After relapse, some patients may benefit from referral to a structured cessation program.

3. Physician Training Programs

Training programs are now available for both physicians-in-training and practicing clinicians (51,52). These programs help provide physicians with the knowledge and skills discussed in the preceding section and help to recruit physicians to function as clinical counselors for smoking cessation.

E. Practical Guidelines for Physicians

The National Cancer Institute recently published a concise reference that summarizes current recommendations on how physicians can help their patients stop smoking (49). The four essential steps are listed in Table 9.

F. Multiple Roles for Physicians in Smoking Cessation

The prevalence of smoking among physicians has decreased from 53% in 1969 to approximately 10% in 1990 (53). Thus, most physicians are nonsmoking role

Table 9 How to Help Patients Stop Smoking

Ask about smoking at every opportunity.
  "Do you smoke?"
  "Are you interested in stopping smoking?"
  "Have you ever tried to stop before? If so, what happened?"
Advise all smokers to stop.
  State advice clearly and repetitively.
  Personalize the message to quit.
Assist the patient in stopping.
  Set a quit date.
  Provide self-help material.
  Consider prescribing nicotine gum.
Arrange follow-up visits.
  Make a follow-up appointment within 1–2 weeks after patient quits
  Reinforce nonsmoker status with telephone call.
  Deal with relapse in a positive and supportive fashion.

Source: Adapted from Ref. 49.

models, and increasing numbers of physicians are helping their patients to quit smoking.

Fiore et al. have suggested that physicians have other opportunities to prevent and control smoking by working in private offices, clinics, and hospitals (39). The National Cancer Institute has prepared an action plan on how to create a smoke-free office (49). Simple steps such as posting no-smoking signs, removing ash trays, providing smoking cessation literature, and eliminating all tobacco advertising from the waiting room can be effective.

Physicians are also needed to work with voluntary nonsmoking coalitions and with government to promote nonsmoking ordinances and legislation (see section on strategies for community and public health efforts).

G. Primary Prevention

More than 75% of smokers start to smoke when they are teenagers. Individuals in this age group tend to underestimate the harmful effects and addicting properties of tobacco products (54). Primary care physicians, especially pediatricians, can play an important role in helping children and teenagers to maintain a nonsmoking status. Promising school-based educational programs teach students to recognize social influences that encourage smoking and to develop behavioral skills to resist these influences (1). Early results from such programs suggest that addiction to tobacco products can be prevented in some teenagers (55,56). Physicians should also work to achieve a strict ban on smoking in all schools (53).

VII. STRATEGIES FOR COMMUNITY AND PUBLIC HEALTH EFFORTS

The multinational tobacco companies are pursuing profit-motivated local, national, and international strategies that, if realized, portend an even greater tobacco-caused epidemic. Government antismoking efforts in the United States have focused on educational programs, taxation, and legal restrictions. U.S. voluntary advocacy and lobbying groups also continue to pursue a broad antismoking agenda. Warner estimates that in the absence of the antismoking efforts, adult per capita cigarette consumption in the United States in 1987 would have been 79–87% higher than the level actually experienced. He also suggests that the antismoking campaign in the United States will result in the postponement or avoidance of 2.1 million smoking-related deaths between 1986 and 2000 (1).

New public health initiatives are needed. For example, a coalition of voluntary advocacy groups recently submitted 76 legislative recommendations to the U.S. Congress including the following: give the Food and Drug Administration authority over all tobacco products, severely restrict tobacco advertising and production, increase excise taxes on tobacco, eliminate tobacco farm price supports, ban distribution of free tobacco samples, and eliminate tax deductions for tobacco advertising (57).

Glynn recommends more public health programs to motivate smokers to quit, to make self-help materials more readily available, and to assist heavier smokers with cessation programs (58). Physicians are needed to work with advocacy and governmental groups in their efforts to confront industry initiatives and to promote a tobacco-free agenda.

VIII. INVOLUNTARY SMOKING

In recent years environmental tobacco smoke has been identified as a cause of disease, including lung cancer, in healthy nonsmokers (59). Glanz and Parmley have reviewed the data on environmental tobacco smoke and CHD (60). They summarized the results of 11 published epidemiologic studies on environmental tobacco smoke exposure and CHD risk. This exposure was associated with a 30% increase in risk for CHD death. They also reviewed a variety of physiological and biochemical data linking environmental tobacco smoke exposure to the development of CHD and concluded that environmental tobacco smoke causes CHD (61).

IX. CONCLUSIONS

Cigarette smoking accounts for one-sixth of all U.S. deaths, and CHD is the cause of a substantial number of these deaths. Cigarette smoking contributes to both the chronic atherosclerotic process and acute ischemic, occlusive, and arrhythmic coronary events. Smoking cessation reduces the risk of CHD for both those without apparent CHD and those with symptomatic CHD.

A behavioral revolution is occurring in the United States, with more than 1 million smokers quitting each year. Physicians can play an important role in assisting their patients to quit smoking by asking about their interest in quitting; strongly advising patients to stop smoking; assisting patients to stop smoking through setting a quit date, providing self-help materials, and prescribing nicotine gum; arranging for follow-up to reinforce the nonsmoker status; and, if necessary, dealing with relapse in a positive and supportive fashion.

Physicians should also take advantage of other opportunities to prevent and control smoking by helping children and teenagers maintain a nonsmoking status. In addition to serving as nonsmoking role models, physicians should work to eliminate smoking from private offices, clinics, and hospitals. Finally, physicians are needed to work with voluntary advocacy groups and public health organizations to confront profit-driven tobacco industry initiatives that, if realized, portend an even greater tobacco-caused epidemic.

REFERENCES

1. U.S. Department of Health and Human Services. Reducing the health consequences of smoking: 25 years of progress. A report of the Surgeon General. Public Health Service, Centers for Disease Control, Center for Chronic Disease Prevention and Health Promotion, Office on Smoking and Health. DHHS Publication No. (CDC) 89-8411, 1989:11–12.

2. Council on Scientific Affairs, American Medical Association. The worldwide smoking epidemic. JAMA 1990; 263:3312–18.

3. U.S. Department of Health and Human Services. Centers for Disease Control. Leads from the Morbidity and Mortality Weekly Report. Tobacco use by adults—United States, 1987. JAMA 1989; 262:2364–9.

4. U.S. Preventive Services Task Force. Guide to clinical preventive services: an assessment of the effectiveness of 169 interventions. Report of the U.S. Preventive Services Task Force. Baltimore: Williams & Wilkins, 1989:289.

5. Holbrook JH. Tobacco. In: Wilson JD, Braunwald E, Isselbacher RF, et al. (Eds). Harrison's principles of internal medicine, 12th ed. New York: McGraw-Hill, 1991:2158–61, chapter 373.

6. Holbrook JH. Physicians and smoking cessation. West J Med 1988; 149: 209–10.

7. American Psychiatric Association. Diagnostic and statistical manual of mental disorders, 3rd ed. Washington, DC, 1980:176–8.

8. American Psychiatric Association. Diagnostic and statistical manual of mental disorders, 3rd ed rev. Washington, DC, 1987:181–2.

9. U.S. Department of Health and Human Services. The health consequences of smoking: nicotine addiction. A report of the Surgeon General, 1988. Public Health Service, Centers for Disease Control, Center for Health Promotion and Education, Office on Smoking and Health. DHHS Publication No. CDC 88-8406, 1988:iv.

10. Hammond EC, Horn D. Smoking and death rates—report on forty-four months of follow-up of 187,783 men. I. Total mortality. JAMA 1958; 166:1159–72.

11. U.S. Department of Health and Human Services. The health consequences of smoking: cardiovascular disease. A report of the Surgeon General. Public Health Service, Office on Smoking and Health. DHHS Publication No. (PHS) 84-50204, 1983:iv–v.

12. Holbrook JH, Grundy SM, et al. Cigarette smoking and cardiovascular diseases. A statement for health professionals by a Task Force appointed by the Steering Committee of the American Heart Association. Circulation 1984; 70:1114–7A.

13. Kaufman D, Helmrich SP, et al. Nicotine and carbon monoxide content of cigarette smoke and the risk of myocardial infarction in young men. N Engl J Med 1983; 308:409–13.

14. Mjos OD. Lipid effects of smoking. Am Heart J 1988; 115:272–5.

15. Hopkins PS, Williams RR, et al. Magnified risks from cigarette smoking for coronary prone families in Utah. West J Med 1984; 141:196–202.

16. Auerbach O, Hammond EC, et al. Smoking in relation to atherosclerosis of the coronary arteries. N Engl J Med 1965; 273:775–9.

17. Strong JP, Richards ML. Cigarette smoking and atherosclerosis in autopsied men. Atherosclerosis 1976; 23:451–76.

18. Weintraub WS, Klein LW, et al. Importance of total life consumption of cigarettes as a risk factor for coronary artery disease. Am J Cardiol 1985; 55:669–72.

19. Fried LP, Moore RD, et al. Long-term effects of cigarette smoking and moderate alcohol consumption on coronary artery diameter. Mechanisms of coronary artery disease independent of atherosclerosis or thrombosis? Am J Med 1986; 80:31–44.

20. Hartz AJ, Anderson AJ, et al. The association of smoking with cardiomyopathy. N Engl J Med 1984; 311:1201–6.

21. Davis JW, Shelton L, et al. Comparison of tobacco and non-tobacco cigarette smoking on endothelium and platelets. Clin Pharmacol Ther 1985; 37:529–33.

22. Asmussen I, Kjeldsen K. Intimal ultrastructure of human umbilical arteries. Observations on arteries from newborn children of smoking and nonsmoking mothers. Circul Res 1975; 36:579–89.

23. Holbrook JH. Cigarette smoking and coronary heart disease. Proceedings of the Eighth International Symposium on Atherosclerosis, Rome. Amsterdam: Excerpta Medica, 1989:487–94.

24. U.S. Department of Health and Human Services. The health benefits of smoking cessation. A report of the Surgeon General. Public Health Service, Centers for Disease Control, Center for Chronic Disease Prevention and Health Promotion, Office on Smoking and Health. DHHS Publication No. (CDC) 90-8416,1990: 192–3.

25. Nowak J, Murray JJ, et al. Biochemical evidence of a chronic abnormality in platelet and vascular function in healthy individuals who smoke cigarettes. Circulation 1987; 76:6–14.

26. Winniford MD, Wheelan KR, et al. Smoking induced coronary vasoconstriction in patients with atherosclerotic coronary artery disease: evidence for adrenergically mediated alterations in coronary artery tone. Circulation 1986; 73:662–7.

27. Allred EN, Bleecker ER, et al. Short-term effects of carbon monoxide exposure on

the exercise performance of subjects with coronary artery disease. N Engl J Med 1989; 321:1426–32.

28. Scholl JM, Benacerraf, et al. Comparison of risk factors in vasospastic angina without significant fixed coronary narrowing to significant fixed coronary narrowing and no vasospastic angina. Am J Cardiol 1986; 57:199–202.

29. Bellet S, Deguzman NT, et al. The effect of inhalation of cigarette smoke on ventricular fibrillation threshold in normal dogs and dogs with acute myocardial infarction. Am Heart J 1972; 83:67–76.

30. Hubert HB, Holford TR, et al. Clinical characteristics and cigarette smoking in relation to prognosis of angina pectoris in Framingham. Am J Epidemiol 1982; 115:231–42.

31. Barry J, Mead K, et al. Effect of smoking on the activity of ischemic heart disease. JAMA 1989; 261:398–402.

32. Martin JL, Wilson JR, et al. Acute coronary vasoconstrictive effects of cigarette smoking in coronary heart disease. Am J Cardiol 1984; 54:56–60.

33. Hallstrom AP, Cobb LA, et al. Smoking as a risk factor for recurrence of sudden cardiac arrest. N Engl J Med 1986; 314:271–5.

34. Friedman GD, Siegelaub AB, et al. Characteristics predictive of coronary heart disease in ex-smokers before they stopped smoking. Comparison with persistent smokers and nonsmokers. J Chron Dis 1979; 32:175–90.

35. Willett WC, Green A, et al. Relative and absolute excess risks of coronary heart disease among women who smoke cigarettes. N Engl J Med 1987; 317:1303–9.

36. The Multiple Risk Factor Intervention Trial Research Group. Mortality rates after 10.5 years for participants in the Multiple Risk Factor Intervention Trial. JAMA 1990; 263:1795–801.

37. Mulcahy R. Influence of cigarette smoking on morbidity and mortality after myocardial infarction. Br Heart J 1983; 49:410–5.

38. Fiore MC, Novotny TE, et al. Methods used to quit smoking in the United States. Do cessation programs help? JAMA 1990; 263:2760–5.

39. Fiore MC, Pierce JP, et al. Cigarette smoking: the clinician's role in cessation, prevention, and public health. Disease-a-Month 1990; 35:4.

40. Centers for Disease Control. Tobacco use in 1986: methods and basic tabulations from adult use of tobacco survey. Rockville, MD: US Dept of Health and Human Services, 1989.

41. Anda RF, Remington PL, et al. Are physicians advising smokers to quit? The patient's perspective. JAMA 1987; 257:1916–9.

42. Ockene JK, Hosmer DW, et al. The relationship of patient characteristics to physician delivery of advice to stop smoking. J Gen Intern Med 1987; 2:337–40.

43. Stokes JF, III, Rigotti NA. The health consequences of cigarette smoking and the internist's role in smoking cessation. Adv Intern Med 1988; 33:431–60.

44. Schwartz JL. Review and evaluation of smoking cessation methods: United States and Canada, 1978–1985. U.S. Department of Health and Human Services, Public Health Service, National Institutes of Health. NIH Publication No. 87-2940, 1987.

45. Kottke TE, Battista RN, et al. Attributes of successful smoking cessation interventions in medical practice. A meta-analysis of 39 controlled trials. JAMA 1988; 259:2883–9.

46. Cummings SR, Rubin SM, et al. The cost-effectiveness of counseling smokers to quit. JAMA 1989; 261:75–9.

47. Prochaska JO, Diclemente CC. Stages and processes of self-change of smoking: toward an integrative model of change. J Consult Clin Psychol 1983; 51:390–5.

48. Orleans CT. Understanding and promoting smoking cessation: overview and guidelines for physician intervention. Annu Rev Med 1985; 36:51–61.

49. Glynn TJ, Manley MW: How to Help Your Patients Stop Smoking—A National Cancer Institute Manual for Physicians. National Cancer Institute, NIH Pub No. 89-3064, 1989:37–39.

50. Fisher EB, Jr, Rost K. Smoking cessation: A practical guide for the physician. Clin in Chest Med 1986; 7:551–565.

51. Ockene JK, Ouirk ME, et al. A residents' training program for the development of smoking intervention skills. Arch Int Med 1990; 148:1039–1045.

52. Cummings SR, Coates TJ, et al. Training physicians in counseling about smoking cessation: A randomized trial of "Quit for Life" program. Ann Int Med 1989; 110: 640–647.

53. Petty TL. Where do we go from here in smoking cessation? Semin Respir Med 1990; 11:115.

54. Leventhal H, Glynn K, et al. Is the smoking decision an "informed choice?" JAMA 1987; 257:3373–6.

55. Perry CL. Results of prevention programs with adolescents. Drug Alcohol Depend 1987; 20:13–9.

56. DuPont RL. Prevention of adolescent chemical dependency. Pediatr Clin North Am 1987; 34:495–505.

57. American Medical Association. Recommendations from the Tobacco Use in America conference, Chicago, Illinois, 1990.

58. Glynn TJ. Methods of smoking cessation—finally, some answers. JAMA 1990: 263: 2795–6.

59. U.S. Department of Health and Human Services. The health consequences of involuntary smoking. A report of the Surgeon General. Public Health Service, Centers for Disease Control. DHHS Publication No. (CDC) 87-8398, 1986.

60. Glantz SA, Parmley WW. Passive smoking and heart disease: epidemiology, physiology, and biochemistry. Circulation 1991; 83:1–12.

61. Pooling Project Research Group. Relationship of blood pressure, serum cholesterol, smoking habit, relative weight and ECG abnormalities to incidence of major coronary events. Final Report of the Pooling Project. J Chron Dis 1978; 31:201–306.

11

Obesity

TIMOTHY G. BUTLER
Intermountain Health Care
Health Plans, Inc.
Salt Lake City, Utah

FRANK G. YANOWITZ
The Fitness Institute
LDS Hospital
and University of Utah School of Medicine
Salt Lake City, Utah

I. INTRODUCTION

Obesity is generally defined as an excess of body fat that frequently results in significant impairment of health. While the medical importance of excess fat weight has been debated for decades, the current consensus was articulated in 1985 by the National Institutes of Health Consensus Development Panel on the Health Implications of Obesity (1): "The evidence is now overwhelming that obesity, defined as excessive storage of energy in the form of fat, has adverse effects on health and longevity."

The term "obesity" is, in a sense, a misnomer and a source of confusion. Its use in common parlance is vague and projects the notion that the condition is basically homogeneous in nature, characterized by a common cause and predictable consequences. In fact, obesity is best thought of as a cluster of disorders that share the common characteristic of excess adiposity. These "obesities" can be differentiated as Stunkard (2) has suggested, on the basis of percentage overweight and, as Bray (3) has proposed, on the basis of fat distribution patterns, anatomical characteristics, age of onset, and causative factors. The complex nature of obesity is such that it is extremely difficult to treat, its health consequences do not extend uniformly to everyone with the condition, and its biological effects are commonly manifested over many years. Furthermore, even mild obesity may be exacerbated or perpetuated by obscure and convoluted psychosocial dynamics as well as independent coexisting medical problems.

A recent review by Kraemer et al. (4) emphasizes the importance of differentiating the medical problems of obesity from the cosmetic and societal problems of fatness. To avoid confusion created by diverse methodologic approaches to studying obesity, researchers have proposed a clarification of terms (4). The term *obesity* should be used in reference to a degree of excess body fat sufficient to impair health. In contrast, *overweight* simply means a weight above some arbitrary standard defined for a particular category of age, height, and gender. *Leanness* can be used to describe the state of body composition that not only lacks excess fat but also is within the range conducive to optimal health and minimal risk. The antithesis of obesity, such as found in anorexia, is *emaciation*, which is the condition of deficient body fat sufficient to impair health. Other terms used in discussions of obesity include *thin* and *fat*, which are based on social standards that vary over time and among cultures. References to weight such as ideal, desirable, average, or relative are terms that have meaning within the context of a specific sample population and its statistical characteristics. Terms such as *ideal* and *desirable* refer to weights, which, for a given combination of age, height, and gender, are associated with the lowest mortality.

Obesity shares some of the characteristics of other chronic diseases. As with diabetes, heart disease, and hypertension, early detection and intervention are required to maximize treatment outcomes. Consistency in following the recommended treatment is essential; periodic evaluations and therapeutic adjustments are also to be expected. Similar to the challenges presented by these other common disorders, those with obesity may be reluctant to enter into treatment, may find the side effects or cost of treatment unacceptable, or may be inconsistent and ultimately unsuccessful in implementing treatment strategies.

In almost all cases the therapeutic objective must be a relatively stable managed remission, in contrast to a cure (5). In addition, the management of obesity must entail modifying lifestyle habits that have been formed over many years and that cannot be restructured quickly or easily. For many, the struggle for change and better health means participating in a personal transformation that at times is arduous and is never fully completed. For some, obesity and familiar patterns of food use represent a powerful and special kind of addiction that will require great perseverance to transcend.

Obesity is also a perplexing and frustrating problem confronting the modern health care professional. Physicians often feel compelled to encourage their obese patients to lose pounds for medical reasons; patients are likewise driven by both a desire for better health and a host of powerful emotional and social concerns. In the United States especially, the past 5 years have been characterized by intensified commercial and professional activities in weight control. Americans are in pursuit of dieting with a vengeance. An estimated 65 million Americans report dieting each year. In the process, they support a mammoth weight loss business, which generated $32 billion in revenues in 1989, and is projected to produce $50 billion by 1995 (6).

A vast array of commercial and medical programs now floods the marketplace, making it more difficult than ever for the consumer to choose from them. Many promise the ultimate quick and easy answer to the struggle for losing and controlling weight, despite the fact that health professionals have long recognized obesity as a complex, chronic disorder that is generally resistant to treatment (7). The multifarious causes of obesity, with its many permutations of contributing factors—age, gender, physical activity level, dietary habits, complicating medical problems, genetic influences, sociocultural and psychological factors—makes effective intervention difficult at best, especially for those who need help the most (8). Brownell contends that if a "cure" for obesity is defined as reduction to desired weight and maintenance of that weight for 5 years, it is more likely that a person will be cured of most forms of cancer than of obesity (9).

Despite its rather dismal history, treatment for obesity now holds new possibilities due to the last several decades of accumulated research and clinical practice. This chapter reviews the nature and scope of the problem, probable causative factors, associated health risks, useful assessment and classification techniques, therapeutic guidelines, and future perspectives.

II. HISTORICAL PERSPECTIVE

Obesity would have been rare among Paleolithic humans as it is today among preindustrial societies. Nevertheless, there is evidence that obesity was part of the prehistoric human experience (10). One of the earliest artifacts indicating obesity is the Venus of Wellendorf, a small Stone Age statue believed to be about 25,000 years old. The statue depicts an obese woman with large pendulous breasts and protruding abdomen. This, along with other similar statues, is believed to represent a mother-goddess figure. It would seem from these and other prehistoric representations, mostly of women, that such fleshy endomorphic physiques were once revered symbols of abundance and fertility.

The obese who lived in times of feast or famine may have had an anatomical advantage over their thin counterparts and an increased chance of survival. Obesity may be seen as unhealthy and maladaptive in the context of modern society in which, for most individuals, there is an abundance of food and a minimum of imposed physical activity. Yet over the course of human history the development of "thrifty" genotypes during the Paleolithic period was most likely a necessary metabolic compromise during times when the food supply depended on the luck and skill of the hunter. This genetic adaptation evolved to enable some of the species to store greater amounts of fat in less time and release it as stingily as possible over the long run. Fat stores would have been especially protective for women during pregnancy and lactation (11). Given the value of such energy storage efficiency over many thousands of years, it should not be surprising that a significant portion of modern populations still carry this once adaptive genetic predisposition (12). Our current struggle against corpulence is likely the vestige of a process of natural selection that has contributed to the survival of the species.

Although prehistoric societies may have revered corpulence, at least among women, there are indications that this view drastically changed in early recorded history. In the 5th century before the Christian era, for example, Hippocrates wrote that

> "sudden death is more common in those who are naturally fat than in the lean. . . . Obese people with laxity of muscle and red complexion because of their moist constitution, need dry food during the greatest part of the year. . . . Obese people and those desiring to lose weight should perform hard work before food. Meals should be taken after exertion and while still panting from fatigue. . . . They should, moreover, eat only once a day and take no baths and sleep on a hard bed, and walk naked as long as possible" (13).

Socrates, in 399 before the Christian era, is said to have warned the overweight to "beware of those foods that tempt you to eat when you are not hungry and those liquors that tempt you to drink when you are not thirsty" (14). Galen, the pre-eminent physician who lived in the 2nd century, was a dominant authority in medicine, setting standards of practice that stood for 1,300 years. He identified two classifications of obesity that he termed moderate and immoderate. The first he regarded as natural; the second, as morbid. He wrote, in a rather judgmental tone, "the hygienic art promises to maintain in good health those who obey it; but those who are disobedient, it is just as if it did not exist at all" (13).

Presaging the contemporary medical consensus, 18th century Scottish physicians viewed obesity as a disease. Malcom Flemyng, M.D., wrote in 1760 that "corpulency when in extraordinary degree, may be reckoned as a disease, as it in some measure obstructs the free exercise of animal functions; and hath a tendency to shorten life, by paving the way to dangerous distempers" (13). Tweedy, at the end of the century, concurred: "Corpulency is in very different degrees in different persons; and may be often considerable without being considered a disease; however, there is a certain degree of it which will generally be allowed to be a disease" (13).

Finally, in 1883, William Beaumont expressed the seeming essence of the struggle that afflicts so many of us today (15): "In the present state of civilized society with the provocation of the culinary art, and the incentive of highly seasoned foods, brandy and wine, the temptation to excess in the indulgences of the table are rather too strong to be resisted by poor human nature."

How ironic that a species that has demonstrated the resiliency to survive over tens of thousands of years, often enduring recurrent food shortages and famine, should now find its health and longevity compromised by a seeming inability to adapt to the consistent abundance available to most postindustrial populations.

III. PREVALENCE AND INCIDENCE

The numbers of overweight adult men and women in the United States have been steadily increasing over the past several decades (16). Recent estimates of overweight people in a national sample of U.S. adults indicate that the prevalence is higher among those 45 years and older (17). The data also suggest that the prevalence has increased most dramatically among women (18).

According to the second National Health and Nutrition Examination Survey completed in 1980, 26% of Americans (34 million) were considered overweight, that is, at least 20% over the desirable weight level. More than 12 million of these people were categorized as severely obese based on measures of skinfold thickness and body mass index (BMI; weight in kg/height in meters^2) (19). For both black and white men between ages 25 and 55, there was an increase in the prevalence of being overweight. This declined for both races after age 55. For women up to age 65 there was a steady increase in prevalence of overweight for both races, after which it tapered off slightly. Sharp increases were noted for black women between ages 25 and 35, and between 45 and 55. In the latter group there were twice as many obese black women as white women. Men below the economic poverty line were only slightly more likely to be overweight than those above the poverty line. By contrast, women below the poverty line had a much higher prevalence of overweight than those of higher economic status.

Recognizing that the prevalence of obesity generally increases with age, it is important to gain an understanding of the incidence of weight gain and overweight in order to elucidate the developmental nature of this chronic disorder over a lifespan. A recent study by Williamson et al. (20) sampled 3,722 men and 6,135 women, ages 25–74 years, to determine the incidence of major weight gain (defined as an increase in BMI >5 kg/m^2) and overweight (BMI >27.8 kg/m^2 for men, >27.3 kg/m^2 for women) over a 10 year period. For persons not overweight at baseline, both men and women were most likely to experience major weight gain between the ages of 35 and 44 years. The incidence of major weight gain was twice as high among women (8.4%) as among men (3.9%) and was highest for persons in the age category 25–34 years, including those classified as overweight at baseline. The highest incidence of major weight gain (14.2%) was found among overweight women ages 25–44 years. For both men and women, nearly 75% of those who were not overweight at baseline were overweight when remeasured at follow-up evaluation.

Ethnic and racial differences similar to those of other studies were also revealed. Black women between ages 25 and 44 had higher baseline BMIs and were 30–40% more likely to have a major weight gain by the end of follow-up.

Among the subgroup of women not overweight at baseline, black women were twice as likely to become overweight by the end of the study (20).

While the second National Health and Nutrition Examination Survey showed that the prevalence of obesity is greatest for middle-aged men and among women over age 60, the incidence data suggest that earlier life periods are more critical for the development of obesity. These findings indicate that among U.S. adults, those in their 20s should be the primary targets for obesity prevention, and that young women, in particular, are most likely to experience major weight gain as they go through midlife.

IV. GENETIC FACTORS

A. Experimental Obesity in Animals

The importance of genetic and constitutional factors in the development of animal obesity has been recognized for many years. Genetic factors have been shown to influence total body weight, body composition, and organ size as demonstrated in studies of "yellow fat" in the laboratory mouse (21).

The genetically obese Zucker "fatty" rat is notorious for its capacity for fat storage (22). The Zucker rat is known to inherit its obesity as a single mendelian recessive gene from the mating of two heterozygous lean rats. The resulting obesity is characterized by near-normal growth accompanied by a massive accumulation of body fat as a consequence of both increase in fat cell size and number. These animals stubbornly resist feeding manipulations designed to reduce their body weight. Thus, the Zucker rat may represent a viable animal model for the resistance to weight loss often seen among humans who display early-onset severe obesity characterized by adipocyte hyperplasia (23). Schemmel and his colleagues (24) showed that even in the absence of such a powerful genetic propensity, among seven strains of rats fed high- and low-fat diets, there were significant differences in food intake, body composition, and body weight, which suggested that genetically transmitted individual differences could influence the degree of obesity across a broad range of weights.

B. Human Obesity

Genetic factors may play a primary or secondary role in the development of human obesity. When genetic factors are primary, obesity manifests as one of a group of rare diseases (3). These diseases are typically associated with characteristic dysmorphic features, often some degree of mental retardation and hypogonadism, and sometimes type II diabetes or congenital heart disease. Obesity in these syndromes usually begins in childhood, may be mild to extreme, and may include a distinctive pattern of fat deposition, such as the truncal obesity characteristic of persons with the Alstrom and Cohen syndromes. These rare diseases demonstrate the potentially powerful role of genetics in the genesis of human obesity, but they are quite easily differentiated from the pervasive obesity that is the common concern of all industrialized societies.

The tendency for obesity to occur in families was documented by Gurney (25) in 1936. This early study showed that if both parents were obese, 73% of the children were obese, whereas only 9% were obese if both parents were lean. With only one obese parent, 41% of the children were obese. While such data are provocative, they can be criticized on the grounds that only weight was used instead of more direct measures of fatness, and little can be said about differentiating environmental from genetic factors.

Since this early work a host of investigations have been conducted in an effort to discern why, under similar environmental conditions, some individuals are likely to become obese while others do not. To answer the question, researchers have explored the influence of inherited aspects of body build, the differential response of individuals to controlled feeding conditions, and variations in weight and body fat among fraternal and identical twins.

1. Genetic Influences on Body Build

Seltzer and Mayer (26), in a study of 180 obese adolescent girls, found the somatype, an inherited constitutional factor, to be strongly associated with the degree of obesity. Compared to nonobese girls, the obese endomorphic subjects (soft and round) were consistently higher in mesomorphy (muscularity) and considerably lower in ectomorphy (linearity and fragility). The authors concluded that obese girls differed from nonobese peers in morphologic features other than differences in amounts of fatty tissue. In terms of the combination of somatype components found in their physiques, the obese girls were judged to be more homogeneous and less variable than nonobese subjects.

It is presumed that persons with strong combined elements of endomorphy and mesomorphy are more predisposed to the layering on of fat unless caloric restriction, vigorous physical activity, or illness supervenes. In contrast, ectomorphic individuals appear to be resistant to obesity and are more able to satisfy their appetites without the fear of becoming fat (26).

2. Differential Responses to Caloric Intake

Marked individual differences in response to overfeeding and underfeeding have been shown repeatedly. These differences are presumed to be due, in part, to genetically transmissible influences on how efficiently the body extracts calories from food and how energy is expended. Sims (27) showed that there was a marked variation in the amount of weight gained by normal volunteers eating a large excess of calories. In addition, subjects who were lean initially required twice as many calories to maintain peak weight compared to those who were overweight at baseline.

Most recently, Bouchard and co-workers (28) studied individual responses to long-term overfeeding in twins to determine the possible role of genetic influences. Mean weight gains in response to overfeeding varied dramatically. There was significantly more similarity with respect to measures of weight gain and changes in subcutaneous fat and muscle mass within each pair than between pairs, suggesting that unspecified genetic factors influence the individual's tendency to store and distribute body fat.

3. Adoption and Twin Studies

Stunkard and his colleagues conducted extensive studies on adoptees and twins to determine the heritability of obesity. One study of adoptees used a sample of 540 adults from the Danish adoption registry (29). These subjects were organized into four classes; thin, median weight, overweight, and obese. Strong correlations were found between the weight class of the adoptees and the BMI of their biological parents but no relation between the adoptees' weight class and their adoptive parents. The correlations were significant across all four weight classes.

More recently, Stunkard et al. (30) studied fraternal and identical twins, classifying them into groups that had been reared apart or together. Identical twins reared apart had intrapair correlation coefficients for BMI of 0.70 for men and 0.66 for women, suggesting strong genetic influences on BMI. These results do not mean, however, that environmental conditions do not influence BMI and obesity. Rather, they underscore the heritability among specific genotypes living in a particular range of environmental conditions. Recent reviews of this subject have emphasized that while there is irrefutable evidence for the heritability of obesity, there is also equally abundant evidence for nongenetic influences (31,32). These reviews discuss numerous studies demonstrating the potentiating effects of changes in socioeconomic status, diet, and activity patterns on the development of obesity.

The high index of heritability found by Stunkard and others is in contrast to more moderate heritability estimates calculated by Bouchard and his colleagues in a study of twins and adoptees (33). In addition to studying BMI in these subjects, Bouchard looked at percentage body fat, skinfold measurements, and fat distribution patterns. Using all these measures of obesity, genetic effects accounted for only 5% of the variance for subcutaneous fat and BMI, but up to 30% for the variance of total body fat, fat free mass, and fat distribution. The authors noted that these heritability estimates differed among subpopulations of obese individuals.

C. Mechanisms of Genetic Influences

In considering the "nature vs. nurture" controversy, these studies point to the particular importance of the genotype–environment interaction. Isolating the role of genes will likely be far less productive than studying the phenotype (i.e., the physical characteristics of individuals) that results from the interaction of their genetic endowment with prevailing environmental conditions. It is now clear that for any given level of body fat, its physical expression can be highly variable and associated with very different clinical implications and health consequences (33). Likewise, for any set of prevailing lifestyle conditions, genetic factors will influence the extent of total body fat developed, the pattern of fat distribution, and the morphologic characteristics of the fat tissue in terms of fat cell hyperplasia or hypertrophy.

In addition, genetic factors are likely to influence the underlying processes that have an impact on energy balance and determine whether fat is stored. For example, it is well known that resting metabolic rate (RMR) accounts for approximately 60% of daily energy expenditure and that, in relation to lean body mass, RMR can vary among subjects by as much as ±20%. Energy expended through the body's thermic effect in response to a meal (TEM) and the thermic effect of exercise (TEE) can vary considerably among individuals (34). Of interest, Sims (35) has reported that obese subjects show a graded thermogenic response to meals that varies inversely with the degree of insulin resistance or impaired glucose tolerance. Bouchard (36) has proposed that at least 40% of the individual differences in RMR, TEM, and TEE are genotype dependent, and that slight genetic effects can be found for the proportion of fat, protein, and carbohydrate in the diet. Genetic influences on physical activity are not as well documented, but individual differences in maximal exercise capacity have been found to be under some genetic control (37).

Schull (38) has described the numerous biochemical pathways by which genetics may influence the development of obesity. Enzymatic defects may affect sodium–potassium pump function which accounts for 20–70% of total cellular thermogenesis. In addition, there are genetic differences in the action of sex hormone-binding-globulin (SHBG) and testosterone, which appear to affect fat distribution pattern and weight gain in both men and women (39). Lipoprotein lipase, the enzyme gatekeeper for the transport of lipid into adipocytes, may also be a mechanism for the genetic influence on obesity. Other biochemical mediators possibly under genetic control include serotonin (40,41), cholecystokinin, glucagon, and somatostatin, factors involved in the regulation of hunger and satiety, cravings for carbohydrates, and changes in mood (38). Clearly the opportunities for genetic influences on the development of obesity are numerous, varied, and complex.

Appreciation of these genotype–environment interactions will allow clinicians in the future to restrict rationally the size of the population targeted for intervention. Those with the greatest inherent susceptibility for particular forms of high-risk obesity can be identified for early and intensive intervention. Those whose excess adiposity is less threatening to health can be educated to deal with their weight concerns through moderate interventions involving nutrition and exercise strategies. In this way the emotional and financial burden on the patient can be minimized while appropriate utilization of health care resources can be optimized.

V. HEALTH IMPLICATIONS OF OBESITY

A. Obesity and Mortality

The fact that severe obesity can shorten life is not disputed. The influence of mild or moderate obesity, characterized by body weights 20–30% above average, on mortality has been controversial. Andres (42) concluded that the health risks of obesity were age-dependent and that the plethora of epidemiologic data relating obesity to increased mortality were inconsistent and inconclusive. Garrison et al. (43) found that cigarette smoking can seriously confound the relationship between body weight and mortality. As part of the Framingham Heart Study, these investigators showed that even modest degrees of overweight, 20% above desirable level, were associated with increased cardiovascular mortality.

More recently Manson et al. (44) reviewed 25 published prospective studies and revealed that each of the studies were flawed by at least one of three major types of biases: 1. failure to control for cigarette smoking, 2. inappropriate control of biological effects of obesity such as diabetes or hypertension, and 3. failure to control for low body weights that may be due to illness or subclinical disease. The authors concluded that these biases underestimate the impact of obesity on premature mortality and preclude a valid assessment of optimal weight from existing data. Nevertheless, available evidence indicates that minimum mortality is associated with relative weights at least 10% lower than the U.S. average weight. Furthermore, there is no convincing evidence for a protective effect of weights above average (44).

Bray (45) has analyzed several large-scale prospective studies that show a J or U-shaped curve relating mortality to body mass index (Fig. 1). Lowest mortality for both men and women occurs at weights somewhat below average. Mortality risk increases gradually between a BMI of 25 and 30 kg/m^2, and above 40 kg/m^2 the curve becomes steep, indicating high mortality risk. Causes of death among subjects below average weight include digestive and pulmonary diseases; those with elevated BMIs are more likely to die from cardiovascular diseases and complications of diabetes mellitus.

Morbid obesity, defined as 100% or more above ideal body weight or 100 lb or more overweight (7), is associated with a significant mortality risk for both men and women (46). Individuals with BMIs of 40 kg/m^2 or greater usually meet these criteria. The level of 60% above ideal body weight appears to be a critical threshold for mortality, since it often corresponds to 100 lb overweight (47).

Drenick et al. (48) evaluated 200 morbidly obese men for over 7.5 years and reported a 1200% excess mortality among subjects between the ages of 25 and 34 years. In the age group 35–44 years there was a 600% excess mortality compared to men in the general population; there was a 300% excess mortality in the age group 45–54 years. Another study of nearly 42,000 morbidly obese women who were candidates for obesity surgery (mean age of 34 years) found a 13-fold greater

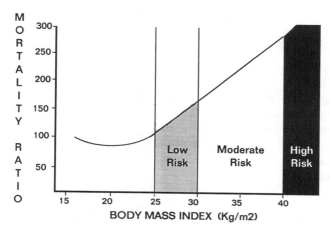

Figure 1 Mortality risk in relation to body mass index. (Adapted from 45.)

increase in sudden death than expected for normal women (46). Heart disease, stroke, and diabetes account for most of the excess mortality found in the morbidly obese population.

B. Obesity and Maternal Risk

Obesity is a proven risk factor for problems related to pregnancy. Garbaciak et al. (49) studied the relationship between overweight and complications of pregnancy in a cohort of 9,667 patients. In subjects classified as >120% or >150% above ideal prepregnancy weights there was a greater incidence of hypertension, diabetes mellitus, urinary tract infections, cesarean deliveries, and perinatal mortality. More recently, Abrams and Parker (50) studied the association between prepregnancy BMI and seven pregnancy complications in a series of 4,100 deliveries. Among this multiracial sample women who were very overweight (>135% over prepregnancy ideal weight) were 7 times more likely to have diabetes, 4.5 times more likely to have essential hypertension, and had twice the risk of developing pregnancy-induced hypertension. This group also had a 42% increased incidence of urinary tract infections, an 85% increase in perinatal mortality, and a 61% increase in cesarean deliveries. In addition to these complications other investigators have noted the increased maternal mortality among the seriously overweight (51–53). In light of the increasing prevalence of obesity among American women, the trend for delaying childbearing, and the common occurrence of increasing weight with age, the concerns regarding obesity and pregnancy are likely to take on greater significance in the future (54).

C. Coronary Heart Disease and Obesity

1. *Studies of Men*

Early research investigating the relationship between obesity and cardiovascular disease was mostly concerned with the male population because of the alarming increase in CHD prevalence in men compared to women. Insurance company data showed that overweight men had a 50% increase in risk of CHD when compared to men of "optimal" weight (56). Subsequent studies confirmed the increased risk associated with extreme obesity, but provided conflicting results on the risks of moderate obesity (BMI < 30 kg/m²) (57–59).

The inconsistent results of many obesity studies were partly due to the lack of long-term follow-up data and the fact that many of the deleterious effects of obesity develop only after many years. Hurbert et al. (60) took this lengthy incubation period into consideration in their 26 year follow-up of 5209 men and women. Their study showed that relative weight was a risk factor for coronary heart disease (CHD), coronary death, and congestive heart failure in men independent of age and other coronary risk factors. In addition, the data revealed that weight gain after age 25 conveyed a risk for CHD that could not be attributed to initial weight or other risk factors.

Much of the CHD risk conferred by obesity, however, is transmitted through other known coronary risk factors. It is well known that increases in body weight are associated with elevated low-density lipoprotein (LDL) cholesterol, low high-density lipoprotein (HDL) cholesterol, increased triglycerides, hypertension, glucose intolerance, hyperinsulinemia, and type II diabetes mellitus (61,62). Prospective studies have demonstrated that weight change in adult life is linearly and directly associated with changes in coronary risk factors (63). The strong association between weight and coronary risk factors is likely due to the fact that most weight gain in men between ages 20 and 50 years is fat, and the percentage of body fat typically increases during this time even if weight does not change (64). Furthermore, weight gain in midlife is associated with an increase in waist/hip ratio and visceral fat deposition, which also confers increased risk of CHD (58,65). (The importance of fat distribution patterns is discussed in the next section.) It has recently been shown by Kannel (66) that a 10% increase in body weight is associated with a 30% increase in CHD risk in men primarily due to obesity's adverse effect on other risk factors.

Obesity exerts its influence on the development of CHD both directly and indirectly. Obesity can be seen as a surrogate or marker for an atherogenic lifestyle characterized by a high-saturated-fat, low-fiber diet, combined with a lack of habitual physical activity (67). These lifestyle factors can induce heart disease through increases in blood pressure, hyperlipidemia, glucose intolerance, and hyperinsulinemia. More directly, obesity can increase the risk of myocardial infarction and sudden death as a result of extreme physical and mechanical burdens placed on an already compromised heart and coronary vasculature (68).

A person's genetic predisposition for CHD and its related risk factors likely interact with both the severity of obesity and its duration. For the individual who has become obese and also has additional CHD risk factors, lifestyle changes to facilitate weight reduction deserve the most serious consideration by both physician and patient. Framingham Heart Study researchers have concluded that "because it reversibly promotes atherogenic traits . . . correction of overweight is probably the most important hygienic measure (aside from avoidance of cigarettes) available for the control of cardiovascular disease" (61).

2. Studies of Women

Studies by Manson et al. (55) indicate that obesity is a significant determinant of CHD in women. These investigators evaluated 115,886 U.S. women, 30–55 years of age, who were initially free of manifest heart disease, cancer, or stroke for 8 years. The data revealed that increasing levels of BMI were associated with increased relative risk of CHD (Fig. 2). BMI at entry into the study was shown to be a more potent determinant of CHD risk than BMI at age 18, suggesting that weight gain during adulthood substantially increased the risk. The distribution of traditional coronary risk factors also varied directly with BMI categories. Women in the heaviest categories had two to five times the reported incidence of hypertension, diabetes, and elevated cholesterol levels. Age-adjusted relative risk for CHD among women in the heaviest category (BMI >29 kg/m^2) was 2.6 times greater than for women in the leanest category (BMI <21 kg/m^2). Since body fat distribution was not assessed in this study, and because BMI is an imperfect

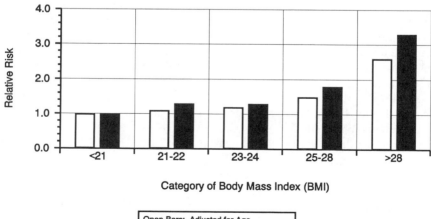

Category of Body Mass Index (BMI)

Open Bars: Adjusted for Age
Solid Bars: Adjusted for Age & Smoking

Figure 2 Relative risks of coronary heart disease in U.S. women, ages 30–55 years, according to body mass index (BMI). (Adapted from Manson (25).)

indicator of body fat composition, these results may underestimate the magnitude of the association between adiposity and CHD risk.

Lew and Garfinkle (56), in a large-scale American Cancer Society study, also found a positive correlation between self-reported weight and mortality from CHD. Subjects more than 40% above average weight for their heights had approximately double the risk of CHD. The risk was further increased after cigarette smoking was controlled for.

D. Psychological and Social Consequences

As severe as the medical consequences of obesity may be, from an individual perspective the psychological and social consequences are often worse. Our contemporary culture's obsession with thinness and physical beauty is likely the root cause of the current mania for dieting as well as the virtual epidemic of eating disorders in the form of anorexia and bulimia (69–72).

It appears that the condition of obesity itself produces much dysphoria, depression, and anxiety; the restrictive dieting people impose on themselves is an additional source of major psychological stress (73,74). Even moderate levels of overweight are commonly associated with substantial levels of emotional distress, restricted activity, and worry (75) as well as compromised functional status. The stigmatization and discrimination associated with obesity is well documented. Allon (76) points out that the visible evidence of obesity itself leads to the person being judged less desirable and differentiated from others.

The cultural conditioning leading to stigmatization of the overweight person begins early in life. Studies have demonstrated that both boys and girls exhibit a distinct preference for the slender (ectomorphic) and well-muscled (mesomorphic) body types, while being aversive to the round, soft, fatter (endomorphic) body build. Children as young as 5 years of age have been shown to discriminate consistently against representations of fatness and show preference for slimmer physiques in responding to photographs of youngsters with varying body types (77). Studies by Staffieri (78) likewise showed that boys and girls ages 6–10 years, both overweight and normal weight, used pejorative labels (sloppy, ugly, stupid, dirty, naughty, lonely, etc.) to describe their thoughts and feelings in response to silhouettes of obese children. The sociocultural conditioning that begins in early childhood produces prejudice that extends into later life (79). Discrimination against obese adults has been found in health care settings (80–82), college admissions (83,84), and at the work site (85).

Despite the abundance of evidence showing that obesity is an extraordinarily complex disorder that often has causative roots in powerful physiological and genetic factors, the obese are nevertheless characteristically treated as if the condition were entirely volitional. The resulting emotional burden of guilt, shame, inadequacy, and even self-hatred may produce a pathologic psychic stress that both complicates attempts at treatment and is itself detrimental to health. In an analysis of the sociocultural influences on obesity Allon (86) has stated that

> the condition of overweight brings with it in our society such a very heavy social pressure to conform that persons who are overweight develop some diseases partly in response to society's condemnation of them. Between overweight as "cause" and disease as "effect" may be the important intervening variable of social stress. Such stress is in part comprised of prejudice and discrimination against fat people. Experiencing the social condemnation of fat certainly may contribute to the physiological problems of the fat person. The strain of dieting and being "fat in a thin world" may add to or even cause medical conditions associated with overweight. (p. 161)

E. Importance of Fat Distribution Patterns

One of the most significant recent developments regarding obesity is the recognition that the pattern of fat distribution is a marker for health risks and metabolic abnormalities (87,88). The potential importance of fat patterning was alluded to in the work on somatypes by Sheldon et al. (89) more than 50 years ago. Some years later the French physician Jean Vague (90) proposed that adipose tissue stored at different locations in the body may have different metabolic functions and prognostic implications. Vague was among the earliest investigators to differentiate between android (upper body) obesity and gynoid (lower body) obesity. He further proposed that the gynoid form, typical of females, was relatively benign, whereas the android form, more common to males, was associated with an increased risk of gout, heart disease, and diabetes mellitus.

Although the original classifications of body fat distribution were based upon skinfold ratios, recent studies have found circumference ratios to be a more meaningful and simple indicator of fat distribution (65,91,92). Waist/hip ratios (WHR) have been shown to be highly correlated with the amount of abdominal or visceral fat, which is implicated in the pathogenesis of several chronic conditions (93). Studies of fat distribution have shown that

> Among middle-aged men, increased WHR is associated with an increased risk for myocardial infarction, stroke, and premature death even when there is a lack of association between these endpoints and generalized obesity as measured by the BMI (94,95).
>
> Those at highest risk may be lean men with a greater concentration of abdominal fat (95).
>
> Among premenopausal women, WHR is a stronger independent risk factor than BMI for myocardial infarction, angina pectoris, and premature death (96,97).
>
> Abdominal obesity is associated with high levels of plasma triglycerides, low levels of high-density lipoproteins and plasma apolipoprotein levels that increase risk for CHD (65,94,96,98,99).

Among obese middle-aged women, high WHR is associated with impaired fibrinolytic activity, especially when associated with hyperinsulinemia and insulin resistance, which commonly coexist with abdominal obesity (100).

The gynoid fat distribution pattern, characterized by a greater concentration of adipose tissue in the gluteal–femoral region, is more likely to be a hyperplastic (increased fat cell number) form of obesity. Hyperplastic obesity in its pure form has not been found to be associated with metabolic derangements or hypertension. Android obesity with fat concentrated in the abdominal region is characterized by fat cell hypertrophy (increased fat cell size), which has been associated with hyperinsulinemia, hypertriglyceridemia, and type II diabetes mellitus (101).

Recent prospective studies have shown that WHR is predictive of subsequent diabetes in men (101,102) and women (96,103). Increased WHR has been shown to be a better predictor of type II diabetes than BMI measures, and its effects are independent of general adiposity (104). Although both general obesity and increased WHR are strongly correlated with the incidence of diabetes, it is speculated that the influence of fat distribution is more likely to reflect an inherited predisposition while the effect of BMI is more controlled by environmental factors (103). The contributions to increased risk from total body fat and abdominal fat appear to be additive. Insulin-dependent (type I) and non-insulin-dependent (type II) diabetes apparently are characterized by distinct body fat distribution patterns. Only type II diabetes is associated with the android fat pattern (104).

In summary, the abdominal fat distribution pattern accounts for a significant portion of the morbidity and mortality previously associated with obesity. The various biological mechanisms by which abdominal obesity contributes to these risks continue to be investigated. In particular, recent studies have focused on the dynamics of the drainage of intra-abdominal tissues by the portal vein. It appears that obese men and abdominally obese women have a large potential for releasing free fatty acids (FFA) from visceral fat depots (105). The increased FFAs released into the portal circulation have the ability to produce several metabolic reactions related to hepatic lipoprotein synthesis and secretion as well as gluconeogenesis. Furthermore, the influx of elevated portal FFAs may inhibit the haptic uptake of insulin (106). Insulin–glucose dynamics are also compromised by impaired insulin sensitivity of the muscle cells.

Evans et al. (107) have shown that among obese women WHR correlated highly with impaired glucose disposal and decreased insulin binding to circulating monocytes. Thus, the enlarged visceral fat depots of abdominal obesity represent an initial causal link explaining the elevations of glucose, lipoproteins, and insulin. These metabolic derangements may also be precursors to hypertension.

The differential anatomical and functional characteristics of fat cells appear to be under the influence of sex hormone balance. In healthy premenopausal women, a strong relationship between WHR and increased androgenic activity has been demonstrated (108). Increased androgenic activity, in turn, is associated with decreased hepatic insulin extraction, hyperinsulinemia, peripheral insulin insensitivity, and increased recruitment and enlargement of abdominal adipocytes in preference to recruitment of gluteofemoral adiposites (108). It is currently theorized that the linkages between sex hormone balance, fat distribution, and metabolic abnormalities may result from or be exacerbated by early developmental or genetic influences (109).

VI. MEASUREMENT OF BODY FAT

Since excess adipose tissue mass, not simply body weight, is the definitive characteristic of obesity, it is essential to assess the relative amount of body fat in order to diagnose obesity. Obesity can be defined as a body fat content greater than 25% in men and greater than 30% in women (110). The only direct way of measuring the body fat component of body composition is through autopsy dissection. Cadaver studies have shown that water is the major constituent of the body, accounting for 60–65% of weight in young adults. Adipose tissue normally accounts for 15–18% of body weight in men and 20–25% in women. After dissection of adipose tissue, men and women are found to have similar proportions of fat-free or lean body mass (87).

While the amount of essential fat required for the maintenance of health and normal endocrine function is not precisely known, it is no doubt higher in women due to their sexual maturation and reproductive function. Early onset of menarche appears to be influenced by the attainment of critical amounts of body fat; conversely amenorrhea is well known to be associated with a low percentage body fat (111). Frisch and McArthur (112) have suggested that 17% body fat is essential for menarche to occur and that 22% fat is necessary for a normal menstrual cycle. Nevertheless, in clinical practice wide variations are seen with respect to menstrual cycle and body fat levels. Some female athletes maintain normal menstrual cycles at high levels of fitness when body fat is as low as 10–15%. In contrast, men, especially highly trained athletes, are able to attain very low levels of body fat, in the range of 5–10%, with no evidence of endocrine dysfunction or other untoward effects.

Since the direct autopsy method of determining body composition is of no practical value to the clinician, a variety of indirect methods have been developed. The most accurate of these methods tend to be costly and inconvenient, while the most economical and practical methods require a compromise in precision. Virtually all of the current research on obesity has relied on some indirect measure of body composition.

A. Laboratory/Research Methods

In recent years the options for measuring body composition have greatly increased and include hydrostatic (underwater) weighing, potassium counting, total body water determination, ultrasound, computed tomography, magnetic resonance imaging, and neutron activation (110). Although potentially very accurate these methods are costly, require expensive equipment and technical skill, and are usually not realistic choices for clinical assessments of obesity.

B. Clinical Methods

1. Visual Assessment

In the case of extreme obesity, with excessive roundness and bulging fat folds, the diagnosis becomes trivial and is frequently labeled as "morbid obesity" (110). Such superficial analysis of fatness, however, becomes highly unreliable when one is assessing individuals whose corpulence is only mild or moderate. Clinicians who frequently perform body composition tests often encounter subjects who carry higher than average amounts of muscle and skeletal mass for their weight and height and are, therefore, leaner than expected. Researchers have also found that subjects who appear visually to be thin may well have considerably more fat than expected (113). In such cases the health risks may be seriously underestimated if their adipose tissue is concentrated in the abdomen (92,95,97,99). For these reasons visual analysis is of limited usefulness in the assessment of obesity.

2. Height/Weight Tables

Height-weight tables have been in wide clinical use for many decades. These tables have been used by life insurance companies for identifying a "desirable," "ideal," or "relative" weight reference associated with the lowest mortality. The first tables, published in the mid-1800s, have been revised numerous times. The Metropolitan Life Insurance Company tables, most recently revised in 1983, are most commonly used in the United States. These tables are not measures of body fat and may, therefore, be very misleading in individual assessments; they should be used cautiously as a diagnostic tool for assessing an individual's optimal weight (114).

Numerous and substantial objections, both conceptual and methodologic, have been raised regarding the utility of these tables for the diagnosis of obesity or the determination of an individual's optimal weight (43,87,114–116). The quality of the data base varies greatly among the various published tables. In many cases heights and weights were not directly measured but were self-reported, or the measurements were not taken under standardized conditions (115). It is also known that although weight and adiposity are correlated, the relationship is not extremely strong, and relative weight does not accurately predict obesity (115,116). In many cases the design of the study that generated the data was flawed by small sample sizes inadequate to detect mortality trends, or did not control for confounding variables such as smoking or subclinical disease (43). Even studies with large sample sizes, such as the American Cancer Society study, the Metropolitan Life studies, and the Framingham Heart Study, may not represent the United States as a whole and should not be used to generalize to specific subpopulations whose characteristics differ from the original sample. The insurance studies also suffer from the bias of only including policy holders in the data base. Another common bias was the tendency to include disproportionate numbers of middle and upper class white men and persons under 60 years of age (114).

Despite these and myriad other technical problems, height/weight tables will continue to be used by physicians and other health professionals since they require measures that are easily obtained and can be accurately repeated. This appeals both to the health professionals and to our weight-conscious society. The height/ weight studies have also highlighted the important relationship between weight levels and health outcomes.

3. BMI

Body mass index is derived from weight (in kilograms) and height (in meters) according to the formula: $BMI = kg/m^2$. Based on criteria of individuality (not requiring reference to a sample population), accessibility, reliability, and measurement validity, BMI is judged to be the preferred indirect measure of obesity (4).

Recommended BMI values are similar for adult men and women, with normal ranges considered to be 20–25 kg/m^2 (117). A BMI of 22 kg/m^2 has recently been proposed as "ideal" since it has been shown to be associated with lowest morbidity (118). As previously discussed (Fig. 1), health risks and mortality appear to increase curvilinearly at BMI levels below 20 kg/m^2 and above 27 kg/m^2 (1,3). Even in the absence of other medical complications, a BMI >35 kg/m^2 is considered "high risk," and > 40 kg/m^2 "very high risk" (117).

It must be emphasized that BMI is not itself a measure of obesity. Currently there is no practical direct or indirect measure of excess fatness without some form of contamination. Since BMI is derived from height and weight, it is subject to problems similar to those encountered with the height/weight tables. For example, two men each weighing 100 kg (220 lbs) and 1.8 m (70 in) in height would have the same BMI of 31.6 kg/m^2, suggesting a medically significant level of obesity. This might be reasonably appropriate for a typical sedentary, middle-aged adult, but for a well-muscled athlete or heavy laborer no obesity with its attendant risks would exist. None of the height/weight indices can differentiate the various contributions of fat, muscle, bone, and water to total body weight.

Nevertheless, the clinical utility of using BMI as a measure of obesity is well established. Kraemer et al. (4) noted the close association between BMI scores and the increased levels of morbidity and mortality correlated with weight in a host of major epidemiologic studies. Of the various weight/height indices, BMI is considered the best because it most strongly correlates with other measures of adiposity and only weakly correlated with height (104,116). Keys et al. (119) have compared BMI with more direct measures of adiposity and reported correlation coefficients in the range of 0.67–0.85. Elevated BMI scores have been shown to be associated with increased risk of diabetes (89,101,103), cardiovascular disease (94,96,99), and premature deaths (93,98). Bray and Gray (117) have recently summarized the health risks associated with various levels of BMI (see Fig. 3).

4. Skinfold Calipers

Skinfold calipers are used to measure specific sites on the body to predict percentage body fat (122). The caliper method has the advantage of being relatively quick, economic, convenient, and portable. Despite these attractions, there are drawbacks that discourage the use of this method as the sole or primary means of diagnosing obesity.

The central assumptions on which the method is based may not be accurate; that is, the portion to total body fat is assumed to be deposited subcutaneously, and fat is distributed uniformly over the body (4,120). It appears that the amount of body fat stored in internal compartments can vary considerably (120). In addition, Lubaski (121) noted that body fat increases with age while the sum of skinfolds remains constant, suggesting that the increase in body fat occurs in areas not measured by the caliper technique. Skinfolds measured on obese subjects are also more error prone. On some very obese patients it may not even be possible to take an abdominal or suprailiac measurement if the thickness of the skin fold exceeds the caliper's capacity.

There is also considerable potential for error if the measurements are not taken with technical precision. Variation in the precise location of the calipers, consistency in the pressure used, and the duration the calipers are left in place can all influence the readings. To maximize accuracy, measurements should be performed by a well-trained technician who also takes any follow-up measurements to avoid interobserver errors (123). Jackson and Pollock have developed generalized equations for estimating percentage body fat from skinfold measurements taken on men and women that take into consideration age, sex, and the curvilinear relationships between body density and skinfold thickness (124). These equations for estimating body composition generally correlate with hydrostatically determined measurements, if experienced personnel perform the measurements.

It is important to emphasize that the regression equations are only valid with the population from which they were derived (117). Thus, equations generated from a sample of white men aged 20–55 years would not be appropriate for women, children, elderly persons, or individuals from other racial backgrounds. It has also been noted by Gray (110) that very few obese subjects were used in studies to derive the regression equations for percentage body fat, which further diminishes the accuracy of this technique in those with the highest levels of body fat.

5. Bioelectrical Impedance

One of the most recent indirect techniques for body composition analysis is bioelectrical impedance plethysmography. This method involves introducing a

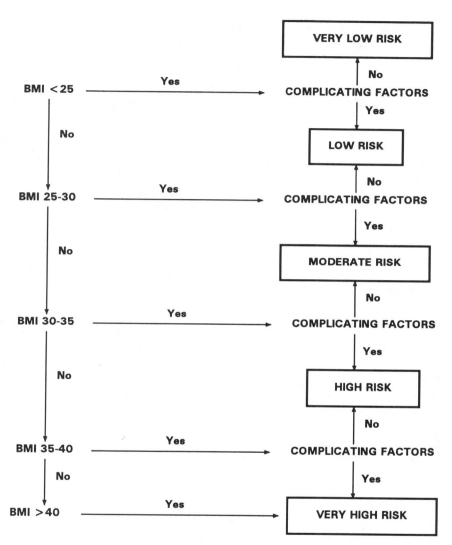

Figure 3 Risk classification based on body mass index (BMI) and the presence or absence of complicating factors including elevated waist/hip ratios, diabetes, hypertension, male sex, and age below 40 years. (Adapted from 117.)

low-voltage, insensible, electrical current between two electrodes attached to distal skin sites on the wrist and ankle and recording the body's resistance in ohms, which is assumed to be highly correlated with total body water (121). Regression equations have been derived that combine the measures of impedance with age, height, weight, and gender to yield a prediction of percentage body fat.

In clinical use our group has found that while the method is quick and convenient for the patient, it yields less consistent results than hydrostatic weighing. Inconsistent or spurious results may be due to variations in total body water secondary to the many factors that influence fluid retention or excretion. This method is also limited by the lack of generalizability of the regression equations due to the nature of the sample populations from which they were derived. Equations currently in use may not give accurate results for children, adolescents, the elderly, the very obese, or the very lean (124,125). However, this method is likely to come into more widespread clinical use as future research resolves these problems.

6. Circumference Measurements

Body circumferences taken with a tape measure provide a simple, noninvasive way of collecting objective data on the patient that can be used to estimate body composition and health risk. Some investigators have proposed the use of circumferences to predict percentage body fat (126–128). Most recently, Fannelli et al. (127) found that circumference measures could provide a better estimate of body density and body fat than ultrasound. This was presumably because circumference measures reflect both the amount of internal and subcutaneous adipose tissue while ultrasound would only provide a measure of subcutaneous fat stores.

The most widespread clinical application of circumference measures has been in determining fat distribution patterns, the importance of which has already been discussed. Of particular importance is the use of waist and girth measurements to calculate a ratio that indicates the presence of an android (male) or gynoid (female) fat distribution pattern. As standard procedure, the waist should be measured at the level of the umbilicus; hip circumference is taken around the widest part of the gluteal region. A high waist/hip ratio (WHR) (>0.8 for women, >0.9 for men) is indicative of the upper body android pattern. Lower values for men and women indicate the lower body gynoid pattern (89). Bray and Gray (117) have published percentile values for men and women by age categories (Fig. 4). Individuals below the 10th percentile (high waist/hip ratios) are considered to be at high risk for cardiovascular disease and a host of additional adverse health consequences.

In summary, while there are many methods for estimating body fat, none of the current methods can be relied upon as completely valid and accurate. Future research is likely to generate improved predictions from some of the more direct chemical methods and an increase in the accuracy and validity of more commonly used indirect field techniques. At the present time, the most clinically useful and

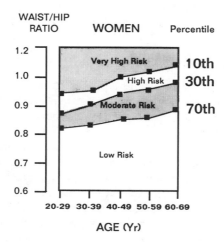

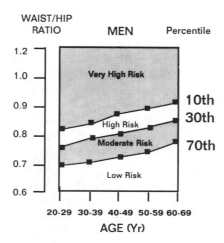

Figure 4   Percentiles and risk classification for men and women based on waist/hip ratios and age (Adapted from 117.)

practical assessment methods seem to be a combination of the BMI as an estimate of the degree of overweight and the WHR as an indicator of fat distribution patterns. In addition, skinfold measurements with calipers could provide useful objective data on fat distribution while bioelectrical impedance would provide an estimate of percentage body fat.

VII. TREATMENT

A. General Expectations of Treatment

The paths to obesity are numerous, as are the paths to weight loss. Ultimately, however, all successful treatments demand lifestyle restructuring with attention to healthy eating habits, physical activity, and psychosocial coping strategies. Often, both therapists and participants begin with shared hope and enthusiasm, only to have their combined morale deflated as they experience the realities of treatment. Most of the attendant frustration and dissatisfaction can be linked to a common set of expectations that clinical experience has shown to be unattainable (Table 1).

No single treatment approach has proven to be a fail-safe way to meet these expectations, and, given the nature of the problem, no such program seems forthcoming. In fact, each of the expectations may actually function as a barrier to favorable outcomes. The word "treatment" itself may trigger a problematic mindset in both the therapist and the patient. "Treatment" generally suggests the power of the therapist consistently to produce enduring change that is physically and medically beneficial. Where weight loss is concerned, the suggestion of medical treatment may even seem to hold out the possibility of a health-enhancing physical transformation without much disruption to other aspects of life (as medicine can sometimes do when it treats other kinds of illnesses). This is rarely the case in the management of obesity, which argues for a re-examination of patients' and therapists' expectations.

First, it is evident that many people who, for medical reasons, need to lose weight are either not internally motivated to do so or have been unsuccessful in translating internal motivation into effective action. For some, health is simply not a high priority, and attention to physical needs seems to conflict with other concerns such as work, school, and family. Successful weight control for those with significant obesity requires major lifestyle restructuring. This inevitably means a steadfast and internal commitment to new priorities with respect to time management, how decisions are made, how problems are solved, and how personal needs are met. Professionals can facilitate this motivation by offering

Table 1 Common Unrealistic Expectations in the Treatment of Obesity

Significantly obese patients will be internally motivated to lose weight.
Those who begin treatment will comply with explicit and implicit program objectives.
Weight loss will be forthcoming at a rate commensurate with the rigor of the treatment used.
Effects of treatment will be uniformly positive.
A single course of standardized treatment will produce both short-term weight loss and
  long-term weight management.

expertise and medical information, but responsibility for resetting priorities must rest with the patient. Too often therapists in weight-control programs imply they can supply the motivation for change, which shifts the responsibility away from the patient and sets the stage for eventual failure (129).

Second, it is the exceptional patient who enters a treatment program, attends consistently, complies perfectly, and continues after the program as an unqualified success. In the experience of many, these rare individuals have worked long and hard at weight control and have come to know themselves well. Such patients lock into the program structure and support services, accept their responsibility for making personal change, and often inspire other participants and therapists. The majority of participants in most programs will enter in a lower state of readiness for change. Many can still achieve a meaningful level of success. Others recognize that they are not ready to comply fully to treatment and will drop out early. Still another subset will be desirous, even desperate, to engage in treatment, yet are plagued with other problems that warrant attention and resolution before success-ful weight loss can occur.

Different program components will be more or less valuable for a given individual. Perfect short-term and long-term compliance is virtually impossible. Persistence through the many vicissitudes of the change process is the prerequisite for success. Ultimately, participants in weight-control programs must use the resources provided to construct for themselves a healthier, balanced lifestyle that meets their personal needs (130).

Third, many patients and therapists are disheartened when weight loss occurs more slowly than expected. This represents a common trap in many programs and exposes the danger in focusing on temporary fluctuations of the scale rather than on permanent lifestyle changes. In the short run, weight loss is not a reliable indicator of conscientious compliance. Even poor compliance itself, which is common to most participants some time during treatment, should not be inter-nalized as inadequacy or weakness in either the patient or the program. The patient is struggling to dismantle an unhealthy lifestyle, and reassemble a healthy one in the face of other demands and stresses. Patients complying with equal rigor to a given treatment will not lose weight at the same rate due to individual physical and metabolic differences. Some patients give up their adipose weight at a relatively slow rate under the best treatment conditions, while others reduce with ease. The challenge for the therapist is to be relentlessly positive in encouraging the patient's efforts and to reinforce increments of healthy behavior change whenever they occur.

Fourth, all results of weight loss and healthy behavior are not positive (131). Clinical experience shows that most patients entering treatment have been over-weight for years, often decades. They have attained a kind of homeostasis that is physical, psychological, and social. Any treatment will upset that homeostasis on all three levels. Many changes patients experience can be distressing, unsettling, or threatening (71,132). Patients should be advised, therefore, to consider the potential consequences of extensive changes for themselves and others. What changes will be predictably and reliably positive? What changes might be negative for the patient? What will change mean to those close to the patient? In practice, the patient will need much guidance and support over a long period of time to deal with extensive changes including their thoughts and feelings about their bodies, the nature of their relationship with food, and the impact changes have on their social and intimate life.

In some cases, patients may panic and sabotage or disengage from treatment. Many patients may conclude that the benefits of weight control are not worth the personal cost. Unfortunately, when that choice is made it is often considered a treatment failure rather than a personal decision made for nonmedical reasons. In response to the context of their lives, people do change their minds about what they want to do about their health. While these personal choices may undermine treatment objectives, they remain beyond the jurisdiction and control of the physician, therapist, or program. These complex issues are thoroughly explored by Stuart and Jacobsen (133).

The fifth erroneous expectation, that a single standardized treatment should be effective for most patients by providing good short-term weight loss and long-term maintenance, oversimplifies the patient and therapeutic process. Obese patients are very heterogeneous in their medical, physical, and psychosocial characteristics, and weight loss and maintenance phases are largely independent processes that deal with different issues and demand different skills (134). Furthermore, since managing obesity shares characteristics with other chronic diseases, it is essential that the potency of treatment be the result of an open-ended therapeutic partnership between patient and therapist, and not be determined solely by suggested treatment protocols.

Wadden and Bell [135] have shown that the high levels of recidivism, historically common in obesity treatment, need not be a cause for pessimism. State-of-the-art programs are multidimensional and of longer duration than earlier treatments. These lengthier programs produce both better weight losses and improved maintenance results [136]. Robust and lengthy approaches are also essential for the successful mastery of psychosocial and behavioral challenges, many of which are similar to those faced by individuals recovering from alcoholism or drug addiction. It is to be expected that for many patients with a long history of significant obesity, especially if characterized by binge eating and food dependency, successful maintenance of weight loss will probably require ongoing external support [137]. Such long-term support could come via periodic phone calls from a therapist, participation in ongoing maintenance classes, or through membership in a group like Overeaters Anonymous or Weight Watchers. With specific respect to the goal of weight control, these ongoing support mechanisms should serve to sustain the individual's motivation and attention to the daily process of lifestyle management. As Bray and Gray (117) have stated: "Pharmacological agents can control hypertension in most patients, but few if any physicians would expect hypertension to remain under control if drug therapy were discontinued. So with obesity, it is unrealistic and unreasonable to expect patients who lose weight to remain thinner when their treatment is terminated."

B. Classification of Obesity

A simple classification system based on the severity of obesity can be useful in selecting appropriate treatment options (Table 2) (2).

1. Mild Obesity

The vast majority of obese individuals are between 20 and 40% above ideal weight. Typically these individuals have a normal complement of fat cells (30–35 billion) and potentially can reach ideal weight through a consistent program of low-fat diet and regular exercise. While the medical complications of this degree of obesity are often either absent or mild, those in the top end of this range may warrant a more aggressive approach if other medical problems such as hypertension, hyperlipidemia, or type II diabetes are present. Most cases of mild obesity can be attributed to chronic exposure to a high-fat diet combined with a sedentary lifestyle (134).

2. Moderate Obesity

In the range of 41–100% above ideal weight, these individuals are more likely to have not only increased fat cell size but also increased fat cell number. While the hypertrophic form of mild obesity is considered to be completely reversible, it has been suggested that those with significant fat cell hyperplasia may be unlikely ever to reach an arbitrarily low level of ideal body weight (138). As weight is lost, fat cells shrink down to a normal size (139). Since fat cell number is considered irreversible, patients with hyperplastic obesity may be left with an increased fat cell mass ranging from 50 to 150 billion. Such patients, at best, may be able to maintain a body weight that remains 50% above height/weight predictions of ideal weight (140). In addition to the essential components of nutrition management, exercise and behavior modification, patients in this category may benefit from pharmacotherapy and participation in a medically supervised very-low-calorie diet program.

3. Severe Obesity

Patients with severe obesity are characteristically more than 100 lb or 100% over ideal weight. As previously discussed, the health risks associated with such extreme adiposity represent a clear and immediate health hazard. Many of the medical complications and health risks that accompany severe obesity can be reduced or eliminated with sustained weight loss. Until recently, however, few

Table 2 Classification of Obesity

	Mild	Moderate	Severe
Approximate lbs over-weight	30–60	60–100	>100
Percentage overweight	20–40	41–100	>100
Approximate BMI (kg/m^2)	25–30	30–45	>45
Prevalence among obese women (%)	90.5	9.0	0.5
Pathologic basis	Hypertrophic	Hypertrophic and hyperplastic	Hypertrophic and hyperplastic
Complications	Dependent on coexisting risk factors and/or morbidities	Exacerbation of coronary risk factors and musculoskeletal problems	Severe cardiovascular risk; sleep apnea, loss of functional capacity
Treatment options	Comprehensive nutrition, exercise, and behavior modification; professional or lay leadership	Lifestyle management program possibly combined with very-low-calorie diet; pharmaco-therapy	Lifestyle management program; pharmacotherapy; very-low calorie diet; gastric surgery

Source: Adapted from Ref. 2.

severely obese persons have demonstrated success at losing weight and maintaining weight loss (7). These cases are often complicated by a combination of factors including extensive fat cell hyperplasia, impairment in functional capacity, co-existing medical problems, and psychosocial dysfunction. Newly developed interventions utilizing drugs, very-low-calorie diets, and gastric surgery hold new promise for the estimated 225,000 Americans who suffer this devastating disorder.

C. Modalities of Treatment

Exhaustive exploration of treatments utilized over the last several decades is beyond the scope of this chapter. Many popular treatments have been largely discredited over time, or have, at least, failed to gain the confidence of credible health professionals and are usually not recommended. These include such single-modality treatments as jaw wiring, hypnosis, acupuncture, starch blockers, amphetamines, intestinal bypass surgery, gastric balloons, and fad diets characterized by unbalanced nutrition and severe calorie restrictions. Since diet, exercise, and behavior modification are essential components of any successful treatment, they will be discussed before we consider more aggressive options incorporating drugs, very-low-calorie diet programs, and surgical techniques.

1. Diet

Some form of dietary management with emphasis on caloric restriction has historically been the cornerstone of obesity treatment. However, recent research has called into question the use of various calorie restrictive diets as a primary approach to achieving successful weight loss and maintenance in most patients (141–148).

The reliance on calorie restrictions stems from the seemingly self-evident notion that most obesity results from chronic overeating or even outright gluttony. While no one disputes that a surfeit of calories above daily energy requirements is necessary to the progressive storage of fat, this must be only part of the story. It is analogous to stating that alcoholics are alcoholics because they drink too much. This comparison is instructive because we know that "drinking" is not the full explanation for alcoholism. Alcoholics can drink many substances without harm to their health, and many people use alcohol without a propensity to abuse it. The problem is with the patient's relationship to alcohol, with a likely biological sensitivity to alcohol, and the particular psychological and social implications of alcohol dependency. In attempts to control body fat, it is likewise essential to resist the temptation to oversimplify the nature of the imbalance between caloric intake and energy expenditure.

Do the obese overeat? There is little evidence that these individuals as a group are eating more than their leaner counterparts. Early reviews by Garrow (141) and Wooley et al. (149) failed to support the assumption that fat people eat more than thin people. Braitman and his colleagues (150), in 1985, studied more than 20,000 people representative of the U.S. population and concluded that the caloric intake, even after physical activity and age were adjusted for, was no higher in obese than in lean people.

Studies comparing eating habits and energy intake of obese and lean subjects have been criticized as being flawed by the likelihood of underestimations in self-reported data (151). On the contrary, recent reports concluded that obese subjects were no less accurate in their recall than thin subjects (152). In fact, there was a slight tendency for obese persons to overestimate their intake. Controlled studies on rats (142) and humans (143,148,153) also support the contention that excess energy intake, in and of itself, is not the principal cause of obesity. Although some obese subjects clearly do take in excess calories, the research suggests that metabolic differences play a crucial role in the development and maintenance of obesity in combination with or in the absence of high caloric intake (155,156). Thus, many obese patients are probably telling the truth when they say they are moderate in their food consumption. To help these patients, treatment recommendations other than caloric restriction will be necessary.

In addition to the lack of convincing evidence for obese persons as "big eaters," there is also little evidence to support chronic calorie-restricted diets as effective therapy (157–159). Stunkard and McFarren-Hume (159) reviewed the obesity treatment literature for the 30 years before 1959 and found that calorie-restricted diets failed to have any enduring results. The average weight loss was 10 lbs among 1,368 patients in 8 different studies. Since most of these subjects were described as "grossly overweight" the reviewers concluded that the results of dietary treatment for obesity were "remarkably similar and remarkably poor" (159).

2. *Behavior Modification*

The 1960s brought the advent of behavior modification to the treatment of obesity. Early studies made a fundamental shift from focusing on a prescription of limited food intake (i.e., a diet) to behavioral strategies for altering the patient's eating style in the interest of calorie control (160–163).

The first published clinical trial of behavior therapy for the control of eating was carried out by Stuart in 1967 (161). This was a lengthy (1 year), comprehensive, highly individualized treatment of 10 obese adult women (average weight of 194 lb). Three subjects lost over 40 lb and six lost over 30 lb, representing the best weight loss results in the literature at that time.

Subsequent studies abandoned Stuart's intensive individual counseling approach in favor of much shorter and simplified group treatment packages. As behavioral techniques became standardized, treatment was usually delivered in groups of 8–12 patients meeting once weekly for 2–3 months. These interventions were basically attempts to reduce caloric intake by attending to how food was eaten rather than focusing on specifically how much and what was consumed. Patients were instructed to concentrate on chewing food more thoroughly, putting their forks down between bites, eating off smaller plates, eating in only one place, controlling food cues, and keeping written records of various aspects of the eating process. These first-generation standardized group treatments were notably ineffective for those who needed help the most (164–166). Few patients lost substantial weight, and sustained significant weight loss was poorest among the most obese subjects with coexisting medical problems.

Wing and Jeffrey (167) reviewed 57 studies carried out between 1966 and 1976 that were either basic diet treatments or a combination of diet and behavior modification. They found that the maximum percentage of weight loss was less than 9%. Bennett (158) reviewed an additional 26 treatment studies between 1976 and 1986 and found a similar small percentage of weight loss, typically representing 12–15 lb at the end of formal treatment. Thus, group treatment programs that use combinations of behavior modification and diet to reduce caloric intake yield only modest amounts of weight loss.

A more important issue, however, is whether weight loss achieved through caloric restriction can be maintained or improved upon over the course of extended follow-up. Typical formalized diet/behavior modification programs last 8–16 weeks. Wing and Jeffrey (167), in analyzing 23 studies that included follow-up statistics, found that, on the average, those who participated in behavioral programs maintained their modest weight loss for at least 6 months. Those who participated in diet only programs had regained about 4 lb after an average follow-up of 32 weeks.

Long-term maintenance of calorie restriction therapies is even less encouraging. Foreyt et al. (165) reviewed the results of 16 studies that provided 1 year follow-up data. The average treatment period was 12 weeks, and weight losses averaged 13 lb after the formal treatment period. Although the average subject evaluated at 1 year maintained the weight loss, mean weight loss for all subjects at 1 year represented only a 5% reduction of the average intake weight of 198 lb. A rare study with a 5-year follow-up found an average weight gain of 1.5 lb above pretreatment weight (168).

These studies indicate that behavior modification strategies and dietary therapies that primarily focus attention on restricting caloric intake are not likely to be effective in the long run. Much more promising, however, is the use of nutrition education (focusing on significant reduction of fat calories and increasing fiber and nutrient density) combined with a strong emphasis on exercise to achieve improvements in fitness and body composition. State-of-the-art behavioral interventions more effectively blend the prerequisite nutrition and exercise components with group support and counseling, so that patients learn how to cope with the psychosocial and emotional aspects of restructuring lifestyle.

3. Nutritional Recommendations

All obese patients, regardless of specific medical or surgical therapies, should receive in-depth nutritional instruction (see Chap. 7), information on exercise programs (see Chap. 12), training in behavioral management strategies (see Chap. 15), and psychological support (see Chap. 14), through attendance at group meetings or individual counseling sessions. The combination of these components, individualized to the patient's specific needs, can make up an effective program of rehabilitative weight management.

Nutritional instruction should emphasize helping the patient to establish a new eating style that is low in sugar, fat, and cholesterol, and high in nutrient density, complex carbohydrates, and fiber. Such a diet can be palatable and result in significant weight loss even in the absence of calorie restriction (144,146,169).

The reduction of dietary saturated fat intake is of major importance as a nutritional strategy (144,145,147,170). Dietary fat can be deposited in adipose tissue at a metabolic cost of 3% of ingested calories, while storing carbohydrate as fat requires 23% of ingested calories (145,171). In animal studies the development of adiposity has been shown to vary in proportion to the amount of fat in the diet (147). Similar observations in humans have also shown that body fat varies in proportion to the habitual fat content of the diet (148,153,172,173). In addition, high-fat diets promote obesity by enhancing taste and stimulating overconsumption. This is most striking when a high-fat diet is combined with increased intake of refined sugar (172,173). In addition to reducing the fat content of the diet, the use of refined sugars should also be decreased. Such added sugars are only empty calories, devoid of vitamins, minerals and fiber, and, when combined with high fat foods, may have addictive properties for many obese subjects. Rarely do obese subjects report overeating foods that are only high in fat or high in sugar; the majority of patients binge on foods high in both fat and refined sugars. It is common for these subjects to report cravings for such foods in the absence of physical hunger and experience withdrawal symptoms (lethargy, headache, agitation, and feelings of deprivation) in the early stages of making dietary changes (137).

Recent studies by Wortman and Wortman (174,175) strongly suggest that high intake of refined sugars may be used by obese subjects as an effective way of altering neurochemistry and regulating moods. The all too common cycles of calorie-restrictive dieting followed by relapses of uncontrolled overeating of high-fat/high-sugar foods may represent a form of substance abuse and dependency (137,175,176). It has been estimated that two-thirds of obese subjects are refined sugar cravers who use food as a drug in reaction to such negative mood states as depression, anxiety, tension, boredom, or mental fatigue (177,178). Recent animal studies indicate that a high-sucrose intake may lead to hyperinsulinemia, adipose cell enlargement, and increases in visceral (intra-abdominal) fat deposits (179). For all these reasons, intake of refined sugars and dietary fat should be greatly reduced.

In the initial stages of weight loss both total daily calorie intake and percentage of fat calories should be reduced. Most women will do well on 1000–1500 kcal/day, and men on 1200–2000 kcal/day. Much of the calorie moderation tends to occur spontaneously as patients focus on higher-quality nutritional choices. Equations for calculating daily energy needs and projecting rate of weight loss are provided by Leon and Hartman (see Chap. 7). A rate of weight loss of 1–2 lb/week or 1% of body weight per week is considered safe (180). Nutritional and mineral supplementation is recommended since it is difficult to ensure nutritional adequacy on diets of less than 1800 kcal (181). In addition, consumption of low-nutrient or "empty calorie" foods (sugars, fats, and alcohol) must be kept to a minimum.

Total daily fat consumption should range from 10 to 25% of calories, divided evenly into saturated, monounsaturated, and polyunsaturated fat constituents. Monitoring the grams of fat intake can be helpful in educating patients regarding common sources of fat. Patients who record food intake, daily calories, and grams of fat consumption can learn over several months how to make the appropriate nutritional adjustments that can be integrated into a stable lifestyle. Popular references are now available as resources for patients working toward modifying their eating habits (182–187).

4. Regulating Meal Frequency

In providing the patient with nutritional recommendations, the pattern and frequency of feedings should be considered (59,188,189). The common habit of eating several large and high-caloric meals each day has been shown to be associated with increases in body weight (190,191), body fat (192), and prevalence of heart disease (193,194).

In animal studies, rats trained to gorge have been compared with control rats who maintained their normal pattern of nibbling throughout the day (195). The rats who ate a few large meals each day became heavier than control rats even though they consumed less food. In addition, gorging rats developed a higher percentage body fat and demonstrated metabolic adaptations in liver and adipose tissue that facilitated the rapid storage of ingested food as glycogen or fat.

Bray (196), in reviewing the effects of nibbling vs. gorging among human subjects, reported that serum cholesterol levels were reduced when equal amounts of food were eaten in several small meals throughout the day instead of one large meal. In contrast, subjects who consumed their food in large meals had higher body weights, thicker skinfolds, more glucose intolerance, and higher serum lipid levels (197–199).

In light of these findings, patients should be counseled to avoid skipping meals and periods of nutritional deprivation and instead adopt a regular eating pattern that begins with breakfast and includes four to six small feedings per day spaced 3 to 4 hours apart. In addition to improving metabolic regulation, this recommended eating pattern eliminates the intense feelings of physical deprivation that characterize erratic, large-meal eaters and commonly lead to indiscriminate food choices and recurrent binges.

5. *Exercise and Physical Activity*

Lack of sufficient exercise and physical activity has been considered by many to play a critical role in the development of obesity in laboratory animals (200), human infants (201,202), school children (203), adolescents (204), and adults (205–210). Despite this abundant evidence, treatment for obesity historically has emphasized regulation of dietary intake much more strongly than energy expenditure. Regular exercise is now considered an essential and powerful component of any successful weight management program (117,130,211–215).

Exercise and physical activity in general can potentiate weight control in a variety of ways that are both individually important as well as synergistically and collectively potent. Exercise can add significantly to the total daily energy expenditure. While the typical sedentary person only expends about 15% of daily calories in physical activity, this portion of energy output has the greatest potential for voluntary manipulation. The addition of a structured exercise program and an increase in other physical activities of daily living can add 250–500 kcal/day of energy expenditure, which, over time, can reduce fat stores. As an example, 300 kcal/day of energy expenditure over 1 year's time would require the caloric equivalent of over 31 lb of body fat.

Exercise also produces favorable alterations in body composition: increases fat free mass and decreases adipose tissue mass even when total body weight does not change. These effects can be achieved without dietary restriction and concomitant reduction in metabolic rate (216). Numerous studies have demonstrated that programs that combine both nutrition management with an exercise regimen produce superior weight loss, greater reduction in percentage body fat, and better preservation of lean body mass compared to diet alone (214,217,218). It should be noted, however, that these results are best obtained on a moderate-calorie diet, high in carbohydrates, and combined with an exercise program of sufficient frequency, intensity, and duration, carried out regularly over extended periods of time (219–221).

For some obese subjects exercise may counteract the decline in resting metabolic rate (RMR) associated with caloric restriction. Since RMR is strongly correlated with lean body mass, better retention of these fat-free tissues will promote higher energy requirements, which make it easier to maintain weight loss (222). The incorporation of resistance weight training is probably necessary to optimize the preservation of lean tissues during weight loss (223,224). Unfortunately, the much touted acute effect of a session of exercise on increasing RMR during the immediate hours after exercise has been overemphasized. It now appears that significant increases in metabolic rate after exercise only occur in more highly trained individuals who engage in high-intensity, long-duration activity. In such subjects metabolic rates remained elevated for 12–72 hours, while deconditioned obese subjects return to baseline within a few hours (225).

Regular exercise may play a role in the suppression of appetite and regulation of food intake (209,226–232). It also appears that lean subjects regulate their caloric intake in response to exercise, while obese subjects often do not. Recent studies have demonstrated that exercise generally does not stimulate an increase in food intake among obese subjects (228,229). Thus, a negative energy balance can be created by the addition of exercise that will be equivalent to the increase in calorie expenditure (230).

Exercise can improve psychological function and help regulate negative mood states (233). Acute physical activity has been shown to reduce anxiety for 2–5 hours after exercise (234,235). Chronic exercise programs of 6–20 weeks have also been associated with decreases in depression (236–238) and enhanced self-esteem (233,237). These effects serve as a significant buffer to emotional stressors. Exercise helps to reduce the intensity of negative moods, promotes a sense of well-being, and provides an alternative noncaloric behavioral response that increases one's perception of self-efficacy. Particularly for the subgroup of obese who are "emotional eaters," such psychological leverage is indispensable.

Regular physical activity can help counteract the ill effects of obesity on health. Exercise has been shown to reduce overall cardiovascular risk through its generally favorable effects on blood lipids, blood pressure, and glucose/insulin regulation (239–243). Exercise and physical activity also counteract the loss of functional capacity and wholesale physical deterioration that accompany inactivity (244–246). For a thorough review of the health enhancing effects of exercise and physical activity, see Chapter 12.

Exercise and physical activity play a central role in promoting long-term maintenance of weight loss and avoidance of weight cycling (227,247). Difficulties in maintaining medially significant weight loss have long been recognized. A number of recent studies indicate that there are potentially numerous negative effects associated with repeated cycles of significant weight loss and regain (248–253). Utilizing subjects and data from the Framingham Heart Study, Lissner and colleagues recently examined the effects of weight cycling in a large number of men and women over a period of 32 years (253). They concluded that subjects with frequent fluctuations of body weight have higher rates of CHD and mortality than do persons with more stable weight patterns. Other epidemiologic data support the association between weight instability and increased CHD risk (254,255). Regular exercise may be a critical factor to counteract the tendency towards weight cycling (247) and has repeatedly been shown to be strongly predictive of successful weight maintenance (211–214). Of particular importance, a number of studies have demonstrated that subjects who maintained their exercise regimens continued to lose weight in follow-up periods of up to 1 year, while nonexercisers exhibited a strong propensity to regain their weight (214,228,256–259).

Any weight control intervention is targeted at the reduction of excess storage fat. The effect of physical training on fat loss will be dependent on the type of activity, its frequency, intensity, and duration, as well as on the qualitative aspects of the body fat in the individual (260). Exercise will likely be most beneficial for those mild to moderately obese subjects whose adipose tissue is characterized primarily by fat cell hypertrophy. Those with severe obesity characterized by fat cell hyperplasia may get little or no fat loss effect from exercise alone (261,262). There is some evidence, however, that exercise may play an important role in the prevention of obesity by retarding fat cell proliferation during the growth periods of childhood and adolescence (262).

Other sex differences in the response to physical training have been recently reviewed by Bjorntorp (261). Exercising males both decrease body fat and increase muscle mass. Females, on the other hand, seem to respond to exercise according to their patterns of fat distribution. Women with android obesity respond similarly to men, with a decrease in body fat and a preservation or slight increase in their lean body mass. In contrast, women with the gynoid fat distribution, with fat stored primarily in the gluteal–femoral regions, show little or no fat loss with physical training. It has been suggested that this may be due to a difference in food intake regulation among women with lower body obesity in an adaptive effort to preserve an energy depot reserved for caloric needs during lactation (226,263).

6. Exercise Guidelines for the Obese Patient

a. *Medical Screening.* Obese subjects, especially those with BMIs in excess of 30 kg/m², often carry additional medical risks related to coexisting hypertension, hyperlipidemia, diabetes, heart disease, or orthopedic problems. Moreover, they are usually in poor physical condition and have a low tolerance for physical activity. For these reasons it is important that the obese patient follow appropriate medical guidelines in initiating an exercise program and have the program designed to meet their individual needs (264,265). Chapter 12 reviews these guidelines for medical screening and fitness assessments.

b. *Program Design.* For best results obese patients should have a program of structured exercises complemented by a plan for increasing activities of daily living. The structured component provides a method for progressively increasing the functional capacity (fitness level) of the individual, making it possible over time to tolerate comfortably activities of higher intensity and longer duration. Increasing activities of daily living such as walking to the store, using stairs instead of elevators, and doing yard work all serve to add to the cumulative daily energy expenditure and, more importantly, help to establish a daily habit for physical activities.

c. *Type of Exercise.* To promote caloric expenditure and improvements in fitness that enhance the ability to mobilize and metabolize fat stores, aerobic activities must provide the foundation of the exercise program. This involves exercises that use a large muscle mass in a rhythmic, continuous fashion for extended periods of time. To minimize stress on the joints, brisk walking, stationary cycling, rowing and cross-country ski machines, stair climbers, and exercising in water are recommended. Jogging should be avoided until significant weight loss and fitness improvements are achieved. Jogging also increases the risk of orthopedic injuries, which may preclude further training for long periods of time. Other high-impact activities such as aerobics classes and various court games should be performed with caution.

d. *Intensity.* The intensity of exercise training should be gauged by a combination of heart rate guidelines and use of the perceived exertion scale (see Chap. 12). When beginning a new exercise program, low-intensity activities performed at or below the 60% level of functional capacity are recommended (i.e, at heart rates at or below 50% of maximal predicted heart rates). These exercises should not be perceived by the individual as any more difficult than "somewhat hard." Initially this low-intensity program should expend 200–300 kcal per session or 1000 kcal per week. Gradually, over several months, the person should increase the duration and intensity to expend 300–500 kcal per session and 1500–2000 kcal per week (220,226).

The duration of the exercise session may initially be as little as 10–20 min, with gradual increases of 5 min/session every two or three weeks until an hour or longer can be tolerated. The emphasis should be on longer, low-intensity sessions to maximize caloric expenditure and other positive effects of exercise (e.g., mood enhancement and appetite suppression) while minimizing the risk of injury and feelings of fatigue.

3. *Frequency.* The frequency of exercise should be three to five sessions per week. Four or five sessions weekly are clearly better for developing the training effect, but the risk of injury is also likely to be proportionally greater. On alternate days some other form of recreational or physical activity is recommended to maximize caloric expenditure and fat utilization. Such a schedule also encourages the development of a "positive addiction" to physical activity, with all its physiological and psychological benefits (223,267).

In summary, the combination of a program of exercise training with a pattern of increased habitual physical activity can greatly increase the likelihood of long-term success in weight management. Clinicians have repeatedly observed that it is rare for a patient to lose a medically significant amount of weight (30–40 lb or more) and maintain the weight loss for more than 1 year in the absence of regular exercise (137,266). Evidence from a host of sources shows that increased exercise and physical activity interact with metabolic, nutritional, and psychological factors that, in totality, create a state of healthful balance conducive to the achievement and maintenance of appropriate weight and body composition. Many of the numerous benefits of exercise cannot be obtained as effectively or at all through alternative means. Furthermore, even in the absence of significant obesity patients should be advised to adopt physically active lifestyles to avoid the litany of unnecessary disabilities and physical deterioration associated with aging (242–246).

7. Very-Low-Calorie Diets

Very-low-calorie diets (VLCDs) are a popular and aggressive form of treatment utilizing either a liquid supplement in the absence of food, a supplement combined with food, or a closely regulated food intake that provides 800 calories or less per day. Such regimens, sometimes referred to as protein-sparing modified fasts or semistarvation diets, are only intended for those who are a minimum of 50 lb overweight or at least 30% above ideal body weight (180).

At present the diet products in widest use (i.e., those marketed to hospitals and physician-based programs) are powdered supplements designed to be mixed with water or other noncaloric beverage and consumed three to five times per day. Protein in these supplements is derived from milk or egg-based sources. Carbohydrate intake is usually 50–100 g day. Vitamin and mineral (especially potassium) supplementation is required and may be included in the powdered formula or taken separately (268). Patients are required to drink at least 2 quarts of additional noncaloric fluid per day. Daily caloric intakes range from 400 to 800 kcal/day. All other caloric intake is prohibited during the initial phase of supplemented fasting.

Currently the best programs have evolved into closely medically supervised, lengthy (duration of 1 year or more), expensive, multidisciplinary treatment programs capable of producing rapid and substantial weight loss in their participants. Properly selected patients can lose 40–80 lb depending on age, sex, height, initial weight, and compliance during the initial 12–16 weeks of VLCD intervention (269). As a result, significant improvement in glucose intolerance, hypertension, and abnormal blood lipid levels are commonly seen as well as improved pulmonary function in morbidly obese patients (268,270,271).

The VLCD treatment regimens have evolved over many years of clinical research, and they should not be confused with the liquid protein diets promoted commercially during the 1970s and early 1980s. The widespread use of these earlier diets, usually without medical supervision and professional support, led to over 60 diet-related deaths mostly attributed to intractible ventricular arrhythmias and severe electrolyte imbalance (268,272,273). While the current VLCDs have been judged to be safe when properly administered and supervised, they are, nonetheless, radical interventions and not without some risk (269,273,277). Of major concern is the amount of body protein and potassium loss resulting from the treatment. To minimize these risks and to promote nitrogen balance, a minimum of 70 g of high biological value protein should be provided. In addition, without close medical monitoring, excessive losses of lean tissue mass combined with dehydration and potassium losses could potentially lead to cardiac arrhythmias, myocardial atrophy, and sudden death (272,273). Other possible complications include cholelithiasis, constipation or diarrhea, headache, postural hypotension, cold intolerance, hair loss, menstrual irregularities, acute gout attacks, dry skin, difficulty concentrating, fatigue, and loss of stamina (274,276,277).

Several recent reviews of VLCDs provide guidelines for their appropriate use in treating obesity (274,275,277,278). A general consensus has developed on the following points:

1. These programs should be conducted under the supervision of physicians who have specialized knowledge of their use, including how to evaluate patients for treatment, how to minimize side effects, adjust medications, and monitor physical and metabolic effects.

2. Patients should be carefully selected and complete a thorough physical examination before entering treatment. Patients should be at least 30% above ideal weight or have a BMI of 30 kg/m^2 or greater. Contraindications to treatment include unstable angina, malignant arrhythmias, active cancer, insulin-dependent diabetes, any muscle-wasting disease (e.g., Cushing's syndrome, lupus erythematosus), any major organ failure, or any disorder requiring high-dosage steroid therapy. VLCDs are not intended for use by children, adolescents, elderly persons, or pregnant women. For a complete review of the medical evaluation process and contraindications, see work by Atkinson (277).

3. Patients should not have any severe psychological disturbances and they should be willing and capable of carrying out a long-term program of lifestyle change. Patients should be advised that successful completion of VLCD treatment will require a strong personal commitment to developing new health habits. Initial treatment is only the first phase of a lengthy process that must extend many months and, for some patients, several years beyond the use of any supplement. After-care services should be provided to support patients as they encounter the many challenges of the maintenance period.

4. Treatment should include phases that deal with medical and psychological evaluation, preparation for change, supplemented fasting, gradual reintroduction to food, training in relapse management and maintenance skills, development of exercise and physical activity habits, and long-term maintenance and support. The initial period of VLCD fasting should not exceed 12–16 weeks.

5. The strongest programs use professional multidisciplinary teams incorporating the services of physicians, nurses, registered dietitians, behavioral counselors, and exercise specialists. As a single modality treatment VLCDs have a very poor track record for compliance and weight maintenance (279,280). As part of a multicomponent program that incorporates

nutrition education, exercise, group support, stress management, behavior modification, and relapse management, VLCDs can be part of a comprehensive, long-term process that can contribute to the successful treatment of obesity (215,274,275).

Programs such as those described above can produce rapid weight loss, averaging 1.5 kg/week for women and 2.0 kg/week for men, during the supplemented fasting phase (275). With good compliance, patients who have not lost all their excess weight in the first several months can continue to show gradual weight loss through the refeeding and maintenance phase. Most patients who participate fully will complete their weight loss during the first 6 months of the program. Thus, for some morbidly obese patients VLCD treatment may be considered as an alternative to gastric bypass surgery or as preparation for surgical treatment.

Despite the potential for such dramatic results, there are still concerns over the long-term maintenance of weight loss (215,281). Some studies have shown substantial improvement in maintenance of weight loss, with an average of two-thirds of the weight loss persisting at 1 year of follow-up (268,282). Other studies, however, have shown a regain of 50–80% of weight loss during the first year after the program (283–285). Also of concern is the high dropout rate characteristic of these demanding programs: 30–50% of patients fail to complete 6 months of treatment (281,284).

One of the pitfalls of this form of treatment is that it is strongly focused on achieving rapid weight reduction through drastic calorie restriction and avoidance of normal food. While the quick weight loss tends to be reinforcing to the patient, it may undermine motivation for following through with the long-term changes required in eating and exercise behaviors. Patients may learn to associate success in regulating intake and weight gain with the use of the supplement rather than their own efficacy in managing their health choices. Dramatic and sudden changes in food use and weight also place the dieter under considerable psychological stress. They must endure rapid behavioral and physical changes, often in the face of social and environmental barriers. Simultaneously they are expected to avoid food consumption, which, in many cases, has served as a primary response strategy for coping with emotions.

In conclusion the current state-of-the-art, comprehensive VLCD programs are potentially safe and effective in the short term for producing substantial weight losses for patients with medically significant obesity. Due to the inherent risks of radical intervention, high costs (typically $2000–$4000 for a 1 year program), and complexity of treatment, VLCDs are best suited for a carefully selected subgroup of the obese population. Continued research and development are needed to refine and strengthen program components, reduce attrition rates, minimize side effects, and enhance long-term retention of weight loss.

8. Surgical Treatment

In response to the lack of effective medical treatments for morbid obesity, a variety of surgical approaches have been utilized for more than 35 years with varying degrees of success. Surgical treatment is considered an appropriate option for those with severe obesity defined as a BMI of 40 kg/m^2 or greater, typically 100 lb or more above ideal weight. An estimated 1.5 million Americans meet these criteria and have unequivocal medical complications secondary to obesity (286). Less severe obesity, characterized by a BMI of 35–40 kg/m^2, may also be an indication for surgery if accompanied by comorbid high-risk conditions such as diabetes, hypertension, cardiomyopathy, or congestive heart failure, and if these conditions are potentially life threatening or seriously compromise the patient's quality of life (287).

Jejunoileal bypass, first introduced in 1955, resulted in rapid and substantial weight losses, but this procedure is no longer performed in the United States because of excessive postoperative morbidity and mortality (288). Since then, surgical procedures have evolved considerably. Kral (287) has noted that more than 27 surgical methods for treating obesity have been used and that further major technical advances are unlikely. Currently two procedures are most widely used: vertical banded gastroplasty and gastric bypass with a Roux-en-Y gastrojejunostomy. The horizontal banded gastroplasty, widely used in the early 1980s, has been largely abandoned due to high failure rates and frequent weight regain (279).

The gastric restriction procedures now in use produce weight loss primarily by limiting food intake. Both gastroplasty and gastric bypass surgically reduce the stomach pouch to 30 ml or less in capacity and create a small outlet of approximately 10 mm (289). Coarse food tends to stop at the stoma, which results in rapid filling of the small stomach and the early onset of sensations of fullness. Patients thus tend to eat smaller amounts of food at more frequent and regular intervals, leading to an overall reduction in daily calorie intake. Gastric bypass involves malabsorption as an additional mechanism, which probably explains its greater effectiveness (290).

Kral and Kissileff (287) have recently proposed that the primary mechanism of weight loss from these surgical methods is aversion. In the case of gastric bypass the rapid passage of liquids from the stomach pouch into the intestine causes lightheadedness, discomfort, and diarrhea (dumping syndrome). With either procedure, overeating and exceeding the pouch capacity can produce pain, nausea, and vomiting. Consequently these surgical methods should not be considered curative but rather a form of "behavioral surgery" that functions by affecting eating behavior rather than removing or reconstructing diseased tissue (289). Combining the predictable aversive influences with intensive education and follow-up will help patients learn to regulate their food intake consistently (291).

Patients should be instructed that untoward side effects can be avoided if they will practice eating slowly, chew food thoroughly, limit amounts to 30–60 ml per meal, eat raw vegetables and high-protein foods, and drink low-calorie liquids. To be avoided are soft calorie-dense foods such as ice cream, chocolate, and cheese; easily dissolvable foods including cookies and cakes; and high-calorie liquids such as whole milk, alcohol, and sodas. Soft breads, red meat, pastas, and citrus fruits should also be used sparingly, since they can cause obstruction of the stoma (292).

Complications from gastric surgery vary with the specific procedure used and the characteristics of the patient. Most common are outlet obstruction, vomiting, gastric leaks, dumping, and wound infections (293). The incidence of postoperative morbidity has been estimated to be 15%, and mortality at 1% or less (180). Failure rates may be as high as 50% if all revisions, reversals, and patients lost to follow-up are considered (117). A common undesirable outcome after surgery is weight gain associated with maladaptive eating. Specifically, patients who fail to lose weight or maintain their weight loss after surgery are most often those who ingest excessive amounts of high-calorie liquids and/or soft foods (290).

Weight loss results are also highly variable. Weight losses at 1 year have been reported to be 75–125 lb, or approximately 75% of excess weight (294). Yale (295) recently published an analysis of long-term results of gastric bypass, vertical banded gastroplasty, and unbanded gastrogastrostomy. In a series of 537 consecutive patients evaluated for 3–5 years the unbanded procedure was considered ineffective for long-term weight control while the gastric bypass and vertical banded gastroplasty were judged effective. Defining success as maintaining a weight loss of at least 20% of the preoperative weight, it was found that after 3 years only a third of the unbanded patients were successful compared to 69% of those who had vertical banded surgery and 84% of those undergoing gastric bypass. Yale concluded that the gastric bypass was the more effective operation for long-term weight control, with the average patient maintaining a weight loss of 31% of preoperative weight or 60% of excess weight (i.e., weight above ideal body weight) (295).

In contrast, Mason (296), who pioneered gastric surgery, now prefers the vertical banded procedure. He and his co-workers reported a 49% loss of excess weight in 22 "super" obese patients and a 61% loss of excess weight in 58 morbidly obese patients 5 years after vertical banded gastroplasty (297). In general it can be said that these current surgical methods produce rapid weight loss for most patients over the first 6 months. Weight loss tapers off and plateaus after 12–18 months, resulting in a loss of about one-third of initial weight. Few patients reach ideal weight, most likely because of the fat cell hyperplasia that characterizes their morbid obesity (297).

In conclusion, contemporary surgical methods are a viable treatment option for the morbidly obese patient who is properly selected, prepared, and evaluated after treatment (293,298). Surgical results are currently far superior to dieting or other treatments for the severely obese patient and can produce major improvements in medical status, quality of life, and psychological disposition (299,300). Nevertheless, these invasive procedures are expensive, averaging $10,000 for uncomplicated cases (286), they carry all the risks associated with major surgery and anesthesia, and they may involve long-term complications not yet revealed in the medical literature. Patients, therefore, should be selected for surgery only after thorough medical evaluation, which includes assessments of behavioral, social, and psychological factors, and only as an integral component of the long-term rehabilitative process (135,300).

9. *Pharmacologic Treatment*

Various drugs have been used as primary or adjunctive therapy for obesity. In the 1950s and 1960s dieters seeking weight control help from their physicians were given prescriptions for anorexiants that later proved to have a high potential for abuse and dependency (180). These frequently used schedule II drugs (amphetamine and methamphetamine) also had undesirable cardiovascular side effects, including increases in heart rate and blood pressure as well as arrhythmias. Furthermore they were ineffective in producing substantial or sustainable weight losses. For these reasons the schedule II appetite suppressants should no longer be used in treating obesity (301).

A new generation of medications is being investigated that may, in the future, prove to have selective utility. Of particular interest are dexfenfluramine (302) and fluoxetine (303). Both of these drugs affect the neurotransmitter serotonin, which has been shown to influence appetite, meal frequency, food intake, and body weight (304,305). Wurtman (41) has recently suggested that enhancement of central serotoninergic transmission by these medications may have particular value for the subgroups of obese patients who display a cluster of characteristics including depression, marked carbohydrate craving, and seasonal affective disorders.

While several studies have documented beneficial short-term effects of fluoxetine and dexfenfluramine on food intake and weight, their long-term effects remain controversial. Two recent placebo-controlled clinical trials have demonstrated the effectiveness of fluoxetine in producing significantly greater weight losses in obese subjects (301,306). A year long, placebo-control trial reported by Darga et al. (301) showed that the superior weight loss of the fluoxetine-treated group faded over the course of the study. The 14 drug-treated subjects achieved a maximal weight loss averaging 12.4 kg at week 29, compared to 4.5 kg lost in the 14 subjects receiving placebo. At the end of the year, however, the placebo-treated group maintained their 4.5 kg of weight loss, while the active-drug-treated patients regained some of their weight to an average loss of only 8.2 kg. Similar short-term efficacy has been demonstrated in studies using dexfenfluramine (307,308).

To investigate the long-term efficacy of dexfenfluramine, Guy-Grand et al. (309) conducted a year long multicenter trial involving over 800 patients who were at least 120% above ideal weight. The drop-out rates for drug- and placebo-treated groups were 37% and 45%, respectively. Patients receiving the active medication reported significantly more side effects related to drowsiness, fatigue, dry mouth, diarrhea, and polyuria, especially during the early stages of treatment. Both groups showed significant weight loss at the end of 1 year, averaging 7.2 kg for the placebo-treated group and 9.8 for the drug-treated group. Given the additional costs and side effects of drug treatment, this study raises serious questions about the long-term effectiveness of this particular medication.

These rather unimpressive results underscore the cautions recently articulated by Cairella (310) that these drugs are only likely to be useful in a small number of carefully selected patients, and then only as an adjunct to comprehensive therapy. There is also the concern that a beneficial treatment outcome might be short lived if the patient attributes the success of treatment to sources other than his or herself. This was dramatically illustrated in a 1-year study by Craighead et al. (311) in which drug therapy with dexfenfluramine was compared to behavioral therapy and a combination of drug plus behavioral therapy in 120 patients averaging 60% above ideal weight. After 6 months, the drug-treated group outperformed the other two groups (−15.3 kg for the drug-treated group vs. −10.9 kg and −14.5 kg for the behavioral and combined treatments, respectively). At 1 year, however, the drug-treated group regained considerable weight, sustaining a loss of only −6.3 kg, compared to sustained losses of −9.0 kg and −4.6 kg for the behavioral and combined treatments, respectively. Thus at 1 year behavioral therapy alone substantially outperformed drug therapy with or without a behavioral component. In fact, the addition of medication to behavioral therapy appears to have compromised the otherwise satisfactory effect of the behavioral intervention. A recent study by Rodin et al. (312) also showed that subjects treated with drugs regained weight substantially faster than those who received cognitive–behavioral therapy alone or with a placebo.

In conclusion, the use of drugs in the treatment of obesity appears to be of limited value at this time. Recent reports showing the influence of fluoxetine and dexfenfluramine on food intake and weight may eventually lead to the development of treatment protocols that utilize such medications for selected patients at specific times during the treatment process. Research to date suggests these serotonin enhancers may be of special benefit to those patients who experience seasonal weight gain, binging, and carbohydrate cravings (41,313). Other developments in pharmacotherapy may eventually provide medications useful for regulating metabolic rate, influencing digestion or absorption, and even mobilizing select regional fat deposits (301,314).

VII. CONCLUSIONS

Obesity continues to be a problem of epidemic proportions. Recent surveys show that the prevalence of obesity is increasing (16,17). According to Pollock and

Wilmore (315), the average American gains approximately 5 lb/year between the ages of 25 and 55 while losing ¼ to ½ lb of lean tissue from bone and muscle each year, predominantly as a result of physical inactivity. Combined with chronic exposure to a high-fat, convenience-oriented diet, the average American will be 45 lb fatter at age 55, having gained 30 lb of scale weight and losing up to 15 lb of lean tissue. This insidious change in body composition can lead to a host of detrimental medical, economic, functional, and psychosocial consequences.

Finding better ways to prevent and treat obesity may soon be seen as not only good medicine but also an economic imperative. The combination of a demographically aging population and spiraling health care costs is likely to spur the interest of government, insurance companies, health care providers, and individuals in creating more effective ways of dealing with obesity and related chronic medical conditions: hypertension, diabetes, heart disease, hyperlipidemia, and orthopedic problems (316).

Our nation's health care expenditures have increased almost 200% in the last decade (317). We now spend over $700 billion yearly, 12.3% of the gross national product (GNP), compared to $380 billion and 9.5% of the GNP in 1980. If current inflationary trends continue unabated to the year 2000, the medical bill will double to $1.6 trillion, making adequate health care accessible to only the very wealthy and placing a crippling financial strain on government agencies, corporations, and American families (318,319).

While health care cost containment is a very complex, multifaceted problem, part of the solution is likely to be in learning how to control obesity and related chronic medical conditions more effectively through lifestyle restructuring (320). Although the search for biomedical solutions to the problems of aging and chronic disease will continue to be important, more research efforts need to focus on the prevention of chronic infirmities such as obesity, in order to minimize and delay the onset of morbid conditions that require increasingly expensive medical care (321).

This chapter has reviewed numerous nutritional, behavioral, pharmacologic, and surgical approaches to the management of obesity. No single treatment modality has been uniformly effective, although several recent approaches, including very-low-calorie diets (VLCDs), surgery, and comprehensive multimodal behavioral therapy have been successful in producing medically significant weight loss in selected patients. The following general conclusions are offered:

1. It is important to recognize that obesity is a potentially serious, chronic medical disorder that develops from a complex, multifarious cause. It is similar in nature to other chronic diseases such as diabetes mellitus, hypertension, and coronary heart disease in that genetic, environmental, behavioral, and psychosocial variables all interact to determine the onset, severity, and duration of the disorder. Obesity should not be approached as if it were a simple linear disorder with a single cause and cure. Patients and

health professionals need to focus more on achieving a state of sustained, stable remission as the primary goal of treatment. Cure is often an unattainable and unrealistic expectation (5,117).

2. Obesity is more easily prevented than treated. Greater efforts need to be made, especially with children, adolescents, and young adults, to promote good nutrition, exercise, and coping skills that would prevent the development of health-compromising obesity.

3. Improved methods of evaluating and classifying patients can lead to more effective treatments individualized to the patient's greatest need (322). Advances are now being made in our understanding of the anatomical and metabolic aspects of obesity, the influence of nutrition and physical activity, and the social and psychological factors that affect both the development and treatment of the disorder. Sufficient knowledge already exists to identify better those obese patients at greatest medical risk who would most likely benefit from aggressive intervention. New information is likely to be forthcoming regarding the psychosocial dynamics critical to the development and maintenance of obesity among certain subgroups of the population. Continued research on the addictive characteristics of obesity and how this disorder is intertwined with social, cognitive, and emotional factors will likely provide a basis for designing more effective treatment interventions. Attrition rates and treatment failures could be substantially reduced if patients who needed psychological counseling were more frequently identified and referred to professionals experienced in the treatment of eating disorders. A subgroup of obese individuals suffer from a substance abuse disorder that has deep psychological underpinnings. This is more commonly recognized in cases of anorexia or purging bulimia, but is often overlooked among the chronically obese who do not purge. The recent insightful work by Stuart and Jacobsen (133) suggests that some obese patients would be better served by participation in marriage counseling or couples therapy than by launching into aggressive treatment of the obesity. The abuse of food and the condition of obesity are, for some, a buffer against intimacy and emotional distress.

4. The role of physical activity has not been fully recognized or utilized in either the prevention or the treatment of obesity. While therapeutic exercise has been used for decades in the rehabilitation of cardiac patients, supervised exercise training has only recently been applied to the problem of obesity. Because physical inactivity is typically a primary causative factor, exercise should be considered an essential component of all treatment approaches. Even when the primary initial therapy is psychosocial in nature, a return to a more biologically normal pattern of physical activity can potentiate the outcome. The obese patient must become intimately reassociated with his or her own physical body. A new relationship to the

physical body characterized by gratitude, appreciation, care, sensitivity, and respect must be developed that will provide an internal desire to carry out a program of self-care. Regular physical activity, in addition to its many physiological benefits, seems to be indispensable to the process of establishing a healthy relationship between the thinking, feeling self and the body it inhabits.

5. Combinations of treatment modalities applied serially over extended periods of time will, in the future, produce much better long-term results than the single-modality approaches of the past. Various subgroups of patients can benefit from different combinations of dietary intervention, exercise, pharmacotherapy, VLCD, surgery, and psychological counseling. Future research needs to focus on treating specific types of obesity with well-conceived combinations of therapies.

6. The dynamics of compliance and maintenance of the treatment regimen should be intensively investigated to help identify the strategies that can most effectively empower the individual to carry out a continuing program of self-care. Social supports, frequent therapist contact, booster sessions, relapse management training, and group exercise sessions have all shown promise for contributing to the desired state of sustainable remission.

REFERENCES

1. National Institute of Health Consensus Development Panel on the Health Implications of Obesity. Ann Intern Med 1985; 103(6pt2):1073–7.
2. Stunkard AJ. The current status of treatment for obesity in adults. In: Stunkard AJ, Stellar E, eds. Eating and its disorders. New York: Raven Press, 1984:157–73.
3. Bray GA. Classification and evaluation of obesities. Med Clin North Am 1989; 73: 161–83.
4. Kraemer HC, Berkowitz RI, Hammer LD. Methodological difficulties in studies of obesity: I. Measurement issues. Ann Behav Med 1990; 12:112–8.
5. Haber S. Effective treatment of obesity produces remission, not cure. Int J Obesity 1980; 4:265–7.
6. Getting Slim. U.S. News and World Report, May 14, 1990, p 32.
7. Van Itallie TB. Morbid obesity: a hazardous disorder that resists conservative treatment. Am J Clin Nutr 1980; 33:358–63.
8. Van Itallie TB, Kral JG. The dilemma of morbid obesity. JAMA 1981; 246:999–1003.
9. Brownell KD. New developments in the treatment of obese children and adolescents. In: Stunkard AJ, Stellar E, eds. Eating and its disorders. New York: Raven Press, 1984.
10. Pontius AA. Obesity types in stone age art. Ann NY Acad Sci 1987; 499:331–4.
11. Brown PJ, Konner M. An anthropological perspective on obesity. Ann NY Acad Sci 1987; 499:29–46.

12. Beller AS. Fat and thin: a natural history of obesity. New York: McGraw Hill, 1977.
13. Bray GA. Obesity: historical development of scientific and cultural ideas. Int J Obesity 1990; 14:909–26.
14. Jordan JA. In defense of body weight. J Am Dietet Assoc 1977; 62:17–21.
15. Beaumont W. Experiments and observations on the gastric juice and the physiology of digestion. New York: Dover Publications, 1959.
16. Simopoulos AP. Dietary control of hypertension and obesity and body weight standards. J Am Dietet Assoc 1985; 85:419–22.
17. Najjar MF, Rowland M. Anthropometric reference data and prevalence of over-weight, United States, 1976–1980. Washington, D.C.: Public Health Service; October 1987. Vital and Health Statistics, Series 11, No. 238. Department of Health and Human Services publication (PHS) 87-1688.
18. Harlen WR, Landis JR, Flegal KM, Davis CS, Miller ME. Secular trends in body mass in the United States, 1960–1980. Am J Epidemiol 1988; 128:1065–74.
19. Van Itallie TB. Health implications of overweight and obesity in the United States (the problem of density). Ann Intern Med 1985; 103(6pt2):1062–7.
20. Williamson DF, Kahn HS, Remington PL, Anda RF. The 10-year incidence of over-weight and major weight gain in U.S. adults. Arch Intern Med 1990; 150:665–72.
21. Carpenter KJ, Mayer J. Physiologic observations on yellow obesity in mice. Am J Physiol 1958; 193:449–54.
22. Zucker LM, Zucker TF. Fatty, a new mutation in the rat. J Hered 1961; 52:275–8.
23. Kelsey RE. A set point theory of obesity. In: Brownell KD, Foreyt JP, eds. Handbook of eating disorders: physiology, psychology and treatment of obesity, anorexia, and bulemia. New York: Basic Books, 1981.
24. Schemmel R, Mickelson O, Gill JL. Dietary obesity in rats. Body weight and body fat accretion in seven strains of rats. J Nutr 1970; 100:1041–8.
25. Gurney R. Hereditary factors in obesity. Arch Intern Med 1936; 57:557–61.
26. Seltzer CC, Mayer J. Body build and obesity—who are the obese? JAMA 1964; 189: 677–84.
27. Sims EA, Danforth E, Horton ES, Bray GA, Glennon JA, Salans LB. Endocrine and metabolic effects of experimental obesity in man. Rec Prog Horm Res 1973; 29: 457–76.
28. Bouchard C, Tremblay A, Despres JP, Nadeau A, Lupien PJ, Theriault G, Dussault J, Moorjane S, Pinault S, Fournier G. The response to long-term overfeeding in identical twins. N Engl J Med 1990; 322:1477–82.
29. Stunkard AJ, Sorensen TIA, Harris C, Teasdale TW, Chakraborty R, Schull WJ, Schulsinger F. An adoption study of human obesity. N Engl J Med 1986; 314:193–8.
30. Stunkard AJ, Harris JR, Pedersen NL, McClearn GE. The body mass index of twins who have been reared apart. N Engl J Med 1990; 322:1483–7.
31. Van Itallie TB. Bad news and good news about obesity. N Engl J Med 1986; 314: 239–40.
32. Sims EAH. Destiny rides again as twins overeat. N Engl J Med 1990; 322:1522–3.
33. Bouchard C, Perusse LA, LeBlanc C, Tremblay A, Theriault G. Inheritance of the amount and distribution of human body fat. Int J Obesity 1988; 12:205–15.
34. Garrow JS. Obesity and related disorders. New York: Churchill Livingstone, 1988.

35. Sims EAH. Storage and expenditure of energy in obesity and their implications for management. Med Clin North Am 1987; 73:97–110.

36. Bouchard C. Genetic factors in human obesity. Med Clin North Am 1989; 73:67–81.

37. Perusse LA, Tremblay A, LeBlanc C, Bouchard C. Genetic and familial environmental influences on level of habitual physical activity. Am J Epidemiol 1989; 129: 1012–22.

38. Schull WJ. Heredity, fitness and health. In: Bouchard C, Shephard R, Stephens T, Sutton JR, McPherson BD, eds. Exercise, fitness and health: a consensus of current knowledge. Champaign, IL: Human Kinetics, 1990: 137–45.

39. De Moor P, Joosens JV. An inverse relation between body weight and the activity of the steroid binding B-globulin in human plasma. Steroidologia 1970; 1:129–36.

40. Cabellero J. Insulin resistance and amino acid metabolism in obesity. Ann NY Acad Sci 1987; 499:84–93.

41. Wurtmann JJ. Disorders of food intake: excessive carbohydrate snack intake among a class of obese people. Ann NY Acad Sci 1987; 499:197–202.

42. Andres R, Elahi D, Tobin JD, Muller DC, Brant L. Impact of age on weight goals. Ann Intern Med 1985; 103:1030–3.

43. Garrison RJ, Feinleib M, Castelli WP, McNamara PM. Cigarette smoking as a confounder of the relationship between relative weight and long term mortality. JAMA 1983; 249:2199–203.

44. Manson JE, Stampher MJ, Hennekins CH, Willet WC. Body weight and longevity: a reassessment. JAMA 1987; 257:353–8.

45. Bray GA. Overweight is risking fate: definition, classification, prevalence, and risks. Ann NY Acad Sci 1987; 499:14–28.

46. Kral JG. Morbid obesity and related health risks. Ann Intern Med 1985; 103: 1043–7.

47. Drenick EJ. Definition and health consequences of obesity. Surg Clin North Am 1979; 59:963–76.

48. Drenick EJ, Gurunanjappa BS, Seltzer F, Johnson DG. Excess mortality and causes of health in morbidly obese men. JAMA 1980; 243:443–5.

49. Garbaciak JA, Richter M, Miller S, Barton JJ. Maternal weight and pregnancy complications. Am J Obstet Gynecol 1985; 152:238–45.

50. Abrams B, Parker J. Overweight and pregnancy complications. Int J Obesity 1988; 12:293–303.

51. Maeder EC, Barno A, Micklenburg F. Obesity: a maternal high-risk factor. Obstet Gynecol 1975; 45:669–71.

52. Gross T, Sokol RJ, King KC. Obesity in pregnancy: risk and outcome. Obstet Gynecol 1980; 56:446–9.

53. Calandra C, Asbell DA, Beischer NA. Maternal obesity in pregnancy. Obstet Gynecol 1981; 57:8–11.

54. Committee on Nutrition and the Mother. National Research Council: Nutritional Services in Perinatal Care. Washington, DC: National Academy Press, 1981.

55. Manson JE, Colditz GA, Stampfer MJ, Willett WC, Rosner B, Monson RR, Speizer FE, Hennekens CH. A prospective study of obesity and risk of coronary heart disease in women. N Engl J Med 1990; 322:882–9.

56. Marks HH. Influence of obesity on morbidity and mortality. Bull NY Acad Med 1960; 36:296–302.
57. Keys A. Overweight, obesity, coronary heart disease and mortality. Nutr Rev 1980; 38:297–307.
58. Kissebah A, Vydelingum N, Murray R, Evans DJ, Hartz AJ, Kalkhoff RK, Adams PW. Relation of body fat distribution to metabolic complications of obesity. J Clin Endocrinol Metab 1982; 54:254–62.
59. Barrett-Connor EL. Obesity, atherosclerosis and coronary artery disease. Ann Intern Med 1985; 103(6pt2):1010–9.
60. Hubert HB, Feinleib M, McNamara PM, Castelli WP. Obesity as an independent risk factor for cardiovascular disease: a 26 year follow-up of participants in the Framingham Heart Study. Circulation 1983; 67:968–77.
61. Kannel WB, Gordon T. Physiological and medical concomitants of obesity: The Framingham Study. In: Bray GA, ed. Obesity in America. Bethesda, MD: N.I.H. Publication No. 79–359. 1979: 125–63.
62. Van Itallie TB. Obesity: adverse effects on health and longevity. Am J Clin Nutr 1979; 32:2723–33.
63. Ashley FW, Kannel WB. Relation of weight change to changes in atherogenic traits: The Framingham Study. J Chron Dis 1974; 27:103–14.
64. Forbes GB, Reina JC. Adult lean body mass declines with age: some longitudinal observations. Metabolism 1970; 19:653–63.
65. Krotkiewski M, Bjorntorp P, Sjostrom J, Smith U. Impact of obesity on metabolism in men and women: importance of regional adipose tissue distribution. J Clin Invest 1983; 72:1150–62.
66. Kannel WB. CHD risk factors: A Framingham Study update. Hosp Pract 1990; July 15:119–30.
67. Newman B, Selby JV, Ovesenberry CP, King MC, Friedman GD, Fabsitz RR. Nongenetic influences of obesity on other cardiovascular disease risk factors: an analysis of identical twins. Am J Public Health 1990; 80:675–8.
68. Heckel DB, Reimen KA. Heart. In: Kissane JM, ed. Anderson's pathology, 9th ed. St. Louis: CV Mosby, 1990: 615–729.
69. Brownell KD. Obesity: understanding and treating a serious, prevalent and refractory disorder. J Consult Clin Psychol 1982; 50:820–40.
70. Brownell KD. The psychology and physiology of obesity: implications for screening and treatment. J Am Dietet Assoc 1984; 84:406–13.
71. Wadden TA, Stunkard AJ. Social and psychological consequences of obesity. Ann Intern Med 1985; 103(6pt2):1062–7.
72. Wooley SC, Wooley OW. Should obesity be treated at all? In: Stunkard AJ, Stellar E, eds. Eating and its disorders. New York: Raven Press, 1984: 185–92.
73. Rodin J, Schank D, Striegel-Moore R. Psychological features of obesity. Med Clin North Am 1989; 73:47–65.
74. Kaplan S. Some psychological and social factors present in the condition of obesity. J Rehab 1979; Oct/Nov/Dec:52–4.
75. Steward AL, Brook RH. Effects of being overweight. Am J Public Health 1983; 73: 171–7.

76. Albon N. Self-perceptions of the stigma of overweight in relationship to weight-losing patterns. Am J Clin Nutr 1979; 32:470–80.
77. Lerner RM, Gilbert E. Body build identification, preference, and aversion in children. Dev Psychol 1969; 5:256–62.
78. Staffieri JR. A study of social stereotyping of body image in children. J Pers Soc Psychol 1967; 7:101–4.
79. Staffieri JR. Body build and behavioral expectancies in young females. Dev psychol 1972; 6:125–7.
80. Goodmen N, Dornbusch SM, Richardson SA, Hastorf AH. Variant reactions to physical disabilities. Am Sociol Rev 1963; 28:429–35.
81. Maddox GL, Liederman VR. Overweight as a social disability with medical implications. J Med Ed 1969; 44:214–20.
82. Breytspraak LM, McGee J, Conger JC, Whatley JL, Moore JT. Sensitizing medical students to impression formation processes in the patient interview. J Med Ed 1977; 52:47–55.
83. Canning H, Meyer J. Obesity—its possible effect on college acceptance. N Engl J Med 1966; 275:1172–4.
84. Canning H, Meyer J. Obesity: an influence on high school performance? Am J Clin Nutr 1967: 20:352–4.
85. Larkin JE, Pines HA. No fat persons need apply. Sociol Work Occup 1979; 6:312–27.
86. Allon N. The stigma of overweight in everyday life. In: Wolman B, ed. Psychological aspects of obesity: a handbook. New York: Van Nostrand Reinhold, 1982: 130–74.
87. Bray GA, Gray DS. Obesity: Part 1—pathogenesis. West J Med 1988; 149:429–41.
88. Hirsch J, Fried SK, Edens NK, Leibel RL. The fat cell. Med Clin North Am 1990; 73:83–96.
89. Sheldon WH, Stevens SS, Tucker WB. The varieties of human physique: an introduction to constitutional psychology. New York: Harper and Row, 1940.
90. Vague J. The degree of masculine differentiation of obesities: a factor determining predisposition of diabetes, atherosclerosis, gout and uric calculous disease. Am J Clin Nutr 1956; 4:20–34.
91. Seidell JC, Bjorntorp P, Sjostrom L, Sannerstedt R, Krotkiewski M, Kvist H. Regional distribution of muscle and fat mass in men—new insight into the risk of abdominal obesity using computed tomography. Int J Obesity 1989; 13:289–303.
92. Bjorntorp P. Classification of obese patients and complications related to the distribution of surplus fat. Am J Clin Nutr 1987; 45:1120–5.
93. Seidell JC, Deurenburg P, Hautvast J. Obesity and fat distribution in relation to health—current insights and recommendations. World Rev Nutr Diet 1987; 50:57–91.
94. Larsson B, Svardsudd K, Welin L, Wilhelmsen L, Bjorntorp P, Tibblin G. Abdominal adipose tissue distribution, obesity and risk of cardiovascular disease and death: 13 year follow-up of participants in the study of men born in 1913. Br Med J 1984; 288:4011–4.
95. Bjorntorp P. Regional patterns of fat distribution. Ann Intern Med 1985; 103 (6pt2):994–5.
96. Lapidus L, Bengtsson C, Larsson B, Pennert K, Rybo E, Sjostrom L. Distribution

of adipose tissue and risk of cardiovascular disease and death: a 12 year follow-up of participants in the population study of women in Gothenburg, Sweden. Br Med J 1984; 288:1401–4.

97. Peiris AN, Sothmann MS, Hoffman RG, Hennes MI, Wilson CR, Gustofson AB, Kissebah AH. Adiposity, fat distribution and cardiovascular risk. Ann Intern Med 1989; 110:867–72.

98. Ducimetiere P, Richard J, Cambien F. The pattern of subcutaneous fat distribution in middle-aged men and the risk of coronary heart disease: the Paris prospective study. Int J Obesity 1986; 10:229–40.

99. Barakat HA, Burton DS, Carpenter JW, Holbert D, Israel RG. Body fat distribution, plasma lipoproteins and the risk of coronary heart disease in male subjects. Int J Obesity 1988; 12:473–80.

100. Landin K, Stigendahl L, Eriksson E, Krotkiewski M, Risberg B, Tengborn L, Smith U. Abdominal obesity is associated with an impaired fibrinolytic activity and elevated plasminogen activator inhibitor-1. Metabolism 1990; 39:1044–8.

101. Ohlson LO, Larsson B, Svardsdudd K, Welin L, Erikson H, Wilhelmson I, Bjorntorp P, Tibblin G. The influence of body fat distribution on the incidence of diabetes mellitus: 13.5 year follow-up of the participants in the study of men born in 1913. Diabetes 1985; 34:1055–8.

102. Haffner SM, Stern MP, Hazuda HP, Pugh J, Patterson JK. Do upper body and centralized adiposity measure different aspects of regional fat distribution? Diabetes 1987; 36:43–51.

103. Lundgren H, Bengtssen C, Blohme G, Lapidus L, Sjostrom L. Adiposity and adipose tissue distribution in relation to incidence of diabetes in women: results from a prospective population study in Gothenburg, Sweden. Int J Obesity 1989; 13:413–23.

104. Kissebah AH, Freedman DS, Peiris AN. Health risks of obesity. Med Clin North Am 1989; 73:111–39.

105. Rebuffe-Serive M, Anderson B, Olbe L, Bjorntorp P. Metabolism of adipose tissue in interabdominal depots in severely obese men and women. Metabolism 1990; 39:1021–5.

106. Svedberg J, Bjorntorp P, Smith U, Lonnroth P. Free fatty acids inhibit insulin binding, degradation and action in the isolated rat hepatocyte. Diabetes 1990; 39:570–4.

107. Evans DJ, Murray R, Kissebah AH. Relationship between skeletal muscle insulin resistance, insulin-mediated glucose disposal and insulin binding: effects of obesity and body fat topography. J Clin Invest 1984; 74:1515–20.

108. Gillum RF. The association of body fat distribution with hypertension, hypertensive heart disease, coronary heart disease, diabetes and cardiovascular risk factors in men and women aged 18–79. J Chron Dis 1987; 40:421–8.

109. Campaigne BN. Body fat distribution: metabolic consequences and implications for weight loss. Med Sci Sports Exerc 1990; 22:291–7.

110. Gray DS. Diagnosis and prevalence of obesity. Med Clin North Am 1989; 73:1–13.

111. Scott EC, Johnston FE. Critical fat, menarche and the maintenance of menstrual cycles. J Adol Health Care 1982; 2:249–60.

112. Frisch RE, McArthur JW. Menstrual cycles: fitness as a determinant of minimum weight necessary for the maintenance or onset. Science 1974; 185:949–51.

113. Durnin JVGA, Rahaman MM. The assessment of the amount of fat in the human body from measurements of skinfold thickness. Br J Nutr 1967; 21:681–9.

114. Weigley ES. Average? Ideal? Desirable? A brief overview of height weight tables in the United States. J Am Dietet Assoc 1984; 84:417–23.

115. Harrison GG. Height weight tables. Ann Intern Med 1985; 103(6pt2):1030–3.

116. Blackburn GL, Kanders BS. Medical evaluation and treatment of the obese with cardiovascular disease. Am J Cardiol 1987; 60:55–8G.

117. Bray GA, Gray DS. Obesity: part II—treatment. West J Med 1988; 149:555–71.

118. Tokunaga K, Matsuzawa Y, Kotani K, Keno Y, Kabataki T, Fujioka S, Tarui S. Ideal body weight estimated from the body mass index with the lowest morbidity. Int J Obesity 1991; 15:1–15.

119. Keys A, Fidanza F, Karvonen MJ, Kimura N, Taylor HL. Indices of relative weight and obesity. J Chron Dis 1972; 25:239–43.

120. Martin AD, Ross WD, Drinkwater DT, Clarys JP. Prediction of body fat by skinfold caliper: assumptions and cadaver evidence. Int J Obesity 1985; 9:31–9.

121. Lukaski HC, Johnson PE, Bolonchuk WW, Lykken GI. Assessment of fat free mass using bioelectrical impedance measurements of the human body. Am J Clin Nutr 1985; 41:810–7.

122. Lohman TG. Skinfolds and the body density and their relation to body fatness: a review. Hum Biol 1981; 53:181–225.

123. Lukaski HC. Methods for the assessment of human body composition: the traditional and the new. Am J Clin Nutr 1987; 46:537–56.

124. Jackson AS, Pollock ML. Steps toward the development of generalized equations for predicting body composition in adults. Can J Appl Sports Sci 1982; 7:187–94.

125. Skinner JS, Baldini FD, Gardner AW. Assessment of fitness. In: Bouchard C, Shephard R, Stephens T, Sutton JR, McPherson BD, eds. Exercise, fitness and health: a consensus of current knowledge. Champaign, IL: Human Kinetics, 1990: 109–17.

126. Roche AF. Body-composition assessments in youth and adults. Columbus, OH: Ross Laboratories, 1985.

127. Fanelli MT, Kuczmarski RJ, Hirsch M. Estimation of body fat from ultrasound measure of subcutaneous fat and circumferences in obese women. Int J Obesity 1988; 12:125–32.

128. Katch FI, Katch VL. Measurement and prediction errors in body composition assessment and the search for the perfect equation. Res Q Exerc Sport 1980; 51: 249–60.

129. Williams GC, Quill TE, Deci EL, Ryan RM. "The facts concerning the recent carnival of smoking in Connecticut" and elsewhere. Ann Intern Med 1991; 115: 59–63.

130. Kayman S, Bruvald W, Stern JS. Maintenance and relapse after weight loss in women: behavior aspects. Am J Clin Nutr 1990; 52:800–7.

131. Stunkard AJ. From explanation to action in psychosomatic medicine: the case of obesity. Psychosom Med 1975; 37:195–236.

132. Stunkard AJ, Rush J. Dieting and depression: a critical review of reports of untoward responses during weight reduction for obesity. Ann Intern Med 1974; 81: 526–33.

133. Stuart RB, Jacobson B. Weight, sex, and marriage: a delicate balance. New York: Simon and Schuster, 1987.

134. Wadden TA. Treatment of obesity in adults: a clinical perspective. In: Keller PA, Ritt GA, eds. Innovations in clinical practice: a source book, IV. Sarasota, FL: Professional Resource Exchange, 1985.

135. Wadden TA, Bell ST. Understanding and treating obesity. In: Bellack AS, Hersen M, eds. International handbook of behavior modification and therapy, 2nd ed. New York: Plenum (in press).

136. Perri MG, Lauer JB, McAdoo WG, McAllister DA, Yancey DZ. Enhancing the efficacy of behavior therapy for obesity: effects of aerobic exercise and a multicomponent maintenance program. J Consult Clin Psychol 1986; 54:670–5.

137. Foreyt JP, Goodrick GK. Factors common to the successful therapy of the obese patient. Med Sci Sports Exerc 1991; 23:292–7.

138. Sjostrom L. Fat cells and body weight. In: Stunkard AJ, ed. Obesity. Philadelphia: WB Saunders, 1980: 72–100.

139. Hirsch J, Bachelor B. Adipose tissue cellularity in human obesity. Clin Endocrinol Metabol 1976; 5:299–311.

140. Mason EE. Morbid obesity: use of vertical banded gastroplasty. Arch Surg 1982; 117:701–6.

141. Garrow JS. Treat obesity seriously. London: Churchill Livingstone, 1981.

142. Oscai LB, Miller WC. Dietary induced severe obesity: exercise implications. Med Sci Sports Exerc 1986; 18:6–9.

143. Miller WC, Lindeman AK, Wallace J, Niederpruem M. Diet composition, energy intake and exercise in relation to body fat in men and women. Am J Clin Nutr 1990; 52:426–30.

144. Prewitt TE, Schmeisser D, Bowen PE, Aye P, Dolecek TA, Langenberg P, Cole T, Brace L. Changes in body weight, body composition, and energy intake in women fed high- and low-fat diets. Am J Clin Nutr 1991; 46:886–92.

145. Flatt JP. Dietary fat, carbohydrate balance, and weight maintenance: effects of exercise. Am J Clin Nutr 1987; 45:296–306.

146. Kendall A, Levitsky DA, Strupp BJ, Lissner L. Weight loss on a low-fat diet: consequences of the imprecision of the control of food intake in humans. Am J Clin Nutr 1991; 53:1124–9.

147. Salmon DMW, Flatt JP. Effect of dietary fat content on the incidence of obesity among ad libitum fed mice. Int J Obesity 1985; 9:443–9.

148. Romieu I, Willett WC, Stampfer MJ, Colditz GA, Sampson L, Rosner B, Hennekens CH, Speizer FE. Energy intake and other determinants of relative weight. Am J Clin Nutr 1988; 47:406–12.

149. Wooley SC, Wooley OW, Danforth SR. Theoretical, practical and social issues in behavioral treatment of obesity. J Appl Behav Anal 1979; 12:3–25.

150. Braitman LE, Adlin EV, Stanton JL. Obesity and caloric intake: the National Health and Nutrition Survey of 1971–5 (HANES I). J Chron Dis 1985; 38:727–32.

151. Andersson I, Rossner S. Energy intake of obese women. Int J Obesity 1989; 13: 247–53.

152. Raymond CA. Do obese persons mirror thin counterparts in calorie intake, recall and food consumed? JAMA 1988; 260:314.

153. Dreon DM, Frey Hewitt B, Ellsworth N, Williams PT, Terry B, Wood PD. Dietary fat: carbohydrate ratio and obesity in middle-aged men. Am J Clin Nutr 1988; 47: 995–1000.

154. George V, Tremblay A, Despres JP, Landry M, Allard L, Leblanc C, Bouchard C. Further evidence for the presence of "small eaters" and "large eaters" among women. Am J Clin Nutr 1991; 53:425–9.

155. Ravussin E, Lillioza S, Knowler WC, Christin L, Freymond D, Abbot WHG, Boyce V, Howard BV, Bogardus C. Reduced rate of energy expenditure as a risk factor for body weight gain. N Engl J Med 1988; 318:467–72.

156. Ravussin E, Bogardus C. Relationship of genetics, age, and physical fitness to daily energy expenditure and fuel utilization. Am J Clin Nutr 1989; 49:968–75.

157. Stunkard A, McLaren-Hume M. The results of the treatment of obesity. Arch Intern Med 1959; 103:79–85.

158. Bennett W. Dietary treatments of obesity. Ann NY Acad Sci 1987; 499:250–68.

159. Weigle DS. Human obesity—exploding the myths. West J Med 1990; 153:421–8.

160. Ferster CB, Nurnberger JI, Levitt EB. The control of eating. J Mathetics 1962; 1: 87–109.

161. Stuart RB. Behavioral control of overeating. Behav Res Ther 1967; 5:357–65.

162. Harris MB. Self-directed program for weight control: a pilot study. J Abnorm Psychol 1969; 74:263–70.

163. Pennick SB, Filion R, Fox S, Stunkard A. Behavior modification in the treatment of obesity. Psychosom Med 1971; 33:49–55.

164. Currey H, Malcolm R, Riddle E, Schacte M. Behavioral treatment of obesity—limitations and results with the chronically obese. JAMA 1977; 237:2829–31.

165. Foreyt JP, Boodrick GK, Gotto AM. Limitations of behavioral treatment of obesity: review and analysis. J Behav Med 1981; 4:159–74.

166. Foreyt JP, Mitchell RE, Garner DT, Gee M, Scott LW, Gotto AM. Behavioral treatment of obesity: results and limitations. Behav Ther 1982; 13:153–61.

167. Wing RR, Jeffrey RW. Outpatient treatments of obesity: a comparison of methodology and clinical results. Int J Obesity 1979; 3:261–79.

168. Stalonas PM, Perri MG, Kerzner AB. Do behavioral treatments of obesity last? A five-year follow-up investigation. Addict Behav 1984; 9:175–83.

169. Hammer RL, Barrier CA, Roundy ES, Bradford JM, Fisher AG. Calorie restricted low-fat diet and exercise in obese women. Am J Clin Nutr 1989; 49:77–85.

170. Sclafani A. Dietary obesity. In: Stunkard A, ed. Obesity. Philadelphia: WB Saunders, 1980: 166–81.

171. Acheson KJ, Schutz Y, Bessard T, Anantharaman K, Flatt JP, Jiguier E. Glycogen storage capacity and denovo lipogenesis during massive carbohydrate overfeeding in man. Am J Clin Nutr 1988; 48:240–7.

172. Lissner L, Levitsky DA, Strupp BJ, Kakwarf HJ, Roe DA. Dietary fat and the regulation of energy intake in humans. Am J Clin Nutr 1987; 46:886–92.

173. Miller WC. Diet composition, energy intake, and nutritional status in relation to obesity in men and women. Med Sci Sports Exerc 1991; 23:280–4.
174. Wurtman RJ. Dietary treatments that affect brain neurotransmitters. Ann NY Acad Sci 1987; 499:177–90.
175. Wurtman RJ, Wurtman JJ. Carbohydrate and depression. Sci Am 1988; 260:68–75.
176. Li T, Lumeng L, McBride WJ, Jurphy JM. Alcoholism: is it a model for the study of disorders of mood and consumatory behavior? Ann NY Acad Sci 1987; 499:239–49.
177. Loro AD, Orleans CS. Binge eating in obesity: preliminary findings and guidelines for behavioral analysis and treatment. Addict Behav 1981; 6:155–66.
178. Lieberman HR, Wurtman JJ, Chen B. Changes in mood after carbohydrate consumption among obese individuals. Am J Clin Nutr 1986; 44:772–8.
179. Keno Y, Matsuzawa Y, Tokunaga K, Fujioka S, Kawamoto T, Kobatake T, Tarui S. High sucrose diet increases visceral fat accumulation in VMH-lesioned obese rats. Int J Obesity; 15:205–11.
180. Kanders BS, Forse RA, Blackburn GL. Obesity. In: Rakel RE, ed. Conn's current therapy. Philadelphia: WB Saunders, 1991: 524–31.
181. Food and Nutrition Board: Recommended dietary allowances, 9th rev. Washington D.C.: National Academy of Sciences, 1980.
182. Remington D, Fisher G, Parent E. How to lower your fat thermostat. Provo, UT: Vitality House International, 1983.
183. Connor SL, Connor WE. The new American diet. New York: Simon and Schuster, 1986.
184. Katahn M. The T-factor diet. New York: Bantam Books, 1990.
185. Pope-Cordle J, Katahn M. The T-factor fat gram counter. New York: WW Norton, 1989.
186. Katahn M. One meal at a time. New York: WW Norton, 1991.
187. Eaton SB, Shostak M, Konner M. The paleolithic prescription—a program of diet and exercise and a design for living. New York: Harper & Row, 1988.
188. Schauf GE. Etiology of obesity—the QQF theory. J Am Geriatr Soc 1973;21:346–9.
189. Weser E, Young EA. Nutrition and internal medicine: obesity. In: Stein JH, ed-in-chief. Internal medicine, 3rd ed. Boston: Little, Brown, 1991: 403–6.
190. Fabry P, Fodor J, Heijl Z, Braun T, Zvolankova K. The frequency of meals: its relation to overweight, hypercholesterolemia, and decreased glucose tolerance. Lancet 1964; 2:614–5.
191. Metzner HL, Lampshiear DE, Wheeler NC, Larkin FA. The relationship between frequency of eating and adiposity in adult men and women in the Tecumseh Community Health Study. Am J Clin Nutr 1977; 30:712–5.
192. Cohn CD, Joseph LB, Alweiss MD. Studies on the effects of feeding frequency and dietary composition on fat deposition. Ann NY Acad Sci 1965; 131:507–10.
193. Fabry P, Fodor Z, Heijl Z, Geizerova H, Balcarova O. Meal frequency and ischemic heart disease. Lancet 1968; 2:190–1.
194. Fabry P, Tepperman J. Meal frequency—a possible factor in human pathology. Am J Clin Nutr 1970; 23:1059–68.
195. Cohn C. Feeding patterns and some aspects of cholesterol metabolism. Fed Proc 1964; 23:67–81.

196. Bray GA. Lipogenesis in human adipose tissue: some effects of nibbling and gorging. J Clin Invest 1972; 51:537–48.

197. Jagannathan SN, Cornell WF, Beveridge JMR. Effects of gorging and semicontinuous eating of equicaloric amounts of formula-type high fat diets on plasma cholesterol and triglyceride levels in human volunteer subjects. Am J Clin Nutr 1964; 15:90–3.

198. Gwinup GR, Byron RC, Roush WH, Kruger FA, Hamwi GJ. Effect of nibbling versus gorging on serum lipids in man. Am J Clin Nutr 1963; 13:209–13.

199. Gwinup GR, Byron RC, Roush WH, Kruger FA, Hamwi GJ. Effect of nibbling versus gorging on glucose tolerance. Lancet 1963; 2:165–7.

200. Mayer J, Marshal NB, Vitale JJ. Exercise food intake and body weight in normal rats and genetically obese adult mice. Am J Physiol 1954; 177:544–8.

201. Rose E, Mayer J. Activity, caloric intake and the energy balance of infants. Pediatrics 1968; 41:18–9.

202. Roberts SB, Savage BA, Coward WA, Chew B, Lucas A. Energy expenditure and intake in infants born to lean and overweight mothers. N Engl J Med 1988; 318: 461–6.

203. Mayer J. Obesity during childhood. In: Wynick M, ed. Childhood obesity. New York: John Wiley, 1975.

204. Dietz WH Jr. Obesity in infants, children and adolescents in the United States. Part I: Identification, natural history, and after effects. Nutri Res 1981; I:117–37.

205. Mayer J, Thomas D. Regulation of food choice and obesity. Science 1967; 156:328–37.

206. Chirico AM, Stunkard AJ. Physical activity and human obesity. N Engl J Med 1960; 263:935–40.

207. Stunkard AJ. Physical activity, emotions and human obesity. Psychosom Med 1958; 5:366–72.

208. Ferraro R, Boyce VL, Swinburn B, Gregorio MD, Ravussin E. Energy cost of physical activity on a metabolic ward in relationship to obesity. Am J Clin Nutr 1991; 53:1368–71.

209. Stern JS. Is obesity a disease of inactivity? In: Stunkard AJ, Stellar E, eds. Eating and its disorders. New York: Raven Press, 1984.

210. Brownell KD, Stunkard AJ. Physical activity in the development and control of obesity. In: Stunkard AJ, ed. Obesity. Philadelphia: WB Saunders, 1980.

211. Colvin RH, Olson SB. A descriptive analysis of men and women who have lost significant weight and are highly successful at maintaining the loss. Addict behav 1983; 8:287–95.

212. Marston AR, Criss J. Maintenance of successful weight loss: incidence and prediction. Int J Obesity 1984; 8:435–9.

213. Gormally J, Rardin D. Weight loss and maintenance and changes in diet and exercise for behavioral counseling and nutrition education. J Counsel Psychol 1981; 28: 295–304.

214. Pavolu KN, Krey S, Stefee WP. Exercise as an adjunct to weight loss and maintenance. Am J Clin Nutr 1989; 49:1115–23.

215. AMA Council on Scientific Affairs. Treatment of obesity in adults. JAMA 1988; 260:2547–51.

216. Hill JO, Thiel J, Heller PA, Markon C, Fletcher G, DiGirolamo M. Energetic and metabolic studies of intragastric infusion of calories before and after exercise training. Int J Obesity 1991; 15:169–79.

217. Hill JO, Schlundt DG, Sbrocco T, Sharp T, Pope-Cordle J, Stetson B, Kaler M, Heim C. Evaluation of an alternating calorie diet with and without exercise in the treatment of obesity. Am J Clin Nutr 1989; 50:248–54.

218. Hill JO, Sparling PB, Shields TW, Heller PA. Exercise and food restriction: effects on body composition and metabolic rate in obese women. Am J Clin Nutr 1987; 46: 622–30.

219. Hill JO, Dorton J, Sykes MN, DiGirolamo M. Reversal of dietary obesity is influenced by its duration and severity. Int J Obesity 1989; 13:711–22.

220. Position Stand of the American College of Sports Medicine: The recommended quantity and quality of exercise for developing and maintaining cardiorespiratory and muscular fitness in healthy adults. Med Sci Sports Exerc 1990; 22:265–74.

221. Pollock ML, Wilmore JH. Exercise in health and disease: evaluation and prescription for prevention and rehabilitation, 2nd ed. Philadelphia: WB Saunders, 1990.

222. Webb P. Direct calorimetry and the energetics of exercise and weight loss. Med Sci Sports Exerc 1986; 18:3–5.

223. Segal KR, Pi-Sunyer FX. Exercise and obesity. Med Clin North Am 1989; 73:217–37.

224. Ballor DL, Katch VL, Becque, Marks CR. Resistance weight training during caloric restriction enhances lean body weight maintenance. Am J Clin Nutr 1988; 47: 19–25.

225. Kolata, G. Metabolic catch-22 of exercise regimens. Science 1987; 236:146–7.

226. Andersson B, Xu X, Rebuffe-Scrive M, Terning K, Krotkiewski M, Bjorntorp P. The effects of exercise training on body composition and metabolism in men and women. Int J Obesity 1991; 15:75–81.

227. Epstein LA, Wing RR. Aerobic exercise and weight. Addict Behav 1980; 5:371–88.

228. Woo R, Garrow JS, Pi-Sunyer XF. Voluntary food intake during prolonged exercise in obese women. Am J Clin Nutr 1982; 36:478–84.

229. Woo R, Garrow JS, Pi-Sunyer XF. Effect of exercise on spontaneous calorie intake in obesity. Am J Clin Nutr 1982; 36:470–7.

230. Saris WHM. Physiological aspects of exercise in weight cycling. Am J Clin Nutr 1989; 49:1099–104.

231. Pi-Sunyer XF. Exercise effects. Ann NY Acad Sci 1987; 499:94–103.

232. Staten MA. The effect of exercise on food intake in men and women. Am J Clin Nutr 1991; 53:27–31.

233. Morgan WP. Affective beneficence of vigorous physical activity. Med Sci Sports Exer 1985; 17:94–100.

234. Raglin JS, Morgan WP. Influence of vigorous exercise on mood states. Behav Ther 1985; 5:179–83.

235. Raglin JS, Morgan WP. Influence of exercise and quiet rest on state anxiety and blood pressure. Med Sci Sports Exerc 1987; 19:456–63.

236. Griest JH, Klein MH, Eischens RR, Faris J, Gurman AS, Morgan WP. Running as a treatment for depression. Comp Psychiatry 1979; 53:20–41.

237. Morgan WP. Psychological effects of exercise. Behav Med Update 1982; 4:25–30.

238. Mellion MB. Exercise therapy for anxiety and depression—part I: does the evidence justify its recommendation? Postgrad Med 1985; 77:59–98.

239. Leon AS. Effects of exercise conditioning on physiologic precursors of coronary heart disease. J Cardiopulmon Rehab 1991; 11:46–57.

240. Wood PD, Stefanick ML, Williams PD, Haskell WL. The effects on plasma lipoproteins on a prudent weight-reducing diet with or without exercise in overweight men and women. N Engl J Med 1991; 325:461–6.

241. Carlucci D, Goldfine H, Ward A, Taylor P, Rippe JM. Exercise: not just for the healthy. Phys Sports Med 1991; 19:46–53.

242. Lampman RM, Schteingart DE, Foss ML. Exercise as a partial therapy for the extremely obese. Med Sci Sports Exerc 1986; 18:19–24.

243. Powell KE, Casperson CJ, Kaplan JP, Ford ES. Physical activity and chronic diseases. Am J Clin Nutr 1989; 49:999–1006.

244. Corcoran PJ. Use it or lose it—the hazards of bed rest and inactivity. West J Med 1991; 154:536–8.

245. Bortz WM. Disuse and aging. JAMA 1982; 248:1203–8.

246. Astrand PO. Exercise physiology and its role in disease prevention and in rehabilitation. Arch Phys Med Rehabil 1987; 68:305–9.

247. Saris WHM. Physiological aspects of exercise in weight cycling. Am J Clin Nutr 1989; 1099–104.

248. Brownell KD, Greenwood MR, Stellar E. The effects of repeated cycles of weight loss and regain in rats. Physiol Behav 1986; 38:459–64.

249. Reed DR, Conrera RJ, Maggio C, Greenwood MRC, Rodin J. Weight cycling in female rats increase dietary fat selection and adiposity. Physiol Behav 1988; 42:389–95.

250. Brownell KD, Steen SN, Wilmore JH. Weight regulation practices in athletes: analysis of metabolic and health effects. Med Sci Sports Exerc 1987; 19:546–56.

251. VanDale D, Saris WHM. Repetitive weight loss and weight regain: effects on weight reduction, resting metabolic rate, lipolytic activity before and after exercise and/or diet treatment. Am J Clin Nutr 1989; 49:409–16.

252. Blackburn GL, Wilson GT, Kanders BS, Stein LJ, Lavin PT, Adler J, Brownell KD. Weight cycling: the experience of human dieters. Am J Clin Nutr 1989; 49:1105–9.

253. Lissner L, Odell PM, D'Agostino RB, Stokes J, Kreger BE, Belanger AJ, Brownell KD. Variability of body weight and health outcomes in the Framingham population. N Engl J Med 1991; 324:1839–44.

254. Lissner L, Bengtsson C, Lapidus L, Larsson B, Bengtsson B, Brownell K. Body weight variability and mortality in the Gothenburg prospective studies of men and women. In: Bjorntorp P, Lassner S, eds. Obesity in Europe. London: John Libbey, 1988: 51–55.

255. Hamm P, Shekelle RB, Stamler J. Large fluctuations in body weight during young adulthood and twenty five year risk of coronary death in men. Am J Epidemiol 1989; 129:312–8.

256. Craighead LW, Blum MD. Supervised exercise in behavioral treatment for moderate obesity. Behav Ther 1989; 20:49–59.

257. Harris MB, Hallbauer ES. Self-directed weight control through eating and exercise. Behav Res Ther 1973; 11:523–9.

258. Stalonas PM Jr, Johnson WG, Christ M. Behavior modification for obesity: the evaluation of exercise, contingency management and program adherence. J Consult Clin Psychol 1978; 46:463–9.

259. Dahlkoetter JA, Callahan EJ, Linton J. Obesity and the unbalanced energy equation: exercise versus eating habit change. J Consult Clin Psychol 1979; 47:898–905.

260. Bray GA. Exercise and obesity. In: Bouchard C, Shephard R, Stephens T, Sutton Jr, McPherson BD, eds. Exercise, fitness and health: a consensus of current knowledge. Champaign, IL: Human Kinetics Publications, 1990: 497–515.

261. Bjorntorp PA. Sex differences in the regulation of energy balance with exercise. Am J Clin Nutr 1989; 49:958–61.

262. Thompson JK, Jarvie GJ, Lahery BB, Cureton KJ. Exercise and obesity: etiology, physiology and intervention. Psychol Bull 1982; 91:55–79.

263. Rebuffe-Scrive M, Bjorntorp PA. Regional adipose tissue metabolism in man. In: Vague J, Bjorntorp PA, Guy-Grand B, Rebuffe-Scrive M, Vague P, eds. Metabolic Complications to Human Obesities. Amsterdam: Elsevier. 1985: 149–59.

264. American College of Sports Medicine. Guidelines for exercise testing and prescription, 4th ed. Philadelphia: Lea & Febiger, 1991.

265. Taylor P, Wood A, Rippe JM. Exercising to health: how much, how soon. Phys Sports Med 1991; 19:95–105.

266. Work JA. Exercise for the overweight patient. Phys Sports Med 1990; 18:113–22.

267. Glasser W. Positive addiction. New York: Harper and Row, 1976.

268. Wadden TA, Stunkard AJ, Brownell KD, Day SC. Very-low-calorie diets: their efficacy, safety, and future. Ann Intern Med 1983; 99:675–84.

269. Timely Statement of the American Dietetic Association: Very low calorie weight loss diets. J Am Dietet Assoc 1989; 89:975–6.

270. Amatruda JM, Richeson JF, Welle SL, Brodow RG, Lockwood DH. The safety and efficacy of a controlled low energy ("very-low-calorie") diet in the treatment of non-insulin dependent diabetes and obesity. Arch Intern Med 1988; 148:873–8.

271. Palgi A, Reed JL, Greenberg I, Hoefer MA, Bistrian BR, Blackburn GL. Multi-disciplinary treatment of obesity with a protein-sparing modified fast: results of 688 outpatients. Am J Public Health 1985; 75:1190–4.

272. Sours HE, Frattali VP, Brand CD, Feldman RA, Forbes AL, Swanson RC, Paris AL. Sudden death associated with very-low-calorie weight reduction regiments. Am J Clin Nutr 1981; 34:101–4.

273. Van Itallie TB, Yang M-U. Cardiac dysfunction in obese dieters: a potentially lethal complication of rapid massive weight loss. Am J Clin Nutr 1984; 39:695–702.

274. Position of the American Dietetic Association. Very-low-calorie weight loss diets. J Am Dietet Assoc 1990; 90:722–6.

275. Wadden TA, Van Itallie TB, Blackburn GL. Responsible and irresponsible use of very-low-calorie diets in the treatment of obesity. JAMA 1990; 263:83–5.

276. Liddle RA, Goldstein RB, Saxton J. Gallstone formation during weight reduction dieting. Arch Intern Med 1989; 149:1750–3.

277. Atkinson RL. Low and very low calorie diets. Med Clin North Am 1989; 73:203–15.

278. Prasad N. Very-low-calorie diets: safe treatment for moderate and morbid obesity. Postgrad Med 1990; 88:179–188.

279. Anderson T. Stokholm KH, Baker OG. Long term (5 year) results after either horizontal gastroplasty or very-low-calorie diet for morbid obesity. Int J Obesity 1988; 12:277–84.

280. Wadden TA, Stunkard AJ. Controlled trial of very low calorie diet, behavior therapy, and their combination in the treatment of obesity. J Consult Psychol 1986; 54:482–8.

281. Friedman RB. Very low calorie diets: how successful? Postgrad Med 1988; 83: 153–61.

282. Lindner PG, Blackburn GL. Multidisciplinary approach to obesity utilizing fasting modified by protein-sparing therapy. Obes Bariatr Med 1976; 5:48–57.

283. Kirschner MA, Schneider G, Ertel NH, Gorman J. An eight year experience with a very-low-calorie formula diet for control of major obesity. Int J Obesity 1988; 12: 69–80.

284. Hovell MF, Loch A, Hofstetter CR, Sipan C, Faucher P, Dellinger A, Borok G, Forsythe A, Feletti VJ. Long term weight loss maintenance: assessment of a behavioral and supplemented fasting regimen 1988; 78:663–6.

285. Wadden TA, Stunkard AJ, Liebschutz J. Three-year follow-up of the treatment of obesity by very low calorie diet, behavior therapy and their combination. J Consult Clin Psychol 1988; 56:925–8.

286. Pollner F. Obesity surgery regaining favor. Med World News May, 1991, 37.

287. Kral JG, Kissileff HR. Surgical approaches to the treatment of obesity. Am Behav Med 1987; 9:15–9.

288. Halmi KA. Gastric bypass for morbid obesity. In: Stunkard AJ, ed. Obesity. Philadelphia: WB Saunders, 1988: 388–94.

289. Yale CE. Surgery for morbid obesity: selecting the patient and their procedure. Postgrad Med 1988; 83:173-80.

290. Linner JH. Comparative effectiveness of gastric bypass and gastroplasty. Arch Surg 1982; 117:695–700.

291. Bukoff Priddy ML. Gastric reduction surgery: a dietitian's experience and perspective. J Am Dietet Assoc 1985; 85:455–9.

292. Kral JG. Surgical treatment of obesity. Med Clin North Am 1989; 73:251–64.

293. Power MA, Pappas TN. Physiologic approaches to the control of obesity. Ann Surg 1989; 209:255–60.

294. Stunkard AJ, Stinnet JL, Smoller JW. Psychological and social aspects of the surgical treatment of obesity. Am J Psychiatry 1986; 147:417–29.

295. Yale CE. Gastric surgery for morbid obesity. Arch Surg 1989; 124:941–6.

296. Mason EE. Vertical banded gastroplasty for obesity. Arch Surg 1982; 117:701–6.

297. Mason EE, Doherty C, Maher JW, Scott DH, Radriguiz EM. Super obesity and gastric restriction procedures. Gastroenterol Clin North Am 1987; 16:495–502.

298. Task Force of the American Society of Clinical Nutrition. Guidelines for surgery for morbid obesity. Am J Clin Nutr 1980; 33:446–51.

299. Hafner RJ, Watts JM, Rogers J. Quality of life after gastric bypass for morbid obesity. Int J Obesity 1991; 15:555–60.

300. Halmi KA, Stunkard AJ, Mason EE. Emotional responses to weight reduction by three methods: gastric bypass, jejunoileal bypass, diet. Am J Clin Nutr 1980; 33:446–51.

301. Weintraub M, Bray GA. Drug treatment of obesity. Med Clin North Am 1989; 73: 237–249.

302. Turner P. Dexfenfluramine: its place in weight control. Drugs 1990; 39:53–62.

303. Darga LL, Carroll-Michals L, Botsford SJ, Lucas CP. Fluoxitine's effect on weight loss in obese subjects. Am J Clin Nutr 1991; 54:321–5.

304. Blundell JE. Serotonin and appetite. Neuropharmacol 1984; 23(suppl3):53–62.

305. Garattini S, Bizzi A, Caccia S, Mennini T, Samanin R. Progress in assessing the role of serotonin in the control of food intake. Clin Neuropharmacol 1988; 11(suppl1): 8–22.

306. Pijl H, Koppeschaar HPF, Willekins FLA, Op de Kamp I, Veldhuis HD, Meinders AE. Effect of serotonin re-uptake inhibition by fluoxetine on body weight and spontaneous food choice in obesity. Int J Obesity 1991; 15:237–42.

307. Enzi G, Crepaldi G, Inelman EM, Bruni R, Baggio B. Efficacy and safety of dexfenfluramine in obese patients: a multicenter study. Clin Neuropharmacol 1988; 11(suppl1):173–8.

308. Finer N, Craddock D, Lavielle R, Keen H. Prolonged weight loss with dexfenfluramine treatment in obese patients. Diabete Metab 1987; 13:598–602.

309. Guy-Grand B, Apfelbaum M, Crepaldi G, Gries A, Lefebvre P, Turner P. International trial of long-term dexfenfluramine in obesity. Lancet 1989; 2:1442–5.

310. Cairella M. Psychological aspects of the drug treatment of obesity. Int J Obesity 1987; 11(suppl3):5–11.

311. Craighead LW, Stunkard AJ, O'Brien RM. Behavior therapy and pharmacotherapy for obesity. Arch Gen Psychiatry 1981; 38:763–8.

312. Rodin J, Elias M, Silberstein LR, Wagner A. Combined behavioral and pharmacologic treatment for obesity: predictors of successful weight maintenance. J Consult Clin Psychol 1988; 56:399–404.

313. Walsh BT, Gladis M, Roose SP. Food intake and mood in anorexia nervosa and bulemia. Ann NY Acad Sci 1987; 499:231–8.

314. Greenway FL, Bray GA. Regional fat loss from the thigh in obese women after adrenergic modulation. Clin Ther 1987; 9:663–9.

315. Pollock ML, Wilmore JH. Exercise in health and disease: evaluation and prescription for prevention and rehabilitation. Philadelphia: WB Saunders, 1990.

316. Schneider EL, Guralnik J. The aging of America: impact on health care costs. JAMA 1990; 263:2335–40.

317. Condition: critical. Time, November 15, 1991: 34–42.

318. How to fight killer health costs. U.S. News and World Report, September 23, 1991; 50–8.

319. Can you afford to get sick. U.S. News and World Report, January 30, 1989; 44–52.

320. Healthy People 2000: National Health Promotion and Disease Prevention Objectives. U.S. Department of Health and Human Services. Public Health Service, Conference edition, 1990: 1–8.

321. Fries JF. Aging, natural death, and the compression of morbidity. N Engl J Med 1980; 303:130–5.

322. Guy-Grand BJP. A new approach to the treatment of obesity: a discussion. Ann NY Acad Sci 1987; 499:313–7.

The Physician's Role in Promoting Physical Activity

TED D. ADAMS
The Fitness Institute
LDS Hospital
and University of Utah
Salt Lake City, Utah

CHAD E. EDGINGTON
The Fitness Institute
LDS Hospital
Salt Lake City, Utah

One specific strategy for improving the health of our nation during the next decade, published in *Healthy People 2000*, recommends that at least 50% of primary care providers "routinely assess and counsel their patients regarding the frequency, duration, type, and intensity of each patient's physical activity practices" (1). In addition, the U.S. Preventive Services Task Force advocates that physicians counsel all patients to "engage in a program of regular physical activity, tailored to their health status and personal lifestyle" (2).

These recommendations have important merit when we consider the fact that 85% of patients surveyed agree that a physician's recommendation to increase their involvement in physical activity would be beneficial (3). A recent meta-analysis, however, showed that physicians provide exercise counseling to only 30% of patients who are sedentary (1,4,5). Reasons why so few patients receive exercise counseling include the fact that doctors often feel uncomfortable about their skill level in suggesting physical activity programs (1) and that the physicians are often pressed for time. For example, a national survey recently indicated that when physicians did advise their patients regarding physical activity, less than 3 min was generally spent discussing the subject (5).

This chapter will assist the physician in providing counsel and advice to patients about physical activity programs. Also, to persuade physicians further of the importance of discussing physical activity the evidence that a sedentary lifestyle is a risk factor for coronary heart disease (CHD) and that physical activity can prevent or control CHD and other chronic diseases is reviewed. The assessment of cardiovascular fitness will be discussed, including the role of exercise electrocardiographic (ECG) testing. The characteristics of and the rationale for the exercise prescription and the basis for promoting leisure time physical activity will also be considered. Sample activity programs are also included.

I. PHYSICAL ACTIVITY: DEFINITION

Caspersen et al. (6) have provided clear definitions for the terms "physical activity," "exercise," and "physical fitness." Physical activity, defined as a "behavior," is considered to be any bodily movement that results in the burning of calories (6). Exercise, also considered to be a "behavior," is a subcategory of physical activity and is defined as physical activity that is "planned, structured, repetitive, and results in the improvement or maintenance of one or more facets of physical fitness" (6). Physical fitness is not a behavior but a "set of outcomes or traits that relates to the ability to perform physical activity" (6). In this context physical fitness can be subdivided into cardiorespiratory endurance (or aerobic capacity), body composition, muscular strength and endurance, and flexibility (7), all of which are components that one is physically endowed with and/or obtains.

Given these definitions, one can view physical activity as behaviors that include exercise (planned, structured activities such as jogging, rowing, swimming, and/ or resistive weight training and flexibility activities) and leisure/occupational activity (less structured and generally less continuous activities such as yard work, stair climbing, housework, and physically demanding occupations). The outcome of physical activity, whether participation in exercise or leisure/occupational activity, is measured as physical fitness.

A final word regarding definitions. A recent update of the *Guidelines for Exercise Testing and Prescription* by the American College of Sports Medicine (ACSM) suggests that Caspersen's (6) definition of physical fitness ("attributes that people have or achieve that relate to the ability to perform physical activity") may not be understood to include those fitness components that relate to health. For this reason, the ACSM has adopted an additional definition developed by Pate (7,8). Health-related physical fitness is defined as "a state characterized by (a) an ability to perform daily activities with vigor, and (b) demonstration of traits and capacities that are associated with low risk of premature development of hypokinetic diseases (i.e., those associated with physical inactivity)" (8).

The inclusion of the expression "health-related physical fitness" implies that individuals with "better status" in the components of physical fitness (cardiorespiratory endurance, body composition, muscular strength and endurance, and flexibility) will also have a reduced risk for disease and functional disability (7).

This concept has great application for the practicing physician because the definition is used to characterize fitness as it relates to disease prevention and health promotion (7).

II. PHYSICAL ACTIVITY: DISEASE PREVENTION AND TREATMENT

The physiological effects of habitual physical activity are many and are listed in Table 1 (9).

Of these factors, the role of physical activity in promoting health has been particularly promising when the following six disease categories are considered: CHD and other cardiovascular disease (CVD), hypertension, non-insulin-dependent diabetes mellitus, osteoporosis, obesity, and mental illnesses such as depression (1). It is important to remember that when reference is made to physical activity as being the vehicle by which these disease states are affected, physical

Table 1   Effects of Habitual Physical Activity

Increase in maximal oxygen uptake, cardiac output, and stroke volume (10–12)
Reduced heart rate at given oxygen uptake (10)
? Reduced blood pressure (13)
Reduced heart rate × blood pressure product (11)
Improved efficiency of heart muscle (10,14)
? Improved myocardial vascularization (15)
Favorable trend in incidences of cardiac mobidity and mortality (15–17)
Increased capillary density in skeletal muscle (18,19)
Increased activity of "aerobic" enzymes in skeletal muscles (19)
Reduced lactate production at given percentage of maximal oxygen uptake (11,20)
Enhanced ability to utilize free fatty acid as substrate during exercise: glycogen saving (19)
Improved endurance during exercise (10)
Increased metabolism: advantageous from a nutritional viewpoint (10,21)
Counteracts obesity (21–23)
Increase in the HDL/LDL ratio (24,25)
Improved structure and function of ligaments, tendons, and joints (26)
Increased muscular strength (19,27)
Reduced perceived exertion at given work rate (10)
Increased release of endorphins (28)
? Enhanced fiber sprouting (29)
Enhanced tolerance to hot environment: increased rate of sweating (10)
Reduced platelet aggregation? (30,31)
Counteracts osteoporosis (32)
Can normalize glucose tolerance (33)

? = There are not general agreements about these effects.
Source: Compiled by P.-O. Astrand, from Ref. 9, with permission.

activity may include either leisure and occupational activities or a more formal structured exercise program. The degree to which these different physical activities influence health is not certain, but clearly evidence exists to support several beneficial correlations.

A. Coronary Heart and Other Cardiovascular Disease

Caspersen has carefully reviewed and listed in tabular form epidemiologic studies examining the relationship of physical activity to CHD (see Table 2) (34).

In addition Powell et al. (90) recently reviewed 43 studies regarding the relationship of physical activity and CHD. Careful attention was given to criteria used in the studies to evaluate physical activity measures, CHD outcome measures, and epidemiologic methods. Powell's review concluded that the lack of physical activity was causally related to the incidence of CHD.

Individuals who are physically inactive appear to have a doubled risk of CHD compared to more physically active people (90). Peters et al. measured the physical work capacity of 2,799 healthy men under the age of 55 years and evaluated them for an average period of 5 years (91). Their findings showed that those with poor physical fitness had an increased risk of 2.2 (95% confidence limits, 1.1 and 4.7) for myocardial infarction, especially among subjects with conventional risk factors.

Ekelund et al. explored the relationship between physical fitness and mortality rates from CHD and other CVD by evaluating a cohort of 4,276 men for an average period of 8.5 years (92). All participants, asymptomatic at baseline, underwent assessment of coronary risk factors and an exercise treadmill test. The duration of the exercise test and the heart rate at the end of stage 2 were used to assess the initial physical fitness level. Based upon the initial exercise test, the men were classified into four fitness categories. Table 3 details the mortality from CHD and CVD during the 8.5 years of follow-up in these men according to the four fitness levels. Subjects in the least-fit category were 6.5 times more likely to die from CHD and 8.5 times more likely to die from other CVD.

A well known study by Paffenbarger et al. examined the physical activity habits of 16,936 Harvard alumni (89). Activity questionnaires, completed by the participants at the start of the study, were used to establish a physical activity index representing an estimate of energy expended in kcal/min for walking, climbing stairs, playing sports, yard work, and other activities. Participants were then evaluated for 12–16 years. Data from this large population study showed physical activity (measured from the activity index) to be inversely related to all-cause mortality, with the primary cause of death reported to be cardiovascular and respiratory diseases. Paffenbarger found the death rates to decline uniformly as reported energy expenditure from physical activity increased from less than 500 kcal per week to 3500 kcal per week. Individuals burning more than 2000 kcal per week had one-quarter to one-third lower death rates than men whose activity habits were in the less active range. This study also suggested that individuals who were physically active (expended greater than 2000 kcal/week) were likely to live 1–2 or more years longer than the less active men (less than 500 kcal/week) by the age of 80 years.

Blair et al. assessed physical fitness by maximal treadmill testing 10,244 men and 3,120 women (93). These participants were then evaluated for an average of 8 years. Based upon the results of the treadmill tests, subjects were classified into fitness categories: the lower 20% were deemed low-fit; the middle 40% were moderate-fit; and the upper 40% were high-fit. Blair concluded that men and women who were in the low-fit group had twice the likelihood of dying from CVD (and all causes combined) when compared to the moderate-fit subjects, and the lowest death rate was found among the high-fit group. This study also concluded that a high level of physical fitness significantly benefitted individuals who had other risk factors for CHD (94).

In the Multiple Risk Factor Intervention Trial (MRFIT) the amount of leisure time physical activity was related to CHD events and overall mortality among 12,138 men who participated in this large primary prevention trial (95). At the start of the study all subjects were free of CHD but were at high risk for CHD based upon levels of cigarette smoking, diastolic blood pressure, and serum cholesterol values. Leisure-time physical activity was determined by questionnaire at baseline and at various intervals during the 7 years of follow-up. Activity levels were classified into low, moderate, and high tertiles. Follow-up data showed that the low-activity level group experienced a CHD death rate of 25:1000, while the moderate- and high-activity groups had 15:1000 and 16:1000 deaths, respectively. In a study of Sobolski et al. (96), 1,734 men were evaluated for 5 years to examine the relationship between physical fitness/physical activity and the development of CHD. Although the estimates of physical activity (work and leisure) were not significantly correlated with CHD, physical working capacity was inversely related to the risk of heart disease.

Many of the citations reviewed by Caspersen and Powell (90,34) and the studies by Blair (93,94), Paffenbarger (89), and Leon (95) previously discussed also suggest a linear relationship between physical activity and health status, such as the risk for CHD and CVD. Furthermore, data found in the MRFIT trial demonstrate that individuals engaging in light or moderate activities had lower rates of CHD death, sudden death, and overall mortality than more sedentary men (95). Data from Sallis et al. based upon the Stanford five-city project, further support the notion that light to moderate physical activity can have positive health benefits, including a reduction of CHD risk (97).

In addition, recent reviews by Wood and Stefanick (98) and Froelicher (99) address potential mechanisms by which physical activity modifies atherosclerosis and CHD as well as the effect of exercise upon cardiac function. Haskell et al.

Table 2 Results of Epidemiologic Studies of Coronary Heart Disease Yielding Statistically Significant and Nonsignificant Associations with Physical Activity

Type of Design	Significant Inverse Association	Nonsignificant Association
Occupational cohort	London postal workers/civil servants (35)	London Transport busmen (36)
	London Transport busmen (35)	London Transport busmen (37)
	U.S. railroad workers (38)	Los Angeles, CA, civil servants (39)
	North Dakota residents (40)	Bell Telephone employees (42)
	Washington, D.C., postal workers (41)	U.S. railroad workers (45)
	Yugoslavia residents (43,44)	Chicago utility company employees (48)
	Italy residents (46,47)	Evans County, GA, residents (52,53)
	Greek islands residents (49,50)	East Finland residents (55)
	Italian railroad employees (51)	
	Israeli kibbutzim, male residents (54)	
	Israeli kibbutzim, female residents (54)	
	West Finland residents (55)	
	San Francisco, CA, longshoremen (56,57)	

Cohorts with various types of physical activity measures	Chicago Western Electric employees (58) Harvard alumni (60,61) British civil servants (62,63) Framingham, MA, male residents (65,66) Framingham, MA, female residents (65,66) Los Angeles, CA, firemen and policemen (68) Gothenberg, Sweden, residents (64) New York health insurance subscribers (70) San Francisco, CA, federal employees (71) Oslo, Norway, residents (work) (72) North Karelina, Finland, male residents (73) Oslo, Norway, workers (74) Belgian male factory workers (fitness) (75) MRFIT men (76) Honolulu, HI, residents (77,78) Puerto Rico residents (80) Finnish men and women (81)	Gothenberg, Sweden, residents (50) Gothenberg, Sweden, residents (64) Gothenberg, Sweden female residents (67) San Francisco corporate employees (69) Oslo, Norway, residents (leisure) (72) North Karalina, Finland, female residents (73) Belgian male factory workers (leisure) (75) Framingham, MA, male residents (work) (79)
Mortality study	Great Britain residents (35) California residents (82) Iowa residents (83)	
Case-control study	Seattle, WA, residents (84,85) Netherlands, male residents (87) Netherlands, female residents (87) Auckland, New Zealand, men (89) Auckland, New Zealand, women (89)	San Francisco, CA, coroner's cases (86) Florida residents (88)

Source: Ref. 34, with permission.

Table 3 Rates of Death (%) from Coronary Heart Disease (CHD) and Cardiovascular Disease (CVD) in Healthy Men over 8.5 Years of Follow-Up, According to Quartile of Stage 2 Heart Rate

Cause of Death	State 2 Heart Rate Quartile[a]				Ratio of Death Rates (4:1)
	1	2	3	4	
CHD	0.26	0.91	0.91	1.69	6.5
	(0.00–0.62)[b]	(0.24–1.58)	(0.24–1.58)	(0.77–2.61)	(1.5–28.7)
CVD	0.26	1.30	1.56	2.21	8.5
	(0.00–0.62)	(0.49–2.11)	(0.68–2.44)	(1.16–3.25)	(2.0–36.7)

[a]1 represents the quartile of the men with the lowest heart rates (most physically fit) and 4 the quartile with the highest heart rates (least physically fit).
[b]Values in parentheses represent 95% confidence interval.
Source: Ref. 92, with permission.

(100) also discuss the influence of exercise on plasma lipid and lipoprotein levels. The relationship between physical activity and CHD risk factors during childhood and adolescence has been reviewed by Despres et al. (101).

B. Hypertension

Participation in a regular exercise program has been shown to decrease blood pressure by an average of 10 mmHg (2,102). Two large population studies have suggested that individuals who are physically inactive have a 35–52% increased risk of developing hypertension compared to a physically active population (103,104). A recently published review by Hagberg (102) details the epidemiologic relationships between physical activity and blood pressure, the effects of a single bout of exercise and habitual exercise training on blood pressure, and the possible mechanisms by which physical activity affects blood pressure. Hagberg concludes that endurance exercise training should be recommended in the nonpharmacologic management of moderate hypertension. For those individuals with excessively elevated pressures (>160/105), moreover, physical activity programs should be recommended following the initiation of drug therapy (102). He also suggests that low-intensity training at 40–60% of maximal oxygen uptake ($\dot{V}O_2$ max) may be as beneficial in lowering blood pressures as more vigorous training (102). This has important implications for the prescription of exercise for the general population and will be considered further below.

C. Obesity

Exercise has long been recognized as a necessary and integral component of successful weight management. Epidemiologic research supports the fact that physical activity is associated with weight control, even when the diet is controlled (2,105). Regular participation in physical activity results in caloric expenditure both during the activity and for a period of time afterwards; habitual exercise can also increase resting metabolic rate (106). Bray has carefully reviewed the relationship between physical activity and obesity (107). He suggests that for the lean or moderately obese subject, physical training does result in a decrease in body fat and may result in a reduction in total body weight (see also a review by Wilmore (108)). A reduction of body fat in the massively obese patient as a result physical training is less certain (107). The explanation for this finding may be related to the high degree of heterogeneity that exists with obesity. In addition, many of the exercise training studies carried out with very obese subjects have been short term (10–12 weeks). Bray recommends walking as a safe and effective form of exercise for the overweight individual. High-intensity activities such as jogging increase the risk of orthopedic injury and result in greater physical discomfort, both of which have negative impact on exercise compliance. In addition to recommending lower intensity physical activity such as walking, Pollock et al. suggest that the frequency of exercise be at least 3–4 days per week (109). Bray concludes his review with the following observation: "Exercise, added to other important forms of treatment for obesity, is important not so much for the extra weight loss during the treatment period but for the fact that at follow-up 3, 6, or 9 months later there appears to be less weight gained in the individuals who exercised than those who did not" (107).

D. Non-Insulin-Dependent Diabetes Mellitus

Physical activity has long been recognized as important in both the prevention and treatment of diabetes. Epidemiologic studies have shown the incidence of non-insulin-dependent diabetes (NIDDM) to be twice as great in sedentary men than in more physically active men (110,111).

The basis for including exercise in the overall care of the diabetic patient is that regular exercise can improve glycemic control by increasing insulin sensitivity and glucose disposal (112), and can reduce cardiovascular risk factors. The later consideration becomes particularly important when one considers that cardiovascular risk factors are accelerated in the patient with NIDDM (110,113). Two recent reviews discuss the acute and chronic effects of physical activity on diabetes and the possible mechanisms by which exercise contributes (110,112). Exercise precautions and guidelines for the diabetic patient have also been outlined by the American College of Sports Medicine (7).

E. Osteoporosis

Several studies have demonstrated that bone resorption can be decreased or even reversed with physical activity, but the specific recommendations regarding the type of activity and the degree of required training to prevent osteoporosis are uncertain (114–116). Smith and colleagues (114) have recommended that efforts directed at preventing bone loss should include physical activities that stress the at-risk areas for fractures such as the hip, spine, femur, and wrist. These should include rhythmic activities that induce greater compressive forces than are normally experienced (114).

Dalsky has suggested that individuals who have had hip fractures, significant bone mineral loss, or a high-risk profile for osteoporosis should consider activities that improve both balance and strength, thereby reducing the likelihood of a fall. Dalsky cautions that the chosen physical activities should not place too great a strain on the bones and that women should progress slowly from non-weight-bearing physical activities gradually to include weight-bearing activities (116). Dalsky also advises that some women may not be able to engage in physical activities that produce weight-bearing effect (116). For those at normal risk for osteoporosis, the physical activity guidelines outlined in this chapter are generally prudent.

F. Enhanced Psychological Well-Being

Brown has carefully reviewed the scientific evidence relating physical activity to mental health or mental illness (117). A recent textbook also reviews and analyzes the available data promoting physical activity to improve mental health (118). The general consensus is that a positive correlation exists between regular physical activity and mental health. One study by Stephens examined four large U.S. and Canadian surveys designed to determine the association of physical activity and mental health (119). Stephens concluded ". . . that the level of physical activity is positively associated with good mental health in the household populations of the United States and Canada, when mental health is defined as positive mood, general well-being, and relatively infrequent symptoms of anxiety and depression" (119).

Although there is considerable uncertainty about the physiological and behavioral mechanisms relating physical activity to mental health, Brown has summarized the potential behavioral and physiological explanations for the beneficial effects of exercise. The behavioral benefits may be derived from a sense of personal control or mastery, a distraction from routine daily stressors, or the obtaining of intrinsic or extrinsic reinforcement. The physiological benefits may stem from a hormonal or metabolic adaptation to physical training, an adjustment in the catecholamine or indolamine neurotransmitter substances, an increased endogenous opiate level, or an enhanced tranquilizer effect resulting from an increased core temperature (117).

III. ASSESSMENT OF HEALTH-RELATED PHYSICAL FITNESS AND EXERCISE ECG TESTING

A. Health-Related Fitness Assessment

Many methods have been explored for assessing physical activity (leisure, occupational, or structured exercise) and physical fitness. Traditional approaches include questionnaires (interview-type or self-report), measurement of movement, monitoring heart rate, or measuring metabolic variables such as maximal oxygen uptake ($\dot{V}O_2$) (120). More recently, health-related fitness assessments have also included body composition analysis, muscular strength and flexibility testing, and periodic screening. Periodic screening generally includes a review of CHD risk factors, the measurement of plasma lipids, and a periodic health examination (see Chap. 6).

Detailed methods used for fitness assessment are beyond the scope of this chapter. Descriptions of these procedures have been published by Pollock and Wilmore (121) and the American College of Sports Medicine (7). Table 4 outlines fitness tests that can be performed in a preventive health center or a physician's office. This table also lists fitness tests that patients can perform themselves. Patients should receive some instruction from the physician or office staff regarding the correct method for performing these home fitness tests.

Table 4 Summary of Health-Related Fitness Tests

Fitness tests to be performed in a preventive medicine center or the physician's examination area

Cardiorespiratory endurance (121)

Maximal test: measurement of $\dot{V}O_2$ max on a treadmill or cycle ergometer
Maximal test: estimation of $\dot{V}O_2$ max on a treadmill or cycle ergometer
Submaximal test: estimation of $\dot{V}O_2$ max on a cycle ergometer or treadmill
Step tests: estimation of fitness using recovery heart rate
Arm ergometer test: estimation of $\dot{V}O_2$ max using an arm ergometer (for patients who are unable to perform treadmill or bicycle tests)

Body composition (121)

Hydrostatic weighing: measurement of % body fat via underwater weighing. Body density is measured and % fat is calculated (122).
Anthropometrics: estimation of % body fat using body diameter measurements.
Skin-fold test: estimation of % body fat by measurement of selected skin fold sites using calipers.
Bioelectrical impedance: estimation of % fat by measuring body resistance and reactance to a very low electrical current (123).
Body mass index (BMI): calculation of weight/height^2. Used to estimate degree of obesity.

Table 4 Continued

Muscular endurance (lower weight resistance with increased testing duration) (121)
  Isokinetic testing: measurement of muscular endurance using isokinetic testing equipment such as Cybex
  Variable resistance testing: measurement of muscular endurance using variable resistance equipment such as Nautilus
  Isotonic testing: measurement of muscular endurance using isotonic resistance equipment such as free weights
Muscular strength (high weight resistance with decreased testing duration) (121)
  Isokinetic testing: measurement of muscular strength using isokinetic testing equipment such as Cybex or hand-held dynamometer
  Variable resistance testing: measurement of muscular strength using variable resistance equipment such as Nautilus
  Isotonic testing: measurement of muscular strength using isotonic resistance equipment such as free weights
  Isometric testing: measurement of muscular strength using static resistance
Flexibility measurement (121,124,125)
  Sit-and-reach test: measures flexibility of low back, hamstrings, and hips.
  Leighton flexometer and electrogoniometer tests: measurement of various joints for assessment of actual range of motion (121,126)
Home fitness tests (to be performed in the patient's environment)
  Cardiorespiratory endurance
    Distance running tests: estimation of $\dot{V}O_2$ max via a timed run (i.e., 1.5 miles)
    Walking tests: Estimation of $\dot{V}O_2$ max via time and/or heart rate associated with 1 mile walk
  Body composition
    Anthropometrics: Estimation of % body fat using body diameter measurements (121)
    BMI: Calculation of weight/height^2. Used to estimate degree of obesity (121,127)
  Muscular endurance (121)
    Push-up test: measurement of muscular endurance using standard full push-up or modified knee push-up
    Curl-up: measurement of abdominal muscular endurance using bent-knee sit-up or curl-up
  Flexibility
    Sit-and-reach test: measures flexibility of low back, hamstrings, and hips (127)
    Behind back hand-touch test: measures shoulder flexibility by measuring distance between hands extended behind back.

The ACSM has delineated the purposes of fitness assessment (7). These include the need to establish data for the generation of an exercise prescription, to collect appropriate baseline and follow-up data for the purpose of assessing progress, to establish goals for motivational purposes, and to enhance participants' understanding of their health-related fitness status.

To ensure further participants' understanding of health-related fitness status, a summary report with a written explanation should be provided following testing. Such reports can be computer generated and customized to include the patient's age and gender and a percentile comparison of their fitness data to other individuals of similar age and gender. This report can also include an activity program and realistic fitness goals.

B. Prescreening Patients for Fitness Testing

Guidelines for exercise testing and participation in physical activity programs have been developed by the American College of Sports Medicine (7) and the American Heart Association (AHA) (128). These guidelines consider the patient's current health status, past medical history with emphasis on previous CHD events and risk factors, age, physical activity habits, and the type of physical activity program the patient wants to undertake (i.e, mild, moderate, or vigorous). Physicians who are performing fitness testing or counseling patients regarding physical activity programs should be familiar with these guidelines (7,128).

As a minimal pretesting or pretraining screening, physicians should consider using a self-administered questionnaire such as the Physical Activity Readiness Questionnaire (PAR-Q) (7,129,130), which is designed to identify individuals who may be at risk for exercise-related cardiovascular or musculoskeletal problems (129). This questionnaire can help to determine the appropriateness of beginning an exercise program and identify any activities that might be contraindicated. Individuals who have positive responses to the PAR-Q can take a follow-up questionnaire, the Physical Activity Readiness Examination (PAR-X), which lists the recommended procedures to be used for medical screening before the patient participates in physical activity, and includes a Physical Activity Prescription form (PAR$_x$) (7). The use of the PAR-Q and the PAR-X has been reviewed by Shephard (129,131). Copies of these questionnaire may be obtained by writing to: Government of Canada, Fitness and Amateur Sport, 365 Laurier Avenue West, Ottawa, Ontario, Canada K1A 0X6.

Additional information about prescreening before physical activity or exercise testing has been published by the AHA and the ACSM (7,128). Sample patient consent forms for use in exercise testing and physical activity participation are also included in these references.

C. Exercise ECG Testing

In 1986, the American College of Cardiology and the American Heart Association published their recommendations regarding exercise testing for the apparently healthy population (132). More recently, guidelines for exercise ECG testing as a prerequisite to participation in physical activity have been published by the ACSM and AHA (7,128). An exercise ECG test is recommended for patients planning to undertake a moderate or vigorous activity program if they have some combination of the following: 1. two or more CHD risk factors; 2. symptoms suggestive of cardiopulmonary or metabolic disease; 3. known cardiac, pulmonary, or metabolic disease; or 4. men over age 40 or women over age 50. A flow chart is provided in Figure 1 to assist physicians in determining when to perform an exercise ECG test on patients who are already physically active or who are interested in beginning a physical activity program. In addition to these recommendations, the ACSM has suggested guidelines for determining whether a physician needs to be present during the exercise ECG stress test (7).

IV. PHYSICAL ACTIVITY PROGRAMS

A. Rationale for the Physical Activity Prescription

Research in physical activity has primarily been limited to the study of exercise, a subcategory of physical activity. Exercise studies have usually been conducted over a period of several months (i.e., 8–16 weeks) and investigations have largely focused on cardiovascular fitness using $\dot{V}O_2$ max to assess fitness changes. This research has focused on advancing our understanding of the "exercise prescription" as it relates to exercise type, duration, intensity, and frequency, and what combination of these variables is necessary to improve $\dot{V}O_2$ max. Thorough reviews of the rationale for prescribing exercise have been published by Pollock and Wilmore (121), Yanowitz (136), and the ACSM (7,137). The ACSM has also published a position statement regarding exercise recommendations for developing cardiorespiratory and muscular fitness (137). These guidelines are an update of the ACSM's 1978 statement and they include the need for regular participation in muscle resistance activities (Table 5).

Efforts have been undertaken more recently to understand the possible distinction between fitness benefits such as increases in $\dot{V}O_2$ max and muscular strength and health benefits of physical activity (137,138). These questions have been raised as a result of studies in which the physical activities associated with a reduced risk for CHD were predominantly of a light to moderate intensity such as walking, stair climbing, and gardening (134–140). In a recent position statement on exercise prescription the ACSM (137) noted that:

> . . . the quantity and quality of exercise needed to attain health-related benefits may differ from what is recommended for fitness benefits. It is now clear that lower levels of physical activity than recommended by this position statement may reduce the risk for certain chronic degenerative diseases and yet may not be of sufficient quantity or quality to improve $\dot{V}O_2$ max.

Evidence suggests that light to moderate physical activity, which can include leisure time and/or occupational physical activity, results in clearly defined health

Resting Electrocardiogram (ECG)

Routine electrocardiogram screening in individuals without symptoms is not recommended. It may be prudent to perform resting electrocardiograms for males over age 40 who have two or more cardiac risk factors or who participate in special occupations (pilots, firemen, police officers, bus or truck drivers, and railroad engineers). [143]

Exercise ECG Stress Test[7, 138, 142, 144]

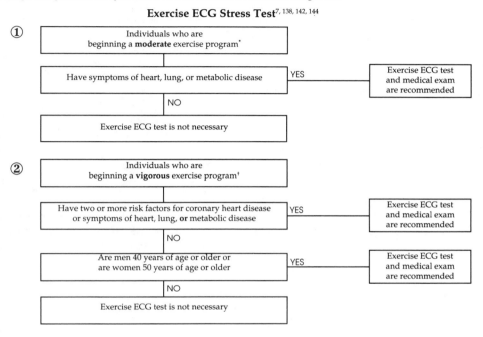

③ Individuals with known heart, lung, or metabolic disease should have an exercise stress test and medical exam prior to beginning an exercise program or before markedly increasing the amount of exercise. [142]

④ It may be prudent for men over the age of 40 who have at least two or more cardiac risk factors to consider undergoing a maximal exercise ECG stress test, or for individuals who participate in special occupations (pilots, firemen, police officers, bus or truck drivers, and railroad engineers) to consider a maximal exercise ECG stress test beginning at age 40. [142]

* A **moderate** exercise program is defined as physical activities such as walking or increasing daily activities. It is also described as activities that can be performed "well within the individual's current capacity" — activities that can be carried out "comfortably for a prolonged period" such as 60 minutes. [7, 145]

† A vigorous exercise routine is described as activitiy "intense enough to represent a substantial challenge" resulting in a significant rise in heart rate and breathing rate. Vigorous activity (intensity greater than 60 percent VO_2 max) such as "training for a marathon or participating in vigorous competitive sports" can generally be sustained by untrained individuals for a period of only 15 to 20 minutes. [7, 145]

The frequency of performing the resting and the maximal exercise ECG stress test for the above guidelines will vary based upon the severity of risk factors and the discretion of your physician.

Figure 1 Guidelines for having a resting or exercise ECG test.

Table 5 American College of Sports Medicine Guidelines for Developing Cardiorespiratory and Muscular Fitness in Healthy Adults

The American College of Sports Medicine (ACSM) makes the following recommendations for the quantity and quality of training for developing and maintaining cardiorespiratory fitness, body composition, and muscular strength and endurance in the healthy adult:

1. Frequency of training: 3–5 days/week

2. Intensity of training: 60–90% of maximum heart rate (HR_{max}), or 50–85% of maximum oxygen uptake ($\dot{V}O_{2max}$) or HR_{max} reserve.[a]

3. Duration of training: 20–60 min of continuous aerobic activity. Duration is dependent on the intensity of the activity; thus, lower-intensity activity should be conducted over a longer period of time. Because of the importance of "total fitness" and the fact that it is more readily attained in longer-duration programs, and because of the potential hazards and compliance problems associated with high-intensity activity, lower- to moderate-intensity activity of longer duration is recommended for the nonathletic adult.

4. Mode of activity: any activity that uses large muscle groups, can be maintained continuously, and is rhythmic and aerobic in nature (e.g., walking–hiking, running–jogging, cycling–bicycling, cross-country skiing, dancing, rope skipping, rowing, stair climbing, swimming, skating, and various endurance game activities).

5. Resistance training: Strength training of a moderate intensity, sufficient to develop and maintain moderate intensity, sufficient to develop and maintain fat-free weight (FFW), should be an integral part of an adult fitness program. One set of 8–12 repetitions of 8–10 exercises that condition the major muscle groups at least 2 days/week is the recommended minimum.

[a]Maximum heart rate reserve is calculated from the difference between resting and maximum heart rate (HR_{max}). To estimate training intensity, a percentage of this value is added to the resting heart rate and is expressed as a percentage of HR_{max} reserve.
Source: Ref. 137, with permission.

benefits (1,95,97). Additional rationale supporting or clarifying the degree of physical activity necessary to obtain health benefits is forthcoming by the ACSM. In concert with this effort, the Department of Health and Human Services in their "year 2000 objectives" has emphasized the importance of reducing the nation's physical inactivity by increasing light to moderate physical activity. The value of this objective is made evident when one considers that light to moderate physical activity is more likely to be adopted and maintained than vigorous physical activity (1). In addition, many individuals are reluctant to follow the ACSM exercise prescription guidelines but are more willing to either maintain or increase their leisure activities. To inform patients that their gardening efforts and their climbing of stairs will have some pay-off in terms of health improvement may further motivate them to remain active.

To assist physicians in differentiating between mild, moderate, or vigorous physical activity, a listing of activities with corresponding energy requirement estimates has been published by the AHA (see Table 6) (128).

B. Physical Activity Prescription

In discussing a physical activity prescription with patients, two approaches can be considered: the structured exercise program and the leisure/occupational time (LOT) program (Figure 2).

The structured exercise program is planned and repetitive and includes activities such as brisk walking, swimming, jogging, rowing, aerobic dance, and stationary cycling performed 3–5 days per week for 30–60 min per session (137). Muscle strengthening activities such as resistive weight training and flexibility exercises should be performed at least 2–3 days per week.

The LOT program is less structured and generally less continuous in nature; it includes stair climbing, yard work, housework, hiking, or sporting activities at least 3 days per week. The amount of cumulative time spent in these activities should be approximately 60 min per day (1 min 60 times a day; 10 min 6 times a day, or other combinations of duration and frequency totaling 60 min) (9). Studies have verified that just being "more active" improves health. Patients should be encouraged to be up and about: moving, climbing the stairs, mowing the lawn, raking the leaves, square dancing, playing tag with the kids, or having a physical demanding occupation. It is recommended that every individual undertake one of these physical activity programs or a combination of each program.

1. Structured Exercise Programs

The structured exercise program consists of three components: cardiovascular, muscle resistance, and stretching.

a. *Cardiovascular Exercises.*   Exercise activities can be defined in terms of type of exercise, intensity, duration, and frequency of exercise along with warm-up and cool-down activities. The type of exercise should involve the use of large muscle groups (primarily the large leg muscles), moving in a rhythmic fashion for a continuous period of time. If these three criteria are met, the activity is considered "aerobic" and will promote cardiovascular fitness. Three methods can be used to determine if an individual is exercising at an appropriate intensity: 1. talk test, 2. perceived exertion, and 3. heart rate. The easiest of these methods is the talk test. If, while exercising, a person is breathing harder but can carry on a conversation, the intensity of exercise is probably not excessive. If, on the other hand, that person is unable to communicate because of marked dyspnea, the intensity is excessive and should be reduced. The old adage "to benefit, it must hurt" could never be further from the truth.

A patient can also rate the level of exertion by using a "perceived exertion scale," developed by Borg (141) and shown in Figure 3. By listening to one's entire body while exercising (such as breathing and muscular effort), a person can determine a perceived exertion level ranging from no effort (6) to maximal effort (20). This roughly correlates in young adults to heart rates of 60 and 200 beats/min. A recommended level for sustained exercise is "13: somewhat hard." Some

Table 6 Estimated Requirements of Selected Activities

Degree of Intensity	Metabolic Equivalents (3.5 ml/kg/min oxygen uptake)
Mild	
Baking	2.0
Billiards	2.4
Bookbinding	2.2
Canoeing (leisurely)	2.5
Conducting an orchestra	2.2
Dancing, ballroom (slow)	2.9
Golf (with cart)	2.5
Horseback riding (walking)	2.3
Playing a musical instrument	
Accordion	1.8
Cello	2.3
Flute	2.0
Horn	1.7
Piano	2.3
Trumpet	1.8
Violin	2.6
Woodwind	1.8
Volleyball (noncompetitive)	2.9
Walking (2 mph)	2.5
Writing	1.7
Moderate	
Calisthenics (no weights)	4.0
Croquet	3.0
Cycling (leisurely)	3.5
Gardening (no lifting)	4.4
Golf (without cart)	4.9
Mowing lawn (power mower)	3.0
Playing drums	3.8
Sailing	3.0
Swimming (slowly)	4.5
Walking (3 mph)	3.3
Walking (4 mph)	4.5
Vigorous	
Badminton	5.5
Chopping wood	4.9
Climbing hills	
No load	6.9
With 5 kg load	7.4
Cycling (moderately)	5.7

Table 6 Continued

Dancing	
Aerobic or ballet	6.0
Ballroom (fast) or square	5.5
Field hockey	7.7
Ice skating	5.5
Jogging (10 min mile)	10.2
Karate or judo	6.5
Roller skating	6.5
Rope skipping	12.0
Skiing (water or downhill)	6.8
Squash	12.1
Surfing	6.0
Swimming (fast)	7.0
Tennis (doubles)	6.0

[a]These activities can often be done at variable intensities, if the intensity is not excessive and the courses are flat (no hills) unless so specified. Categories are based upon experience of tolerance; if the activity is perceived to be more than indicated, it should be judged accordingly.

Source: Ref. 128, with permission.

individuals may want to exercise at a greater intensity than this level. This is permissible, providing the person has met the medical guidelines for safely proceeding with a more vigorous exercise program.

The heart rate during exercise is the most precise indicator of how hard a person is working. Research has shown that individuals can expect similar training effects if their exercise results in a comparable amount of caloric expenditure during the activity (127). This concept allows for a table of training heart rates to be used based on age (Table 7).

A person's maximal heart rate is determined by subtracting age from 220. Exercising at 60–90% of maximum heart rate is recommended to attain and maintain optimal fitness (134). This range is often referred to as the "target zone." Listed in Table 7 are the target zones corresponding to age ranges. Midway through the exercise session, the pulse should be counted for 10 sec right after momentarily stopping exercise. If the count is above the target zone, exercise intensity should be reduced. If it is below, the intensity can be increased appropriately. Sedentary individuals should consider exercising in a lower heart rate range (60–75%) for the first 2–4 weeks of their exercise program. Thereafter, depending on the type of activity chosen, they can continue in this range or increase to the 75–90% range.

Problems with this method include the wide range of variation for maximal

```
┌─────────────────────────────────────────┐
│              Programs                     │
└─────────────────────────────────────────┘
```

Exercise Program
- Structured, planned, repetitive

Leisure/Occupational Time (LOT) Activity Program
- Less structured (may include leisure, occupational, household activities)

Examples:
- Walking
- Jogging
- Aerobic dance
- Stationary cycling

Plus
- Muscle-resistance exercises
- Flexibility exercises

Examples
- Walking
- Yard work
- Stair climbing
- Hiking
- Housework

Guidelines
- 3–5 days/week for 20–60 minutes (cardiovascular activity)
- 8–10 muscle resistance exercises (at least 2 days/week)
- 4–5 stretching exercises (at least 3–5 days/week)

Guidelines
- At least 3 days/week (preferably 3–5 days/week) for at least 60 minutes per day

Benefits

1. Decreased risk of death from coronary heart disease (physically inactive people are twice as likely to develop heart disease).
2. Lower death rate.
3. Prevention or control of high blood pressure, osteoporosis, obesity, mental health problems, and diabetes.
4. Improvement in structure and function of ligaments, tendons, and joints.
5. Increased muscular strength.
6. Continued independent living with increasing age.

Figure 2 Physical activity programs.

6	No Effort
7	
8	
9	Very Light
10	
11	
12	
13	Somewhat Hard
14	
15	Hard
16	
17	Very Hard
18	
19	
20	Maximal Effort

Figure 3   Borg Perceived Exertion Scale. The rating of perceived exertion (RPE) scale was developed by Borg (151).

heart rates (plus or minus 20 beats/min), and the difficulty some individuals find in locating or counting the pulse. In addition, this method cannot be used in patients taking heart-rate-lowering medications such as a beta-blocker and some calcium channel blockers. For these reasons, the talk test and perceived exertion scales are often more appropriate techniques for monitoring exercise intensity. Individuals

Table 7   Taking Your Heart Rate

Age (years)	Average Maximum Heart Rate (beats/min)	60–75% Target Zone (beats/10 sec)	(beats/min)	75–90% (beats/10 sec)	(beats/min)
20	200	20–25	120–150	25–30	150–180
25	195	20–24	117–146	24–29	146–176
30	190	19–24	114–143	24–29	143–171
35	185	19–23	111–139	23–28	139–167
40	180	18–23	108–135	23–27	135–162
45	175	18–22	105–131	22–26	131–158
50	170	17–21	102–128	21–26	128–153
55	165	17–21	99–124	21–25	124–149
60	160	16–20	96–120	20–24	120–144
65	155	16–19	93–116	19–23	116–140
70	150	15–19	90–113	19–23	112–135
75	145	15–18	87–109	18–22	109–131
80	140	14–18	84–105	18–21	105–126

who choose to use the heart rate method are encouraged to take their heart rates during the early weeks of the exercise program (halfway through the exercise session). Most people soon learn to associate a particular "perceived exertion" with the appropriate training heart rate and thereby avoid taking the pulse during every exercise session.

The duration of the exercise session depends to some degree on the intensity of the activity. For example, the recommended duration of walking is longer than the time suggested for jogging or riding a stationary bike. Although the target heart rate zone will be lower with walking than jogging, the same cardiovascular benefits can be realized by increasing the duration of the walk. The exercise duration is short when starting an exercise program, and is gradually increased every week or 2, as is discussed later in the detailed sample exercise programs. The minimum number of exercise sessions per week for cardiovascular fitness is three, preferably every other day. We recommend 4–5 days per week as an optimal number of exercise sessions.

A very important component of each exercise session is the warm-up and cooldown. A 5–7 min warm-up allows the body to adjust to the fitness activity gradually. The warm-up should include some light stretching followed by the same activity that will be performed during the exercise session, but at a reduced intensity. For example, if the activity is stationary cycling, several minutes of light stretching should be done before getting on the bike. After stretching, the bike should be pedaled without any tension being applied; the tension is then gradually increased over the next 4–5 min until the target heart rate is reached. A proper warm-up will help to reduce the strain on the cardiovascular and musculoskeletal systems of the body. The 5–7 min cool-down permits the body's machinery to readjust to the reduced activity. A gradual cool-down keeps the large leg muscles working and prevents blood from pooling in the lower extremities. Failure to cool down may result in lightheadedness, dizziness, or fainting. An example of proper cool-down with stationary cycling would include releasing the bike's tension and pedaling freely for several minutes until normal breathing is restored. If the activity has included brisk walking, cool-down should include a slower walk.

Many individuals perform stretching activities following the exercise session. We encourage this procedure because the muscles are warm and less likely to experience "muscle pulls."

Two sample 16 week cardiovascular exercise programs (for all ages) are provided in Tables 8 and 9. If participants are already involved in a structured exercise program, they can begin at their current duration, as listed on the charts.

The program outlined in Table 8 is for lower-intensity activities such as brisk walking, jumping on a minitrampoline, and riding a stationary cycle with very little or zero tension. A blank column is included in the table for entering the 10 sec target heart rate (60–75%, taken from Table 7). As an alternative to using heart rate for exercise intensity, subjects can use the talk test or perceived exertion scale, as previously discussed.

Table 8 Cardiovascular Exercise Programs: Lower-Intensity Activities, Such as Brisk Walking, Minitrampolining, Country Bicycling, Roller Skating, Stationary Cycling (Very Little or Zero Tension)

Week	% of Maximal Heart Rate Target Zone	Heart Rate (Beats/10 sec) Target Zone	Warm-Up	Duration (exercise time, min)	Cool-Down	Frequency (days/week)
1–2	60–75		5 min	15–20	5 min	3–4
3–4	60–75		5 min	20–25	5 min	3–4
5–6	60–75		5 min	25–30	5 min	4–5
7–8	60–75		5 min	30–35	5 min	4–5
9–10	60–75		5 min	35–40	5 min	4–5
11–12	60–75		5 min	40–45	5 min	4–5
13–14	60–75		5 min	45–50	5 min	4–5
15–16	60–75		5 min	50–55	5 min	4–5

Every 2 weeks adjustments in the exercise program should be made. The first 2 weeks include a warm-up (5 min), 15–20 min of exercise, and a cool-down (5 min). After this period the person should increase the exercise time (duration) by about 5 min every 2 weeks until a goal of 50–60 min is reached. The exercise time can be divided into two 30 min sessions, if time will not allow for a continuous hour of activity. The frequency of exercise is initially set for 3–4 days per week, with an eventual increase to 4–5 days per week. Lower intensity exercise activities such as brisk walking can be performed daily.

Table 9 Cardiovascular Exercise Programs: Higher-Intensity Activities, Such as Jogging, Swimming, Aerobic Dancing, Cross-Country Skiing, Stationary Cycling (with Tension)

Week	% of Maximal Heart Rate Target Zone	Heart Rate (Beats/10 sec) Target Zone	Warm-Up	Duration (exercise time, min)	Cool-Down	Frequency (days/week)
1–2	75–90		5 min	10–15	5 min	3–4
3–4	75–90		5 min	15–20	5 min	3–4
5–6	75–90		5 min	20–25	5 min	4–5
7–8	75–90		5 min	25–30	5 min	4–5
9–10	75–90		5 min	30–35	5 min	4–5
11–12	75–90		5 min	30–35	5 min	4–5
13–14	75–90		5 min	30–35	5 min	4–5
15–16	75–90		5 min	30–35	5 min	4–5

After the subject reaches a goal of 50–60 min of lower-intensity exercise, this duration may be maintained indefinitely or the person may consider a more intense exercise program outlined in Table 9 and discussed in the next paragraph. Because more intense activities may fall into the category of "vigorous activities," it is important to determine the need for an exercise treadmill test before any subject begins this program (Fig. 1).

Table 9 is for the more intense activities such as jogging/running, aerobic dance, or stationary cycling (with moderate tension), which require a higher target heart rate (75–90% of maximum). The person's training range should be a 10 sec pulse count taken from Table 7.

As suggested in Table 9, the duration of exercise should be 10–15 min for the first 2 weeks, in addition to the warm-up and cool-down. Every 2 weeks thereafter the duration should be increased by 5 min until a goal of 30–35 min is attained. After 16 weeks, recommendations listed in the "15–16 week" column can be followed indefinitely.

An exercise log will generally help individuals remain consistent with their exercise program. Patients should be encouraged to keep a log for at least 16 weeks. The Appendix includes a sample exercise log.

b. *Muscle Resistance Exercises.* The popularity of muscle resistance training is increasing among both men and women. Women are realizing that weight resistance training will not produce large, bulky muscles. Instead, the exercises improve their attractiveness by decreasing body fat, increasing lean body mass, and improving muscle tone. Daily weight resistance activities have been shown to improve the structure and function of ligaments, tendons, and joints (9,142), decrease lower back pain, and increase muscular strength (9,10,143). Conversely, inadequate muscular strength can result in serious musculoskeletal problems that can lead to poor posture, excessive pain, disability, and early retirement (121). Lack of weight resistance activities can also lead to bone loss that can eventually lead to osteoporosis (121).

The ACSM has recently recommended that all individuals include weight resistance training as part of their regular training program (see Table 5) (137). This section discusses how to strengthen skeletal muscle using primarily the person's own weight.

If patients have a history of heart disease, they should be advised to avoid heavy resistance weight training. In addition, all patients should be told to start and progress slowly. Individuals should never hold their breath while performing weight resistance exercises; instead, they should breathe freely during each repetition of the resistance exercise. Also, someone should be present with the person who is lifting.

The Appendix includes photographs of the basic muscle resistance exercises that can be performed using the body's weight. These exercises should be done at least 3 days per week. The muscle resistance program begins with 3–5 repetitions of each exercise for the first week, and then progresses by 2 or 3 each week until 25 repetitions per exercise session are done.

When using weights to perform muscle resistance activities, the "overload principle" is employed. There are two basic methods to use this principle: 1. heavy weights can be lifted a few times (3–6 repetitions) emphasizing muscular strength; or 2. lighter weights can be lifted more times (15–20 repetitions) emphasizing muscle endurance and tone. The later approach is generally recommended to most people as part of a structured exercise program.

To use weights effectively for strengthening the skeletal muscles, individuals should purchase weight-lifting equipment for the home (e.g., dumb-bells and a chin-up bar), or visit a local health club. The manufacturer of the weight equipment will usually provide weight training instructions, or a fitness expert at the health club will recommend a weight training regimen. It is important to advise patients to begin lifting weights that are appropriate for their initial strength and to progress slowly as they increase the amount of weights.

    c. *Stretching or Flexibility Exercises.*   Flexibility is measured by the ability to move a joint through its full range of motion. Individuals are likely to have a lower risk for orthopedic injuries and lower back problems if they have normal flexibility. Loss of flexibility, on the other hand, may result in serious musculoskeletal problems that can lead to poor posture and excessive pain (121). As people properly and regularly stretch major muscle groups, their body movements will seem easier. We recommend that four to five stretching exercises be performed at least three to five times per week, or daily.

All stretching should be slow and deliberate. Patients should be encouraged not to bounce or force joint movements; bouncing makes the muscles respond with a reflex contraction that may injure the muscle being stretched. When stretching, individuals should move slowly to the suggested position until mild tension is felt. At this point, they should hold that position for 10–15 sec and then gradually move forward about one-quarter of an inch. The new position should then be held for 10–15 sec before returning to the original position, and each stretching exercise should be repeated for 2 or 3 min. The entire time spent on stretching will vary from person to person. Patients should spend at least 10–15 min stretching, preferably after cardiovascular exercises when the muscles are warm. Listed in the Appendix are the recommended stretches.

2. *LOT Program*

The secret to this program is simply to be more active. The LOT program should include at least 60 min of activity for 3 days or more per week. This amount of LOT activity should be adequate for achieving and maintaining at least an average fitness level. Home fitness tests such as the Rockport Fitness Walking Test will permit patients to monitor their fitness levels occasionally (144). If a person falls below the average fitness level, he or she may need to increase the leisure time activity and/or consider the structured exercise program discussed earlier.

Astrand recommends that people follow a combination of the structured and LOT activity programs. He encourages people to be up and about, on their feet, walking, climbing stairs, moving, for 60 min a day (9). Astrand also recommended 30–45 min 3 days per week, of exercise such as brisk walking, jogging, swimming, or aerobic dance. Just being more active can pay off in terms of calories burned and health benefits gained.

V. CONCLUSION

The Department of Health and Human Services recommended in its "year 2000 objectives" that at least 50% of primary care physicians counsel their patients about physical activity programs (1), and the US Preventive Services Task Force strongly suggests that all physicians give such counsel to their patients (2). Justification for such recommendations can be found in scientific investigations that relate health benefits to participation in physical activity programs. Because of the high percentage of the population who are physically inactive, physical inactivity can now be viewed as a risk factor for CHD that is more important than hypertension, hypercholesterolemia, or cigarette smoking (1).

Physicians can discharge these recommendations by encouraging patients to engage in a structured exercise program or leisure/occupational time program. These physical activity programs can be easily described to the patient. In addition to informing the patient about the mechanics of beginning a physical activity program, efforts should also be made by physicians and their clinical staffs to inform patients of the potential health benefits to be derived just by being more physically active.

REFERENCES

1. Department of Health and Human Services. Healthy people 2000: national health promotion and disease prevention. U.S. Dept of Health and Human Services, Public Health Service 1990. Conference Edition, pp. 96–112.
2. U.S. Preventive Services Task Force. Exercise counseling. In: Guide to clinical preventive services: report of the U.S. preventive Services Task Force. US Dept. of Health and Human Services, Prepublication Copy, p. 198.
3. Harris L and Associates, Inc. The prevention index '89: summary report. Emmaus, PA: Rodale Press, 1989.
4. Lewis CE. Disease prevention and health promotion practices of primary care physicians in the United States. Am J Prev Med 1988; 4(4):9–16.
5. American College of Physicians. Results of the American College of Physicians membership survey of prevention practices in adult medicine. Ann Intern Med, in press.

6. Caspersen CJ, Powell KE, Christenson GM. Physical activity, exercise, and physical fitness: definitions and distinctions for health related research. Public Health Rep 1985; 100:126–31.

7. American College of Sports Medicine. Guidelines for exercise testing and prescription, 4th ed. Philadelphia: Lea & Febiger, 1991.

8. Pate RR. The evolving definition of physical fitness. Quest 1988; 40:174–9.

9. Astrand PO. Exercise physiology and its role in disease prevention and in rehabilitation. Arch Phys Med Rehab 1987; 68:305–9.

10. Astrand P-O, Rodahl K. Textbook of work physiology, ed. 3, New York: McGraw-Hill, 1986.

11. Blomquist CG, Saltin B. Cardiovascular adaptations to physical training. Annu Rev Physiol 1983; 45:169–89.

12. Saltin B, Blomquist G, Mitchell JH, Johnson RL Jr, Wildenthal K, Chapman CB. Response to exercise after bed rest and after training. Circulation 1968; 38(Suppl 7): 1–78.

13. Seals DR, Hagberg JM. Effect of exercise training on human hypertension: review. Med Sci Sports Exercise 1984; 16:207–15.

14. Kitamura K, Jorgensen CR, Gobel FL, Taylor HL, Wang Y. Hemodynamic correlates of myocardial oxygen consumption during upright exercise. J Appl Physiol 1972; 32:516–22.

15. Hammond HK. Exercise for coronary heart disease patients: is it worth the effort? J Cardiopulmonary Rehab 1985; 5:531–9.

16. Paffenbarger RS Jr, Hyde RT, Hsieh C-C, Wing AL. Physical activity, other lifestyle patterns, cardiovascular disease and longevity. In: Astrand P-O, Grimby G (eds). Physical activity in health and disease. Acta Med Scand Symposium Series no 2. Stockholm: Almqvist and Wiksell International, 1986, 85–91.

17. Shepard RJ. Exercise in coronary heart disease. Sports Med 1986; 3:26–49.

18. Henriksson J, Reitman JS. Time course of changes in human skeletal muscle succinate dehydrogenase and cytochrome oxidase activities and maximal oxygen uptake with physical activity and inactivity. Acta Physiol Scand 1977; 99:91–7.

19. Saltin B, Gollnick PD. Skeletal muscle adaptability: significance for metabolism and performance. In: Peachey LD, Adrian RH, Geiger SR (eds). Handbook of physiology, section 10. Skeletal muscle. Baltimore: Williams & Wilkins, 1983; 555–631.

20. Hurley BF, Hagberg JM, Allen WK, Seals DR, Young JC, Cuddihee RW, Holloszy JO. Effect of training on blood lactate levels during submaximal exercise. J Appl Physiol 1984; 56:1260–4.

21. Durnin JV. Muscle in sports medicine–nutrition and muscular performance. Int J Sports Med [Suppl 1] 1982; 3:52–7.

22. Garrow JS. Effect of exercise on obesity. 1986; In ref 1:67–73.

23. Tremblay A, Despres J-P, Bouchard C. Effects of exercise-training on energy balance and adipose tissue morphology and metabolism. Sports Med 1985; 2:223–33.

24. Haskell WL. The influence of exercise training on plasma lipids on lipoproteins in health and disease. In: Astrand P-O, Grimby G (eds). Physical activity in health and disease. Acta Med Scand Symposium Series no 2. Stockholm: Almqvist & Wiksell, 1986; 25–37.

25. Wood PD, Terry RB, Haskell WL. Metabolism of substrates: diet, lipoprotein metabolism, and exercise. Fed Proc 1985; 44:358–63.

26. Tipton CM, Vailas AC, Matthes RD. Experimental studies on the influences of physical activity on ligaments, tendons and joints: a brief review. In: Astrand P-O, Grimby G (eds). Physical activity in health and disease. Acta Med Scand Symposium Series no 2. Stockholm: Almqvist & Wiksell, 1986; 157–68.

27. Atha J. Strengthening muscle. Exercise Sport Sci Rev 1981; 9:1– 73.

28. Dearman J, Francis KT. Plasma levels of catecholamines, cortisol and beta-endorphins in male athletes after running 26.2,6, and 2 miles. J Sports Med Phys Fitness 1983; 23:30–8.

29. Stebbins CL, Schultz E, Smith RT, Smith EL. Effects of chronic exercise during aging on muscle and end-plate morphology in rats. J Appl Physiol 1985; 58:45–51.

30. Rauramaa R. Physical activity and prostanoids. In Astrand P-O, Grimby G (eds). Physical activity in health and disease. Acta Med Scand Symposium Series no. 2. Stockholm: Almqvist & Wiksell, 1986; 137–42.

31. Rauramaa R, Salnen JT, Kukkonen-Harjula K, Seppanen K, Seppala E, Vapaatalo H, Huttunen JK. Effects of mild physical exercise on serum lipoproteins and metabolites of arachidonic acid: controlled randomized trial in middle aged men. Br Med J 1984; 288:603–6.

32. Smidt EL, Raab DM. Osteoporosis and physical activity. In Astrand P-O, Grimby G (eds). Physical activity in health and disease. Acta Med Scand Symposium Series no 2. Stockholm: Almqvist & Wiksell, 1986; 149–56.

33. Holloszy JO, Schultz J, Kusnierkiewicz J, Hagberg JM, Ehsani AA. Effects of exercise in glucose tolerance and insulin resistance. In Astrand P-O, Grimby G (eds). Physical activity in health and disease. Acta Med Scand Symposium Series no 2. Stockholm: Almqvist & Wiksell, 1986; 55–65.

34. Caspersen CJ. Physical activity epidemiology: concepts, methods, and applications to exercise science. In: Pandolf KB (ed). Exercise and sport sciences reviews, vol. 17. Baltimore: Williams & Wilkins, 1989; 423–74.

35. LaPorte RE, Adams LL, Savage DD, Rrenes E, Dearwater S, Cook T. The spectrum of physical activity, cardiovascular disease and health: an epidemiologic perspective. Am J Epidemiol 1984; 120:507–17.

36. Fidanza F, Puddu V, del Vecchio A, Keys A. Men in rural Italy. Acta Med Scand (Suppl) 1966; 460:116–46.

37. Kriska AM, Sandler RB, Cauley JA, LaPorte RE, Hom DL, Pambianco G. The assessment of historical physical activity and its relation to adult bone parameters. Am J Epidemiol 1988; 127:1053–63.

38. Rosenman RH, Bawol RD, Oscherwitz M. A 4-year prospective study of the relationship of difficult habitual vocational physical activity to risk and incidence of coronary heart disease in volunteer federal employees. Ann NY Acad Sci 1977; 301: 627–41.

39. Caspersen CJ. Physical inactivity and coronary heart disease (guest editorial). Physician Sportsmed 1987; 15:43–4.

40. Siscovick DS, Weiss NS, Hallstrom AP, Inui TS, Peterson DR. Physical activity and primary cardiac-arrest. JAMA 1982; 248:3113–7.

41. Gayle RH, Montoye HJ, Philpot J. Accuracy of pedometers for measuring distance walk. Res Q 1977; 48:632–6.

42. LaPorte RE, Cauley JA, Kinsey DM, Corbett W, Robertson R, Black-Sandler R, Kuller LH, Falkel J. The epidemiology of physical activity in children, college students, middle aged men, menopausal females and monkeys. J Chron Dis 1982; 35:787–95.

43. Bradfield RB. A technique for determination of usual daily expenditure in the field. Am J Clin Nutr 1971; 24:1148–54.

44. Brand RJ, Paffenbarger RS Jr, Sholtz RI, Kampert JB. Work activity and fatal heart attack studied by multiple logistic risk analysis. Am J Epidemiol 1979; 110:52–62.

45. Ross CE, Hayes D. Exercise and psychologic well-being in the community. Am J Epidemiol 1988; 16:403–7.

46. Dauncey MJ, Murgatroyd PR, Cole TJ. A human calorimeter for direct and indirect measurement of 24-h energy expenditure. Br J Nutr 1978; 39:557–66.

47. DeBacker G, Dornitzer M, Sobolski J, Dramaix M, Degre S, deMarneffe M, Denolin H. Physical activity and physical fitness levels of Belgian males aged 40–55 years. Cardiology 1981; 67:110–28.

48. Pooling Project Research Group. Relationship of blood pressure serum cholesterol, smoking habit, relative weight and ECG abnormalities to incidence of major coronary events: final report of the pooling project. J Chron Dis 1978; 31:202–306.

49. Aloia JF, Cohn SH, Ostuni JA, Cane R, Ellis K. Prevention of involutional bone loss by exercise. Ann Intern Med 1978; 89:356–8.

50. Aloia JF. Exercise and skeletal health. J Am Geriatr Soc 1981. 29:104–7.

51. Klein PD, James WP, Wong WW, Irving CS, Murgatroyd PR, Cabrera M, Dallosso HM, Klein ER, Nichols BL. Calorimetric validation of the doubly-labeled water method for estimation of energy expenditure in man. Hum Nutr Clin Nutr 1984; 38C:95–106.

52. Caspersen CJ, Christenson GM, Pollard RA. Status of the 1990 physical fitness and exercise objectives-evidence from NHIS 1985. Public Health Rep 1986; 101: 587–92.

53. Kiburz D, Jacobs R, Reckling F, Mason J. Bicycle accidents and injuries among adult cyclists. Am J Sports Med 1987; 14:416–9.

54. Bouchard C, Lesage R, Lorti G, Simoneau JA, Hamel P, Boulay MR, Perusse L, Theriault G, LeBlanc C. Aerobic performance in brothers, dizygotic and mono-zygotic twins. Med Sci Sports Exercise 1986; 18:639–46.

55. Montoye HJ, Washburn R, Servais S, Ertle LA, Webster JG, Nagle FJ. Estimation of energy expenditure by a portable accelerometer. Med Sci Sports Exercise 1983; 15: 403–7.

56. Blair SN, Lavey RS, Goodyear N, Gibbons LW, Cooper KH. Physiology responses to maximal graded exercise testing in apparently healthy white women aged 18–75 years. J Cardiac Rehab 1984; 4:459–68.

57. Lie H, Mundal R, Erikssen J. Coronary risk factors and incidence of coronary death in relation to physical fitness. Seven-year follow-up study of middle-aged and elderly men. Eur Heart J 1985; 6:147–57.

58. Magnus K, Matroos A, Strackee J. Walking, cycling, or gardening, with or without

seasonal interruption, in relation to acute coronary events. Am J Epidemiol 1979; 110:724–33.

59. Sallis JF, Haskell WL, Wood PC, Fortmann SP, Rogers T, Blair SN. Paffenbarger RS Jr. Physical activity assessment methodology in the Five-City Project. Am J Epidemiol 1985; 121:91–106.

60. Loosli AR, Requa RK, Ross W, Garrick JG. Injuries in slow-pitch softball. Physician Sportsmed 1988; 16:110–8.

61. Lorentzon R, Wedren H, Pietila T, Gustavasson B. Injuries in international ice hockey. A prospective, comparative study of injury incidence and injury types in international and Swedish elite ice hockey. Am J Sports Med 1988; 16:392–6.

62. Cassel J, Heyden S, Bartel AG, Kaplan BH, Taylor HA, Coroni JC, Hames CG. Occupational and physical activity and coronary heart disease. Arch Intern Med 1971; 128:920–8.

63. LaPorte RE, Cauley JA, Link M, Bayles C, Marks B. The assessment of physical activity in older women: analysis of the interrelationship and reliability of activity monitoring, activity surveys and caloric intake. J Gerontol 1983; 38:394–7.

64. Schoeller DA, Webb P. Five day comparison of the doubly labeled water method with respiratory gas exchange. Am J Clin Nutr 1984; 40:153–8.

65. Gerhardsson M, Norrell SE, Kirviranta H, Pedersen NL, Ahlbam A. Sedentary jobs and colon cancer. Am J Epidemiol 1986; 123:775–80.

66. Glagor S. Heart rate during 24 hours of usual activity for normal men. J Appl Physiol 1970; 29:799–805.

67. Janda DH, Wojtys EM, Hankin FM. Softball sliding injuries. A prospective study comparing standard and modified bases. JAMA 1988; 259:1848–50.

68. Maughan Rj, Miller JDB. Incidence of training-related injuries among marathon runners. Br J Sports Med 1983; 17:162–5.

69. Morris JN, Everitt MG, Pollard R, Chave SPW. Vigorous exercise in leisure-time: protection against coronary heart disease. Lancet 1980; 2:1207–10.

70. Paffenbarger RS Jr, Hyde RT, Wing AL, Steinmetz CH. A natural history of athleticism and cardiovascular health. JAMA 1984; 252:491–5.

71. Morris JN, Crawford MD. Coronary heart disease and physical activity of work: evidence of a national necropsy survey. Br Med J 1958; 2:1485–96.

72. Frisch RE, Wyshak G, Albright NL, Albright TE, Schiff I, Jones KP, Witschi J, Shiang E, Koff E, Marguglio M. Lower prevalence of breast cancer and cancers of the reproductive system among former college athletes compared to non-athletes. Br J Cancer 1985; 885–91.

73. Mueller JK, Gossard D, Adams F, Taylor CB, Haskell WL. Assessment of pre-scribed increases in physical activity: application of a new method for micro-processor analysis of heart rate. Am J Cardiol 1986; 57:441–5.

74. Kannel WB, Belanger A, D'Agostino R, Israel I. Physical demand on the job and risk of cardiovascular disease and death: the Framingham Study. Am Heart J 1986; 112:820–5.

75. Pettrone FA, Ricciardelli E. Gymnastic injuries: the Virginia experience 1982–1983. Am J Sports Med 1987; 15:59–62.

76. Kahn HA. The relationship of reported coronary heart disease mortality to physical activity of work. Am J Public Health 1963; 53:1058–67.

77. Chapman JM, Goerke LS, Dixon W, Loveland DB, Phillips E. The clinical status of a population group of Los Angeles under observation for two to three years. Am J Public Health 1957; 47:33–42.

78. Siconolfi SF, Garger CE, Lasater TM, Carleton RA. A simple valid step test for estimating oxygen uptake in epidemiologic studies. Am J Epidemiol 1985; 121: 382–90.

79. Halpern B, Thompson N, Curl WW. High school football injuries: identifying the risk factors. Am J Sports Med 1987; 15:316–20.

80. Durin JVGA. Energy consumption and its measurement in physical activity. Ann Clin Res 1982; 14(suppl. 34):6–11.

81. Mueller FO, Blyth CS. North Carolina high school injury study: equipment and prevention. J Sports Med 1974; 2:1–10.

82. Blair SN. Risk factors and running injuries. Med Sci Exercise 1985; 17:12.

83. Menotti A, Puddu V. Ten-year mortality from coronary heart disease among 172,000 men classified by occupational physical activity. Scand J Work Environ Health 1979; 5:100–8.

84. Patrick JM, Bassey ES, Irving JM, Blecher A, Fentem PH. Objective measurements of customary physical activity in elderly men and women before and after retirement. Q J Exp Physiol 1986; 71:47–58.

85. Paul O, Lepper MH, Phelan WH, Dupertuis GW, MacMillan A, McKean H, Park H. A longitudinal study of coronary heart disease. Circulation 1963; 28:20–31.

86. Donahue RP, Abbot RD, Reed DM, Yano K. Physical activity and coronary heart disease in middle-aged and elderly men: the Honolulu Heart Program. Am J Public Health 1988; 78:1–3.

87. Kannel WB, Sorlie P. Some health benefits of physical activity: the Framingham Study. Arch Intern Med 1979; 139:857–61.

88. Foster FG, McPartland RJ, Kupfer DJ. Motion sensors in medicine: a report on reliability and validity. J Inter-Am Med 1978; 3:4–8.

89. Paffenbarger RS Jr, Hyde RT, Wing AL, Hsieh C-C. Physical activity, all-cause mortality, and longevity of college alumni. N Engl J Med 1986; 314:605–14.

90. Powell KE, Thompson PD, Caspersen CJ, Kendrick JS. Physical activity and the incidence of coronary heart disease. Annu Rev Public Health 1987; 8:253–87.

91. Peters RK, Cady LD, Bischoff DP, Bernstein L, Pike MC. Physical fitness and subsequent myocardial infarction in healthy workers. JAMA 1983; 249(22):3052–6.

92. Ekelund LG, Haskell WL, Johnson JL, Whaley FS, Criqui MH, Sheps DS. Physical fitness as a predictor of cardiovascular mortality in asymptomatic North American men. N Engl J Med 1988; 319(21):1379–84.

93. Blair SN, Kohl HW, Paffenbarger RS, Clark DG, Cooper KH, Gibbons LW. Physical fitness and all-cause mortality: a prospective study of healthy men and women. JAMA 1989; 262(17):2395–2401.

94. Blair SN. Exercise and health. In: Sports science exchange, vol. 3(29). Chicago: Gatorade Sports Science Institute, 1990.

95.   Leon AS, Connett J, Jacobs DR, Rauramaa R. Leisure-time physical activity levels and risk of coronary heart disease and death. JAMA 1987; 258(17):2388–95.

96.   Sobolski J, Kornitzer M, DeBacker G, Dramaix M, Abramowicz M, Degre S, Denolin H. Protection against ischemic heart disease in the Belgian Physical Fitness Study: physical fitness rather than physical activity? Am J Epidemiol 1987; 125: 601–10.

97.   Sallis JF, Haskell WL, Fortmann SP, Wood PD, Vranizan KM. Moderate-intensity physical activity and cardiovascular risk factors: the Stanford five-city project. Prev Med 1986; 15:561–8.

98.   Wood P, Stefanick ML. Exercise, fitness, and atherosclerosis. In: Bouchard C, Shephard RJ, Stephens T, et al. (eds). Exercise, fitness, and health: a consensus of current knowledge. Champaign, IL: Human Kinetics Books, 1988; 409–24.

99.   Froelicher VF. Exercise, fitness, and coronary heart disease. In: Bouchard C, Shephard RJ, Stephens T, et al. (eds). Exercise, fitness, and health: a consensus of current knowledge. Champaign, IL: Human Kinetics Books, 1988; 429–50.

100. Haskell WL, Stefanick ML, Superko R. Influence of exercise on plasma lipids and lipoproteins. In: Horton ES, Terjung RL (eds). Exercise, nutrition, and energy metabolism. New York: Macmillan, 1988; 213–27.

101. Despres JP, Bouchard C, Malina RM. Physical activity and coronary heart disease risk factors during childhood and adolescence. In: Pandolf KB (ed). Exercise and sports sciences reviews, vol. 18. Baltimore: Williams and Wilkins, 1990, 243–62.

102. Hagberg JM. Exercise, fitness, and hypertension. In: Bouchard C, Shephard RJ, Stephens T, et al. (eds). Exercise, fitness, and health: a consensus of current knowledge. Champaign, IL: Human Kinetics Books, 1988; 455–66.

103. Paffenbarger RS Jr, Wing AL, Hyde RT, et al. Physical activity and incidence of hypertension in college alumni. Am J Epidemiol 1983; 117:245–7.

104. Blair SN, Goodyear NN, Gibbins LW, Cooper KH. Physical fitness and incidence of hypertension in healthy normotensive men and women. JAMA 1984; 253:487–90.

105. Epstein LH, Wing RR. Aerobic exercise and weight. Addict Behav 1980; 5:371–8.

106. LeBlanc J. Exercise training and energy expenditure. In: Bray GA, LeBlanc J, Inoue S, Suzuki M (eds.). Diet and obesity. Tokyo: Japan Scientific Societies Press, 1988; 181–90.

107. Bray GA. Exercise and obesity. In: Bouchard C, Shephard RJ, Stephens T, et al. Exercise, fitness, and health: a consensus of current knowledge. Champaign, IL: Human Kinetics Books, 1988, 497–510.

108. Wilmore JH. Body composition in sport and exercise: directions for future research. Med Sci Sports Med 1983; 15:21–31.

109. Pollock ML, Miller HS, Linnerud AC, Copper KH. Frequency of training as a determinant for improvement in cardiovascular function and body composition of middle-aged men. Arch Phys Med Rehab 1975; 56:141–5.

110. Vranic M, Wasserman D. Exercise, fitness, and diabetes. In: Bouchard C, Shephard RJ, Stephens T, et al. Exercise, fitness, and health: a consensus of current knowledge. Champaign, IL: Human Kinetics Books, 1988, 467–90.

111. Taylor R, Ram P, Zimmet P, Raper LR, Ringrose H. Physical activity and prevention of DM in Melanesian and Indian men in Fiji. Diabetologia 1984; 27:578–82.

112. Kanj H, Schneider SH, Ruderman NB. Exercise and diabetes mellitus. In: Horton ES, Terjung RL, eds. Exercise, nutrition, and energy metabolism. New York: Macmillan, 1988: 228–41.

113. Schneider SH, Vitug A, Ruderman NB. Atherosclerosis and physical activity. Diabetes Metab Rev 1986; 1:513–53.

114. Smith EL, Smith KA, Gilligan C. Exercise, fitness, osteoarthritis, and osteoporosis. In: Bouchard C, Shephard RJ, Stephens T, et al. Exercise, fitness, and health: a consensus of current knowledge. Champaign, IL: Human Kinetics Books, 1988, 517–28.

115. Dalsky GP, Stocke KS, Ehsani AA, et al. Weight-bearing exercise training and lumbar bone mineral content in postmenopausal women. Ann Intern Med 1988; 108: 824–8.

116. Dalsky GP. The role of exercise in the prevention of osteoporosis. Comp Ther 1989; 15:30–7.

117. Brown DR. Exercise, fitness, and mental health. In: Bouchard C, Shephard RJ, Stephens T, et al. Exercise, fitness, and health: a consensus of current knowledge. Champaign, IL: Human Kinetics Books, 1988; 607–26.

118. Morgan W, Goldston SE, Eds. Exercise and mental health. Washington, DC: Hemisphere, 1987.

119. Stephens T. Physical activity and mental health in the United States and Canada: evidence from four population surveys. Prev Med 1988; 17:35–47.

120. Durin JVGA. Assessment of physical activity during leisure and work. In: Bouchard C, Shephard RJ, Stephens T, et al. Exercise, fitness, and health: a consensus of current knowledge. Champaign, IL: Human Kinetics Books, 1988; 63–70.

121. Pollock ML, Wilmore JH. Exercise in health and disease. Philadelphia: W.B. Saunders, 1990.

122. Behnke AR, Wilmore JH. Evaluation and regulation of body build and composition. Englewood Cliffs, NJ: Prentice-Hall, 1974.

123. Lukaski HC. Methods for the assessment of human body composition: traditional and new. Am J Clin Nutr 1987;46:537–56.

124. Kraus H. Clinical treatment of back and neck pain. New York: McGraw-Hill, 1970.

125. Melleby A. The Y's way to a healthy back. Piscataway, NJ: New Century Publishers, 1982.

126. Leighton J. An instrument and technique for the measurement of joint motion. Arch Phys Med Rehab 1955; 36:571–8.

127. American College of Sports Medicine. Guidelines for exercise testing and prescription, 4th ed. Philadelphia: Lea & Febiger, 1991.

128. Fletcher GF, Froelicher VF, Hartley LH, Haskell WL, Pollock ML. Exercise standards: a statement for health professionals from the American Heart Association. AHA Medical/Scientific Statement. Circulation 1990; 82(6):2286–322.

129. Gledhill N. Discussion: assessment of fitness. In: Bouchard C, Shephard RJ, Stephens T, et al. Exercise, fitness, and health: a consensus of current knowledge. Champaign, IL: Human Kinetics Books, 1988: 121–6.

130. Chisholm DM, Collis ML, Kulak LL, Davenport W, Gruber N. Physical activity readiness. Br Columbia Med J 1975; 17:375–8.

131. Shephard RJ. PAR-Q, Canada Home Fitness Test and exercise screening alternatives. Sports Med 1988; 5:185–95.
132. American College of Cardiology/American Heart Association: Guidelines for exercise testing. Circulation 1986; 74:653–67A.
133. U.S. Preventive Services Task Force. Screening for asymptomatic coronary artery disease. In: Guide to clinical preventive services: report of the U.S. Preventive Services Task Force. US Dept. of Health and Human Services, 1989: 3–7.
134. Grundy SM, Greenland P, Herd, A, et al. Cardiovascular and risk factor evaluation of healthy American adults. Circulation 1987, 75(6):1340–60A.
135. American College of Sports Medicine. Health appraisal, risk assessment, and safety of exercise: a committee report (in press).
136. Yanowitz FG. Exercise prescription and cardiovascular screening. In: Mellion M, ed. Office management of sports injuries and athletic problems. Philadelphia: Hanley & Belfus, 1987: 11–22.
137. American College of Sports Medicine. The recommended quantity and quality of exercise for developing and maintaining cardiorespiratory and muscular fitness in health and disease: position stand. Med Sci Sports Exercise 1990; 22(2):265–74.
138. Haskell WL. Physical activity and health: need to define the required stimulus. Am J Cardiol 1985; 55:4D–49.
139. Rose G. Physical activity and coronary heart disease. Proc R Soc Med 1969; 62: 1183–6.
140. Morris JN, Pollard R, Everitt MG, Chave SPW. Vigorous exercise in leisure time: protection against coronary heart disease. Lancet 1980; 206:1207–10.
141. Borg GAV. An Introduction to Borg's RPE—scale. Ithaca, NY: Mouvement Publications, 1985.
142. Tipton CM, Vailas AC, Matthes RD. Experimental studies on the influences of physical activity on ligaments, tendons, and joints: a brief review. In: Astrand P-O, Grinmby G, eds. Physical activity in health and disease. Acta Med Scand Symposium Series no. 2 Stockholm: Almqvist & Wiksell, 1986: 157–68.
143. Atha J. Strengthening muscle. Exercise Sport Sci Rev 1981; 9:1–73.
144. Rippe JM, Ward A. Dr. James M. Rippe's complete book of fitness. New York: Prentice Hall Press, 1990.

APPENDIX 1: SAMPLE PHYSICAL ACTIVITY LOG

Days	Date	Physical Activity Type	Minutes			Distance (optional)	Activity Heart Rate (10 sec.)	Weight (pounds)	Meditation/ Relaxation (Yes or No)	Did Some-thing For Self (Yes or No)
			Warm-up	Exercise	Cool-Down					

APPENDIX 2: MUSCLE RESISTANCE EXERCISES

STRENGTHENING SKELETAL MUSCLES USING YOUR OWN WEIGHT

Located on the following pages are photographs of the basic muscle resistance exercises. Eight to 10 of these exercises should be done at least two days per week. For each exercise you choose, begin by doing one set of three to five repetitions for the first week. Increase the number by two or three each week until you reach eight to 12 repetitions. Eventually you may want to increase the number of sets.

Listed below are one or more muscle-resistant exercises that can be used to strengthen the appropriate body parts. The numbers correspond to the **numbered** photographs on the following pages.

Shoulder	1a, 1b, 1c, 3, 4
Abdomen	5,6
Chest	1a, 1b, 1c
Legs	9, 10a, 10b, 11, 12
Back.	3, 4, 7, 8
Biceps	1a, 1b, 1c, 2
Triceps	1a, 1b, 1c, 3

You may want to ask your physician or a physical therapist about other muscle resistance exercises that might be appropriate for your specific needs.

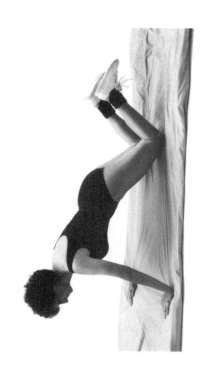

1b. Push-Up (Knee Pivot Position): Keeping hips and back straight, bend elbows to bring the chest to the floor and then return to starting position.

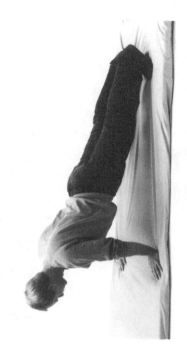

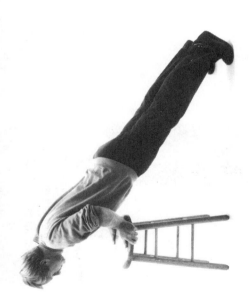

1a. Chair (or Bench) Push-Up: Keeping body straight, lower chest to level of hands and push back up.

1c. Standard Push-Up: Keep body straight from shoulders to ankles, bend elbows to bring the chest to the floor and then return to starting position.

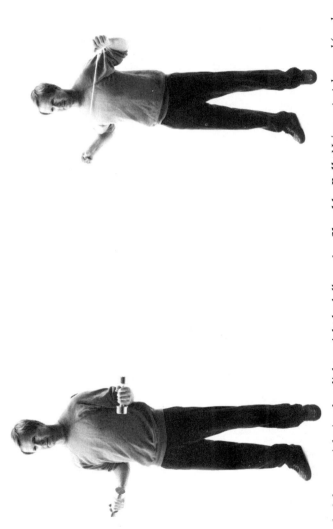

2. **Biceps Curl:** *Select a weight (such as light-weight barbell or soup cans) that can be easily lifted for three to five repetitions. Start with the arms to the side, elbows straight. Bend the elbow, pulling the hand up to the shoulder.*

4. **Shoulder Pull:** *Using a stretchy cord (such as Theraband, surgical tubing or elastic cord) held between the hands, pull the hands apart, bringing the elbows back and down and the shoulder blades together.*

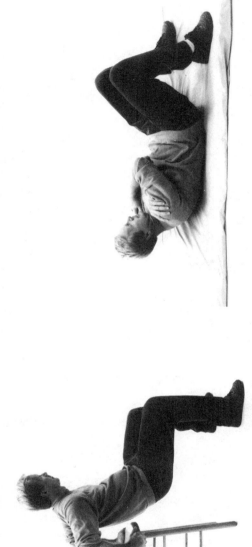

3. **Chair Dip:** *Placing the hands on the edge of a sturdy chair or the edge of a counter, lower your hips toward the floor as far as you feel comfortable. (Note: To adjust the degree of difficulty of this exercise, use chairs or counter of varying heights. The higher the chair surface is from the ground, the less difficult the exercise.)*

5. **Partial Trunk Curl:** *Lying on your back with knees bent (and not anchored), flatten the low-back onto the floor, using abdominal muscles. Holding this position throughout the exercise, curl the head and shoulders up until the shoulder blades clear the ground. Continue holding the low-back flat as you return to the starting position.*

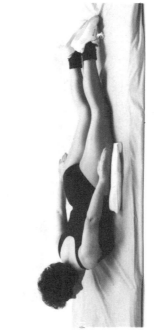

8.   **Chest Raise:** Lying face down (with a pillow under your hips, if desired), raise the head, chest, and arms up, squeezing the shoulder blades down and together.

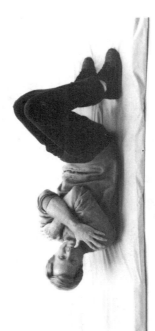

6.   **Side Curl:** Using the instructions given in the exercise #5, add a rotation as you curl up, bringing left shoulder towards right knee and vice versa.

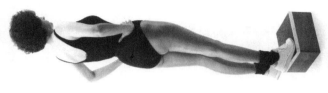

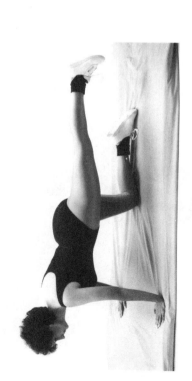

7. *Kneeling Leg Raise:* *From an all-fours position, raise one leg straight behind you from the floor to a horizontal position, and back down to the ground.*

9. *Toe Raise:* *Standing with the toes on the edge of a step, push yourself upwards onto your toes.*

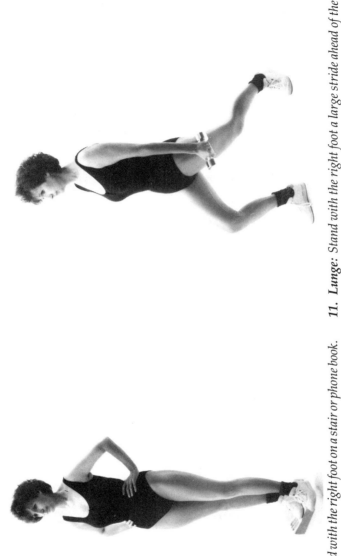

10a. Step Up: *Stand with the right foot on a stair or phone book. Keeping the left leg straight, push up with the right leg as in Figure 10b. Repeat the exercise with the left leg on the step.*

11. Lunge: *Stand with the right foot a large stride ahead of the left. Keeping the right knee over the right toe, bend the right leg forward, lowering the body towards the ground.* **Do not** *go past a 90-degree angle at the knee. To increase the difficulty of the exercise, you may hold weights in your hands. Alternate legs.*

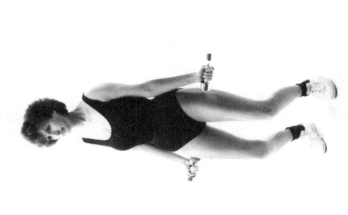

12. ***Partial Squats:*** *Stand with the feet shoulder-width apart; bend the knees forward over the toes (about a 40-degree angle), and straighten up again.*

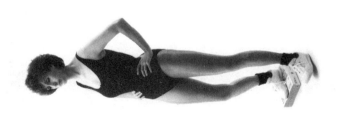

10b. ***Step Up.***

The entire time spent on stretching will vary from person to person. Try to spend at least 10–15 minutes stretching (preferably after physical activity when the muscles are warm).

SUGGESTED FLEXIBILITY (STRETCHING) EXERCISES

Listed in this section are recommended stretches. For each body part listed, there are one or more exercises that can be used to stretch the appropriate muscles. The numbers correspond to the **numbered** photographs on the following pages.

Low back	1, 2, 3
Quadriceps	11
Hamstrings	5
Upper back	4, 6
Trunk rotators	4
Shoulders	6, 7
Achilles Tendon	3, 10
Chest	7, 8, 9
Hip flexor	2, 3
Groin	3, 12

You may want to ask your physician or a physical therapist about other body stretches that might be appropriate for your specific needs.

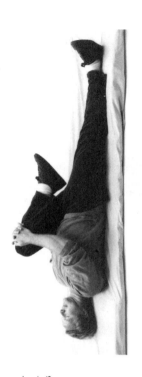

2. **Single Knee-to-Chest:** *Repeat exercise #1, using only one leg. Keep the leg that is not brought to the chest flat to the floor. A modification of this exercise can be performed by bringing the knee across diagonally towards the opposite shoulder.*

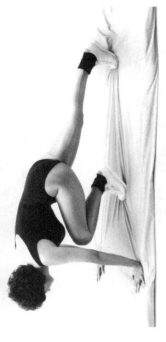

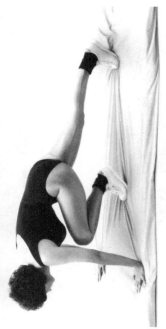

1. Double Knee-to-Chest: Lying on your back, bring your knees upward, grasp them with your hands, and pull them towards your chest.

3. Lunge: Stand with the left foot a large stride ahead of the right. Keeping the left knee over the left toe, bend the left leg forward, lowering the body towards the ground. Place the hands on the floor and lower the hips towards the ground. Alternate feet.

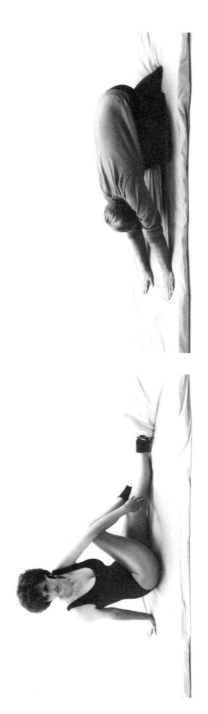

4. *Twist:* Sitting as shown, rotate the torso and head to the right and then to the left.

6. *Prayer Stretch:* Sit on the heels of your feet and stretch the hands out in front of you, placing your chest on your knees.

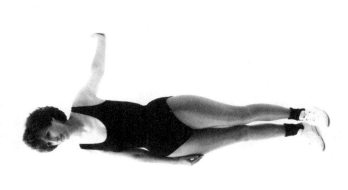

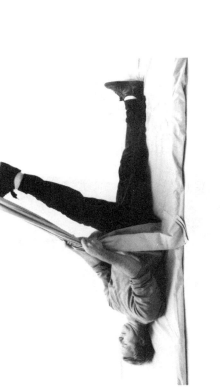

5. **Hamstrings:** *Placing a rolled sheet or rope across the ball of the right foot, raise the right leg with the knee straight. Alternate legs.*

7. **Corner Stretch:** *Place the left hand on a door jamb or a wall corner below shoulder height, and turn the body to the right. Alternate positions.*

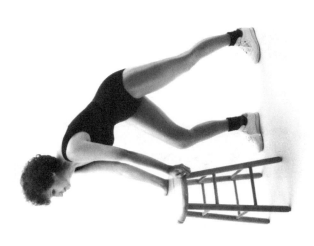

10. Achilles Tendon: Place the right foot ahead of the left foot, toes pointing straight ahead, and bend forward at the ankle. Lean against a wall with your arms outstretched. Alternate legs.

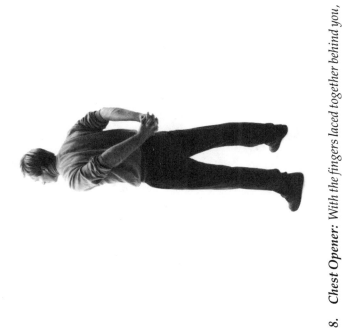

8. Chest Opener: With the fingers laced together behind you, straighten the elbows and raise the arms up.

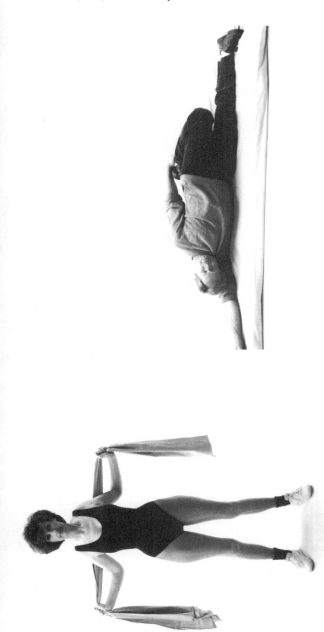

9. Pull Down: *Using a rolled sheet or rope between your hands, pull the arms and sheet down behind your back.*

11. Quadriceps: *Lie on the right side, grasp the left ankle, and pull the heel towards the buttock. Keep the left knee down and avoid arching the back. Alternate legs.*

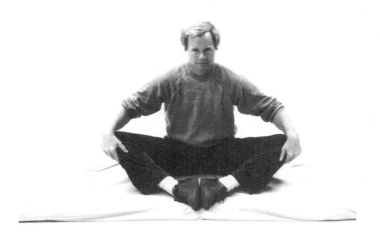

12. Groin: *Sit with the soles of the feet together and allow the knees to drop outward. Bring the feet as close to the groin as feels comfortable. Be certain to keep the back erect.*

13

Cardiac Rehabilitation and the Prevention of Recurrent Coronary Heart Disease

PAUL S. FARDY
Queens College
Flushing, New York

FRANK G. YANOWITZ
The Fitness Institute
LDS Hospital
and University of Utah School of Medicine
Salt Lake City, Utah

I. INTRODUCTION

In the modern era of interventional cardiology, with its increasing reliance on such innovative catheter devices as "crackers, breakers, stretchers, drillers, scrapers, shavers, burners, welders, and melters" (1), it is important not to lose sight of the comprehensive rehabilitation needs of patients with advanced coronary heart disease (CHD). The treatment of advanced CHD will always require these modern interventional techniques to remove or remodel atherosclerotic plaque in an effort to restore myocardial blood flow. Nevertheless, the long-term prognosis in these patients will ultimately be determined by the success, if any, of those measures directed toward slowing, halting, or reversing the progression of coronary atherosclerosis.

This chapter addresses the comprehensive rehabilitation of patients with known and often advanced CHD. The interventions to be discussed are directed toward achieving three long-term therapeutic objectives (2):

1. Restoring individuals with cardiovascular disease to their optimal physiological, psychosocial, and vocational status.

2. Prevention of progression or reversal of the underlying atherosclerosis process in patients with CHD or at high risk for CHD.
3. Reduction of risk of sudden death and reinfarction and alleviation of angina pectoris in CHD patients.

Cardiac rehabilitation should be a multidisciplinary service that includes exercise training, education, and lifestyle modification to improve health and fitness in patients with CHD. In reality, however, many patients do not have the opportunity to participate in formal hospital-based or independent cardiac rehabilitation programs. The primary focus of this chapter, therefore, is on rehabilitative and preventive strategies applicable to primary care physicians who often play pivotal roles in the long-term management of patients with coronary disease. In addition, the components of formal cardiac rehabilitation will be discussed, in order to familiarize physicians with the rationale for these multidisciplinary services.

"Secondary prevention" refers to programs designed to prevent recurrences of coronary disease complications in patients with diagnosed disease. In many respects, these programs are a continuation of strategies found to be effective in the primary prevention of coronary disease, namely interventions dealing with smoking cessation, hyperlipidemia, hypertension, and stress management. Studies published in recent years have shown that the progression of coronary atherosclerosis leading to CHD morbidity and mortality is strongly determined by levels of established coronary risk factors (3–6). Furthermore, interventions that favorably alter the coronary risk profile have been associated with a reduction of coronary morbidity and mortality and, in some cases, with a slowing, halting, or regression of atherosclerotic lesions (7–10). For these reasons it is imperative for physicians managing patients with CHD to emphasize exercise and lifestyle changes known to reduce risk, enhance function, and improve quality of life. Details regarding the management of specific coronary risk factors are discussed in other chapters of this book and will not be considered further here.

II. SCIENTIFIC BASIS FOR EXERCISE

The potential benefits of exercise training and other aspects of cardiac rehabilitation are listed in Table 1. Because of the nature and extent of the scientific evidence, which is often conflicting and controversial, these benefits are categorized as "definite" or "possible." Possible benefits are still unproven, and they may only be realized in a small subset of patients with CHD. Although definite benefits occur in most patients, the range of improvement varies considerably and depends on the quality and length of the prevention program.

Improved physical work capacity is the most clearly established benefit of exercise training and occurs in practically all patients. In patients who have experienced myocardial infarction (MI), however, almost all of the functional

Table 1 Benefits of Exercise Training in CHD

Definite	Possible
Improved physical work capacity	Improved cardiac function and contractility
Reduction in myocardial ischemia	Improved myocardial perfusion
Reduction in coronary risk factors	Reversal or slowed progression of atherosclerosis
Psychological benefits	Antiarrhythmic benefits
	Reduction in mortality and morbidity

improvement during the first 6–12 months is secondary to peripheral conditioning of skeletal muscles, with only minimal improvement in cardiac function or contractility (11). In fact, a recent and disturbing study suggested that there may even be a deterioration in ventricular function due to infarct expansion when exercise training is begun too soon after a large anterior wall infarction (12). For most patients recovering from acute coronary events, however, exercise training begun shortly after hospital discharge has been found to be both safe and beneficial. In some patients with small infarcts, parameters of ventricular function may eventually improve if exercise training is continued for 1 year or longer (11,13,14).

The second well-established benefit of exercise training is reduction in anginal symptoms and other ischemic manifestations (15). This results from physiological adaptations that occur with training and lower myocardial oxygen demands during submaximal work. After training, the more efficient heart can deliver the same cardiac output at lower heart rates and greater stroke volumes than before training. Because heart rate is a more important determinant of myocardial oxygen demands than stroke volume, the training effect improves the efficiency of cardiac work as it enables "more miles per gallon of gas." Myocardial oxygen requirements are further reduced by peripheral adaptations to training, which include a lowering of systemic vascular resistance and improved oxygen extraction by skeletal muscles (16). Reduction in ischemic manifestations may also reflect improved myocardial perfusion, although more evidence is required to address this important question (13).

Coronary risk factors are often reduced during cardiac rehabilitation, but these benefits are more a result of the enhanced physical and psychological well-being than any direct effects of the exercise training. It is sometimes easier for patients to give up bad habits after succeeding with a positive behavioral change such as an exercise habit. There are, however, several direct, albeit small, exercise effects on cardiac risk factors (17). Patients with hypertension may experience a lowering of blood pressure because of the fall in peripheral resistance that occurs with training. There is also a modest increase in high-density lipoprotein (HDL)-cholesterol and a decrease in triglyceride levels with training.

Exercise training is an effective strategy for dealing with the psychological and social disabilities associated with recovery from recent coronary events. Measures of depression and anxiety are sometimes reduced in patients who train when compared to nonexercising patients (18). Return-to-work statistics are also improved after exercise training (19). The restoration of confidence so frequently seen in patients who regain or even surpass their previous level of functioning should be regarded by both patients and physicians as an important prerequisite for returning to productive roles in society. These benefits, although difficult to measure and frequently overlooked, cannot be underestimated.

The other benefits listed as "possible" in Table 1 are more speculative but certainly deserve consideration. The evidence that exercise training in patients with CHD reduces morbidity and mortality is not substantial. Oldridge and his colleagues (20) recently performed a meta-analysis of previously reported randomized controlled trials of cardiac rehabilitation and concluded that all-cause and cardiovascular mortality were significantly lower (by 25%) in the rehabilitation group compared to controls. The same analysis, however, showed no difference in nonfatal recurrent myocardial infarction. Reduction or slowed progression of atherosclerosis, although difficult to document, may actually occur in some patients who participate in exercise programs combined with intensive efforts to modify other risk factors (21).

Antiarrhythmic benefits are purely speculative, although there are several theoretical reasons to suggest that this may occur. As already discussed, training may reduce myocardial ischemia during submaximal work and, therefore, minimize the likelihood of ischemic arrhythmias (15). The trained state is also associated with reduced sympathetic tone and lower circulating levels of catecholamines, therefore decreasing the arrhythmogenic potential of these states.

III. EXERCISE PROGRAMS FOR CARDIAC PATIENTS

Cardiac rehabilitation programs are traditionally classified into three phases: phase I, the inpatient program; phase II, the early posthospitalization program; and phase III, the improvement phase leading to long-term maintenance. Phase IV is sometimes used to describe the long-term maintenance program, although this phase is clearly beyond rehabilitation. The specific components of each of these phases will vary considerably depending upon availability of services, size of program, and financial considerations, including insurance reimbursement issues.

A. Phase I

Phase I is the inpatient program in which cardiac rehabilitation services are provided during hospitalization. Eligible patients include those recovering from acute myocardial infarction, coronary artery bypass surgery, and coronary angioplasty procedures. Patients recovering from other cardiac events such as valve surgery, congestive heart failure, and cardiac transplantation are also appropriate candidates for phase I. Phase I services include self-care activities, bedside activities, education, and a progressive ambulation schedule. A typical seven-step program designed for an average 7–10 day hospitalization is illustrated in Figure 1. Phase I exercise activities have been shown to be safe (22,23), feasible (24), and beneficial (25).

The progressive exercise program is designed to minimize problems associated with bed rest, to reassure patients that they are not likely to become permanently disabled, and to prepare them for a more active lifestyle after hospital discharge. Levels 1 and 2 (Fig. 1) are usually carried out while the patient is still in the intensive care unit, and the remaining levels on the hospital wards or in a hospital-based cardiac rehabilitation center. Each level includes self-care and bedside activities as well as light calisthenics and breathing exercises. More advanced levels may also include supervised treadmill, bicycle, and stair exercises with continuous electrocardiographic (ECG) monitoring. Exercises are generally conducted once or twice daily for each patient.

The rate of advancement through these levels is determined by the patient's clinical condition and the response to the current level's activities. Older and sicker patients should progress more slowly than younger patients with uncomplicated conditions. Contraindications for exercise are presented in Table 2. Careful monitoring of blood pressure, heart rate, ECG rhythm, and symptoms is required during the early phases of this program to ensure that there are no adverse hemodynamic or arrhythmic findings associated with physical activity.

The attending physician is ultimately responsible for advancing the patient through each level, although, in practice, the nursing or rehabilitation staff follow a standard routine based on the patient's daily progress. The actual supervision of activities is done by nurses, physical therapists, or cardiac rehabilitation specialists. It is important that the rehabilitation staff have a good understanding of cardiac hemodynamics and ECG rhythm analysis when working with high-risk cardiac patients. The supervising staff should review each patient's progress daily to provide appropriate feedback to the patient and physician.

Patient education, an important component of phase I services, is designed to enhance the recovery process and provide a foundation for lifestyle modification. Education is initiated early during hospitalization and should involve, in addition to the patient, significant family members or friends (26). A variety of different formats are available for patient education, including self-help reading materials, audiovisual materials, bedside teaching, and group classes. The subject matter includes such topics as cardiac risk factors, exercise training, nutrition, psychosocial adjustments, sexual activities, and general information about coronary artery disease. The teaching approach is multidisciplinary and usually involves physicians, nurses, psychologists or social workers, physical therapists, and other members of the cardiac rehabilitation staff.

The most important goal of phase I is to enhance the patient's mental and

Daily Activity Levels for Patients

During your hospital stay, your activity will gradually increase with the supervision of the medical staff. This is to facilitate your recovery and subsequent discharge from this hospital. Self-care and activity levels, along with suggested exercises, are listed here so that you know exactly what you may do. Help us with your progress by doing only what your physician, nurses, and exercise therapists feel is allowable for your individual condition.

	Self-Care	Bedside Activities	Calisthenics	Ambulation and Exercise Post MI	Post Surgery
1	• Feed self • Use bedside commode • Wash hands/face • Brush teeth	• Sit in bed with firm back support	• Passive ROM, all extremities • Active plantar and dorsiflexion • Ankle circles • Diaphragmatic breathing	**MET Level:** none **Ambulation:** none	none
2	• Bathe self at bedside	• Dangle legs at bedside • Sit up in chair for 20 minutes (not right before or after another activity such as bathing or walking) • Light reading	Same as above, plus: • Active assisted ROM, all extremities • Shoulder shrugs	**MET level:** none **Ambulation:** none	1.5 100-200 ft. (1-5 min.)
3	• Bathe self at bedside or sitting in chair in front of sink (nurse assists with back and legs)	• Walk to bathroom in room with assistance • Sit up in chair as tolerated • Sit in bedside chair for meals	Same as above plus: • In supine position, flex knees to 75° • Sitting knee extensions • Sitting knee lifts • Sitting arm extensions	**MET level:** none **Ambulation:** none	1.5 200-400 ft. (2-5 min.)
4	• Take warm shower if appropriate	• Same as above	• Same as above, repeated 3-4 times a day, especially before walking	**MET level:** 1.5-2.0 **Ambulation:** 100-400 ft. (2-5 min.) **Treadmill/bike:** none	1.5-2.0 400-600 ft. 3-7 min.
5	• Take shower if desired	• Increased bedside chair sitting time as tolerated	• Same as above	**MET level:** 1.5-2.0 **Ambulation:** 400-600 ft. **Treadmill/bike:** 3-7 min. **Stairs:** 3-6	1.2-2.5 up to 1000 ft. 5-8 min. 3-12
6	• Continue as above, plus standing self-care	• Continue with bedside chair and bathroom privileges	• Same as above	**MET level:** 1.5-2.5 **Ambulation:** up to 1000 ft. **Treadmill/bike:** 5-8 min. **Stairs:** 6-12	1.2-2.5 up to 2000 ft. 8-10 min. 6-12
7	• Up ad lib	• Up ad lib	• Same as above	**MET level:** 1.5-2.5 **Ambulation:** up to 2000 ft. **Treadmill/bike:** 8-12 min. **Stairs:** 12	2.0-3.0 up to 3000 ft. 10-15 min. 12

Additional Notes on Supervised Exercise

- Blood pressure is recorded before and immediately after each walk or calisthenics session.
- Heart rate is recorded before, during, and approximately one minute after each exercise session.
- Exercise therapists will supervise calisthenics, treadmill, stationary cycle, and stairs two times each day. During these sessions, patients are EKG-monitored and blood pressure is recorded during each activity.
- Home preparation will generally begin at level 6.

Figure 1 Seven-step progressive ambulation schedule used in the phase I cardiac rehabilitation program at LDS Hospital, Salt Lake City, Utah.

Table 2 Contraindications for Phase I Exercise Activities

Chest discomfort, dyspnea, or palpitations
Heart rate below 50 beats/min or above 120 beats/min[a]
Appearance of frequent abnormalities in cardiac rhythm
Increased ischemic-looking ST segment displacement
Systolic blood pressure decreased by more than 10–15 mmHg with exercise
Orthopedic problems that would prohibit exercise
Moderate to severe aortic stenosis
Recent embolism
Thrombophlebitis

[a]Patients on beta-adrenergic blocking drugs should not increase heart rate more than 15–20 beats/min above resting levels.

emotional outlook. Expectations of increased physical work capacity and decreased hospital stay are unrealistic from low-level exercises and an already shortened hospitalization. Complete bed rest is seldom prescribed for more than several days after myocardial infarction, and hospital stays are now typically less than 10 days. Patient education objectives must also be put into perspective, since the amount of real learning that occurs during a short hospital stay is questionable.

Predischarge or early postdischarge exercise ECG or thallium testing is routinely performed in patients recovering from acute coronary events. These tests are useful for risk assessment as well as for determining safe home activities and enhancing self-efficacy (27–30).

Some patients may recuperate at home for several weeks before entering a formal phase II cardiac rehabilitation program. During this time a progressive home exercise program should be initiated to improve strength and stamina. A typical early at-home walking program is described in Table 3. It is important during this initial period at home that patients not exceed their prescribed heart rates (usually <20 beats/min above resting), and not exercise for at least 30 min after eating. Patients should also be encouraged to commence other preventive health behaviors while at home, including dietary modifications and stress management.

B. Phase II

Phase II programs are designed to meet the needs of outpatients recovering from acute myocardial infarction (MI), heart surgery, coronary angioplasty procedures, and other acute heart disease events. Some patients with stable angina pectoris are also candidates for phase II programs. A major area of controversy in the cardiac rehabilitation literature is the question of medical supervision during this phase. Do all patients recovering from acute coronary events require supervised, mon-

Table 3 Six Week Home Walking Program

Week	No. Sessions per day	Duration (min/session)	Indications for Stopping
1	Twice	10	Chest discomfort
2	Twice	15	Lightheadedness
3	Twice	20	Dyspnea
4	Once	30	Undue fatigue
5	Once	35	Numbness/tingling in extremities
6	Once	40–45	Visual disturbance
7+	3–5 days/wk	45–60	Excessive cold or sweating Nausea or vomiting

itored exercise programs to restore function? This is unlikely to be the case, since most patients recovering from MI without complications spontaneously recover functional capacity within 3 months without formal exercise training (31). Although it is true that a supervised exercise program may result in somewhat greater improvement in physical work capacity compared to spontaneous recovery, this increased function is not large enough to justify the expense of providing cardiac rehabilitation services for all patients.

Given the evidence supporting the role of exercise for patients recovering from acute coronary events, how is this best accomplished? Ideally, although this is not always cost effective, patients should be encouraged to join comprehensive phase II programs whenever possible. Such programs offer considerable assistance to physicians hoping to improve their patients' lifestyles and reduce their risk for recurrent disease complications. These programs are also very motivational for some patients, because of the group psychology effect. However, because of the increasingly serious financial issues facing the various medical reimbursement plans, future cardiac rehabilitation programs are likely to be restricted to a subset of patients at increased risk of exercise-related complications.

In an effort to develop realistic guidelines for cardiac rehabilitation services, the Health and Public Policy Committee of the American College of Physicians (ACP) has published recommendations (32) based on a comprehensive review of the cardiac rehabilitation literature by Greenland and Chu (17). Three categories of post-MI patients were defined in these recommendations: 1. low-risk patients, 2. intermediate-risk patients, and 3. high-risk patients. These categories could also be applied to other cardiac patients who might benefit from exercise therapy, such as those recovering from surgery and angioplasty procedures.

Low-risk patients are those recovering from uncomplicated acute coronary events who already have an adequate functional capacity, defined as 8 metabolic equivalents (METS) or greater at 3 weeks after the event. One MET refers to a person's resting energy requirements and is defined as 3.5 ml O_2/kg/min. Eight METS, or eight times the resting oxygen uptake, represents a level of functional capacity adequate for most occupational or recreational activities engaged in by sedentary individuals. In the exercise testing laboratory 8 METS is approximately the end of stage 7 of the modified Naughton protocol (29) or the first minute of stage III of the Bruce protocol (33). The use of METS to classify risk should be approached cautiously, however, since these units are not precise measurements. Nevertheless, the ACP position paper indicates that these patients may not need supervised exercise programs (32), although such programs are likely to provide additional benefits beyond functional improvement.

Intermediate-risk patients are those who have a moderate risk for recurrent cardiac events or who have functional capacities less than 8 METS. These are patients who may have had complications of heart failure during hospitalization or ischemic ECG changes (less than 2 mm ST segment depression) on exercise testing. They may also be patients who cannot adequately monitor their own heart rates during exercise. The ACP position paper suggests that these patients may benefit from a shortened phase II program, in which the need for ECG monitoring is left to the supervising physician's discretion (32). Patients should remain in the program long enough to develop self-monitoring skills and achieve an adequate functional capacity to allow their return to normal activities.

High-risk patients generally require ECG-monitored exercise programs because of the greatly increased risk of recurrent cardiac events and exercise-related complications. Patients in this group usually have one or more of the clinical features listed in Table 4. Exercise activities should be closely supervised by cardiac rehabilitation specialists, and continuous ECG monitoring must be provided. Individually prescribed aerobic exercises based on exercise test findings are carried out for 30–40 min, 3 times a week for at least 12 weeks. The specific requirements for organized phase II programs are discussed in the cardiac rehabilitation literature and will not be covered in this chapter (26,34).

Table 4 High-Risk Patients After Myocardial Infarction

Severely depressed left ventricular function with ejection fractions <30%
Complex ventricular arrhythmias at rest
Ventricular arrhythmias increasing in severity with exercise
Systolic blood pressure fall of 15 mmHg or more with increasing exercise
Recent MI complicated by serious ventricular arrhythmias
Severe ischemia (>2 mm ST segment depression or angina during exercise testing)
Survival after sudden cardiac death

C. Home Exercise Training

For those patients who do not need formal cardiac rehabilitation services or who are unable to attend such programs, a safe exercise prescription should be provided to meet their occupational and recreational needs. There are five major components to the exercise prescription (34): 1. type of exercise, 2. intensity, 3. duration, 4. frequency, and 5. mode of progression. The specific details will depend on age, the patient's clinical status, the results of exercise testing, and the particular interests of the patient. To qualify for unsupervised home exercise training, however, patients should not have any of the high-risk characteristics described previously (Table 4).

1. *Type of Exercise*

Any exercise activity that uses large muscle groups, such as the legs, in a repetitive, rhythmic manner is acceptable for exercise training, provided the remaining requirements in the exercise prescription are met. Examples of activities include walking, cycling, stair climbing, jogging, use of rowing machines, rope jumping, swimming, and many recreational games. Light-weight resistance exercises are also recommended for most patients to build up strength in the upper extremities. When beginning an exercise program, however, it is best to avoid competitive games because of the difficulty in staying within the guidelines of safe intensity. More strenuous activities may be permitted once the patient's functional capacity has improved and their safety has been established in the exercise testing laboratory.

2. *Intensity*

The safety of exercise is primarily assessed by heart rate monitoring and perceived exertion. Before undergoing an exercise assessment, patients should be encouraged to continue those activities begun in the hospital and at heart rates no greater than 20 beats/min above resting heart rate (Table 3). After a symptom-limited exercise test, performed 3–6 weeks after the cardiac event, the intensity of exercise can be calculated as a heart rate range representing 60–85% of either the maximal heart rate achieved or the heart rate within which ischemic manifestations such as angina, ST segment depression, or arrhythmias occurred.

During the first several weeks of training, the patient should remain at the lower end of this heart rate range to ensure comfort and minimize the risk of exercise complications. Later in the program patients may choose to increase the intensity toward the higher end of the training range. It must be emphasized, however, that low-intensity exercise training is all that is necessary to improve cardiovascular fitness when one is first starting an exercise program (34). This is especially important for older patients, as well as those with more compromised ventricular function.

The widespread use of beta blockers after myocardial infarction complicates the prescription of exercise intensity. One approach is slowly to taper and discontinue use of the drug before exercise testing. Although controversial, it is reasonable to discontinue use of beta blockers permanently if the exercise test shows good functional recovery and no ischemia (35). A second approach is to perform the exercise test while the patient is taking beta blockers and use the blunted heart rate response to calculate the training range, as described previously. In some patients who are taking high dosages of beta blockers, this may not be an adequate training range to improve functional capacity (36,37). Under these circumstances cautious increments in the exercise heart rate are reasonable, providing there are no ischemic manifestations during exercise testing.

After several months of exercise training, patients often learn to associate a particular perception of exertional symptoms with the training heart rate range. Substituting this level of perceived exertion in place of frequent pulse checks is permissible, providing that the patient's clinical condition is stable and that there were no significant ischemic manifestations on exercise testing.

3. Frequency and Duration

There is still much to be learned about the proper balance between frequency and duration of exercise relative to the patient's functional capacity. Initially after hospital discharge, patients may exercise for 5–15 min several times a day at heart rates <20 beats/min above resting. After the training heart rate range is established, based on exercise test findings, patients should gradually increase the duration of exercise and decrease the frequency. The goal for most patients during the first 3 months is to achieve a duration of 45 min 3–5 days a week, avoiding more than 2 days between exercise sessions. The 45 min sessions should include a 5–10 min warm-up, 20–30 min of aerobic exercise within the training heart rate, and a 5–10 min cool-down period. Warm-up and cool-down activities consist of lower-intensity aerobic activities as well as stretching, range-of-motion exercises, and use of light weights, especially for the upper extremities. Some patients who have limited functional capacities will not be able to follow these guidelines. For them, more frequent exercise sessions of shorter duration are recommended.

4. Mode of Progression

An exercise program can be seen as involving three distinct phases: initial, improvement, and maintenance. The rate of progression through these phases depends upon the patient's age, functional capacity, overall clinical status, and specific needs or goals.

The initial phase for patients with CHD should last at least 3 months, the usual duration for phase II cardiac rehabilitation. This is a most critical time for the patient, since a bad experience during this period is likely to result in noncompliance with further exercise recommendations. For these reasons, the emphasis is on a slowly progressive and gentle program, as previously discussed. A major behavioral goal during this phase is to develop the exercise habit. This involves not only learning the various exercise routines but also restructuring daily activities to include the exercise program.

After 3 months of training, patients are usually anxious to assess their progress. Repeat exercise testing is often performed at this time. In addition to documenting improved functional capacity, the exercise test offers an opportunity to revise the exercise prescription. Many patients who have regained confidence will push to a higher symptom-limited maximal heart rate, which results in an increase in the target heart rate for training.

The improvement phase is designed to increase the patient's functional capacity to a level compatible with long-term occupational and recreational needs. The target level of function varies considerably with each patient's clinical status and capabilities. This phase of exercise training leading up to a maintenance level of function is often called phase III cardiac rehabilitation and may be carried out in an organized program under minimal supervision. Again, the emphasis is on slow progression, making small increments in duration and/or intensity every few weeks. A reasonable goal for most patients is 30–60 min of aerobic exercise, 3–5 days a week at 70–85% of maximal achieved heart rate during exercise testing. During this period patients may substitute endurance sports for other aerobic activities in order to enhance enjoyment, if the clinical disease states are stable and compatible with these exercise activities. Nonendurance sports such as volleyball are also recommended to complement aerobic training.

The final phase is long-term maintenance and is sometimes called phase IV by cardiac rehabilitation specialists. This phase should be continued as long as the patient remains in a stable clinical condition. Since changes in clinical status are common in patients with chronic CHD, patients need to maintain close relationships with their personal physicians. New symptoms of chest discomfort, unusual dyspnea, palpitations, lightheadedness, extreme fatigue, and weight gain need to be quickly recognized, evaluated, and treated appropriately. Periodic exercise testing every 6–12 months or whenever there is a questionable change in clinical status provides useful information for subsequent therapeutic decisions and revisions in the exercise prescription.

IV. SUMMARY AND FUTURE DIRECTIONS

In 1985 the American College of Cardiology's Position Report on Cardiac Rehabilitation (38) stated the goals of cardiac rehabilitation services to be:

1. To return the individual to optimal physiological and psychological function.
2. To reverse the adverse effects of physiological deconditioning resulting from a sedentary lifestyle that is accelerated by bed rest.
3. To prepare the individual and his or her family for a lifestyle that may

reduce the risk of coronary heart disease and hypertensive cardiovascular disease. This will involve activities to control smoking, blood pressure, diabetes mellitus, lipid disorders, and emotional stress. It will also involve discussion and clarification of the disease, vocational guidance, and the importance of a regular program of physical activity.

4. To assist the individual with heart disease to return to activities that were important to the quality of his or her life prior to onset of cardiac illness.
5. To reduce the emotional disorders frequently accompanying serious health disorders.
6. To reduce the cost of health care through shortened treatment time and reduced use of drugs.
7. To prevent premature disability and lessen the need for institutional care of elderly patients.

There are many potential mechanisms for achieving these goals, including programs that are supervised or unsupervised, organized or individually carried out, ECG monitored or not-monitored, and so on. Scientific studies are needed to define the optimal rehabilitative and preventive strategies for specific subsets of patients with CHD based on risk classification and other clinical variables.

It is unfortunate that the driving force behind much of today's specific program content is the issue of insurance reimbursement rather than the optimal delivery of services. Medical services that are reimbursed are generally well provided, whereas those not covered are likely to be given superficial attention or completely omitted. For example, nutrition and stress reduction programs are seldom of the quality recommended to provide patients with real benefits. Because the current system of medical service payments does not reimburse for all important features of cardiac rehabilitation, many programs do not achieve their full potential. A major challenge for the future is to provide an adequate scientific basis for meeting the comprehensive rehabilitation needs of patients with chronic CHD.

Continuous ECG monitoring and patient supervision are expensive, and insurance companies and others concerned with cost savings want to reduce this expense. For these reasons risk assessment has become an important aspect of the evaluation process, in order to select patients who require these more expensive rehabilitation services. It is also important to identify lower-risk patients who might benefit just as well from a carefully designed home program and return to productive life more quickly than in the past.

Outcome studies are required for us to learn more about the long-term effectiveness of both supervised, monitored programs and home-based programs. For example, while group dynamics are considered to be important in motivation and in enhancing compliance, it is not yet known if long-term adherence to preventive lifestyles is influenced by being part of a group. Another area of concern is that psychosocial issues are generally not considered when determining who can best exercise at home. There is a great need for studies on the psychosocial ramifications of CHD relative to its treatment and prevention. Some patients classified clinically as being at low risk, but with particular psychosocial maladjustments, might have a much better outcome in an organized rehabilitation program because of the group dynamics. While the cost of cardiac rehabilitation is an important consideration, the more important question is how to provide the best rehabilitation program to sustain long-term preventive behaviors in patients with CHD.

Although exercise is certainly important and the focus of cardiac rehabilitation services, it is essential to give attention to all modifiable risk factors and promote a lifetime commitment to heart-healthy behaviors. It is unfortunate that during the early post-hospitalization period, when patients are most likely to be receptive to making behavioral changes, adequate risk-factor modification programs are seldom available due to lack of reimbursement. This may be an excellent opportunity for volunteer organizations such as the American Heart Association and others to provide valuable preventive services in those environments where reimbursement is unavailable.

The primary care physician is in the best position to influence patient behaviors and should assume a significant role in the promotion of good health. To do this, however, may require a conceptual shift from the traditional biomedical paradigm to a more encompassing model that considers the patient, the disease, and the therapeutic process in biopsychosocial terms rather than purely biomedical (mechanistic) terms (see Chap. 1).

REFERENCES

1. Waller BF. "Crackers, breakers, stretchers, drillers, scrapers, shavers, burners, welders, and melters"—the future treatment of atherosclerotic coronary artery disease? A clinical-morphologic assessment. J Am Coll Cardiol 1989; 13:969–87.
2. Leon AS, Certo C, Comoss P, et al. Position paper of the American Association of Cardiovascular and Pulmonary Rehabilitation. Scientific evidence of the value of cardiac rehabilitation services with emphasis on patients following myocardial infarction—Section I: exercise conditioning component. J Cardiopulmon Rehab 1990; 10:79–87.
3. Schlant RC, Forman S, Stamler J, et al. The natural history of coronary heart disease: prognostic factors after recovery from myocardial infarction in 2789 men. Circulation 1982; 66:401–9.
4. The Coronary Drug Project Research Group. The natural history of myocardial infarction in the Coronary Drug Project: long-term prognostic implications of serum lipid levels. Am J Cardiol 1978; 42:489–98.
5. The Coronary Drug Project Research Group. Cigarette smoking as a risk factor in men with a prior history of myocardial infarction. J Chron Dis 1979; 32:415–24.

6. Jenkins CD, Zyzanski SJ, Roseman RH. Risk of new myocardial infarction in middle-aged men with manifest coronary heart disease. Circulation 1976; 53:342–47.

7. Blankenhorn DH, Nessim SA, Johnson RL, et al. Beneficial effects of combined colestipol–niacin therapy on coronary atherosclerosis and coronary venous bypass grafts. JAMA 1987; 257:3233–40.

8. Selvester R, Sanmarco M, Blessey R. Risk reduction and coronary progression and regression in humans. In: Roskamm H (ed). Myocardial infarction at young age. Berlin/Heidelberg/New York: Springer, 1981: 196–200.

9. Arntzenius AC, Kromhout D, Barth JD, et al. Diet, lipoproteins, and the progression of coronary atherosclerosis. The Leiden International Trial. N Engl J Med 1985; 318:805–11.

10. Nash DT, Gensini G, Esente P. Effect of lipid-lowering therapy on the progression of coronary atherosclerosis assessed by scheduled repetitive coronary angiography. Int J Cardiol 1982; 2:53–5.

11. Paterson DH, Shephard RJ, Cunningham D, et al. Effects of physical training on cardiovascular function following myocardial infarction. J Appl Physiol 1979; 47: 482–9.

12. Jugdutt BI, Michorowski BL, Kappagoda CT. Exercise training after anterior Q-wave myocardial infarction: importance of regional left ventricular function and topography. J Am Coll Cardiol 1988; 12:362–72.

13. Froelicher V, Jensen D, Genter F, et al. A randomized trial of exercise training in patients with coronary heart disease. JAMA 1984; 252:1291–7.

14. Ehsani AA, Martin WH III, Heath GW, et al. Cardiac effects of prolonged and intense exercise training in patients with coronary artery disease. Am J Cardiol 1982; 50: 246–56.

15. Redwood DR, Rosing DR, Epstein SE. Circulatory and symptomatic effects of physical training in patients with coronary artery disease and angina pectoris. N Engl J Med 1972; 286:959–65.

16. Clausen JP. Circulatory adjustments to dynamic exercise and effect of physical training in normal subjects and in patients with coronary artery disease. Prog Cardiovasc Dis 1976; 18:459–95.

17. Greenland P, Chu JS. Efficacy of cardiac rehabilitation services with emphasis on patients after myocardial infarction. Ann Intern Med 1988; 109:650–63.

18. Taylor CB, Houston-Miller N, Ahn DK, et al. The effects of exercise training programs on psychosocial improvement in uncomplicated postmyocardial infarction patients. J Psychosom Res 1986; 30;581–7.

19. Krasemann EO, Jungmann H. Return to work after myocardial infarction. Cardiol 1979; 64:190–6.

20. Oldridge NB, Guyatt GH, Fisher ME, et al. Cardiac rehabilitation after myocardial infarction. Combined experience of randomized clinical trials. JAMA 1988; 260: 945–50.

21. Ornish D, Brown SE, Scherwitz, et al. Can lifestyle changes reverse coronary heart disease? The Lifestyle Heart Trial. Lancet 1990; 336:129–33.

22. West RR. Early mobilization after uncomplicated myocardial infarction. Am Heart J 1982; 103:311–2.

23. Wenger NK, Hellerstein HK, Blackburn H, Castronova SJ. Physician management of patients with uncomplicated myocardial infarction: changes in the past decade. Circulation 1982; 65:421–7.

24. Graber AL, Manley MV. Cardiovascular disease prevention programs in a community hospital. J Tenn Med Assoc 1977; 70:95–6.

25. Wenger NK. Rehabilitation of the coronary patient: status 1986. Prog Cardiovasc Dis 1986; 23:181–204.

26. Fardy PS, Yanowitz FG, Wilson PK. Cardiac rehabilitation, adult fitness, and exercise testing, 2nd ed. Philadelphia: Lea & Febiger, 1988.

27. DeBusk RF, Kraemer HC, Nash E, et al. Stepwise risk stratification soon after acute myocardial infarction. Am J Cardiol 1983; 52:1161–6.

28. Sullivan ID, Davies DW, Sowton E. Submaximal exercise testing early after myocardial infarction. Prognostic importance of exercise induced ST segment elevation. Br Heart J 1984; 52:147–53.

29. Starling MR, Crawford MH, Kennedy GT, O'Rourke RA. Exercise testing early after myocardial infarction: predictive value for subsequent unstable angina and death. Am J Cardiol 1980; 46:909–14.

30. Ewart CK, Taylor CB, Reese LB, DeBusk RF. Effects of early postmyocardial infarction exercise testing on self-perception and subsequent physical activity. Am J Cardiol 1983; 51:1076–80.

31. DeBusk RF, Houston N, Haskell W, et al. Exercise training soon after myocardial infarction. Am J Cardiol 1979; 44:1223–9.

32. Health and Public Policy Committee, American College of Physicians. Cardiac rehabilitation services. Ann Intern Med 1988; 109:671–3.

33. Bruce RA, Kusumi F, Hosner D. Maximal oxygen intake and normographic assessment of functional capacity. Am Heart J 1973; 85:346–51.

34. American College of Sports Medicine. Guidelines for exercise testing and prescription, 4th ed. Philadelphia: Lea & Febiger, 1991.

35. Griggs TR, Wagner GS, Gettes LS. Beta-adrenergic blocking agents after myocardial infarction: an undocumented need in patients at lowest risk. J Am Coll Cardiol 1983; 1:1530–3.

36. Hossack KF, Bruce RA. Altered exercise ventilatory responses by apparent propranolol-diminished glucose metabolism: implications concerning impaired physical training benefit in coronary patients. Am Heart J 1981; 102:378–82.

37. Vanhees L, Fagard R, Amery A. Influence of beta-adrenergic blockade on the hemodynamic effects of physical training in patients with ischemic heart disease. Am Heart J 1984; 108:270–5.

38. Recommendations of the American College of Cardiology on cardiovascular rehabilitation. J Am Coll Cardiol 1986; 7:451–3.

14

Stress Reduction in the Prevention and Management of Coronary Heart Disease

TIMOTHY W. SMITH and PAULA G. WILLIAMS
University of Utah
Salt Lake City, Utah

I. INTRODUCTION

Decades of clinical and epidemiologic research have delineated an invaluable list of risk factors for coronary heart disease (CHD). This list not only provides important information on the causes of the modern epidemic of CHD but also forms the outline of intervention strategies. As detailed in the preceding chapters in this volume, pharmacologic and behavioral interventions for reducing plasma cholesterol levels, elevated blood pressure, excess body weight, and smoking, as well as interventions intended to increase physical fitness, have great potential value in the prevention and management of CHD.

Although quite useful, the traditional list of modifiable CHD risk factors may be incomplete. For centuries, medical and behavioral scientists have suspected that prolonged or intense emotional stress can contribute to the development of coronary artery disease (CAD) and the precipitation of acute coronary events. The eminent 18th century cardiovascular surgeon and pathologist John Hunter aptly described the association between his temper and his angina in noting, "my life is at the mercy of any rascal who chooses to put me in a passion" (1). Hunter is alleged to have died suddenly after a vigorous argument in the Royal College of Physicians. In the late 19th century, Sir William Osler suggested that CHD is caused by "the high pressure at which men live and the habit of working the machine to its maximum capacity" (2). These and many other early physicians anticipated the considerable interest of recent years in the role of stress in CHD. A variety of animal, human epidemiologic, and intervention research has indicated that stress may indeed be an important CHD risk factor.

This chapter has three aims. First, we will review the research indicating that stress can contribute to the progression of CAD and the expression of CHD. Second, we will discuss the findings of recent studies on the effectiveness of stress management interventions for changing CHD risk factors and the prevention of coronary events. Finally, we will discuss issues in the general design and implementation of stress reduction procedures in the prevention and management of CHD. A brief review of the concept of stress and its physiological correlates will be useful before we review the role of stress in CHD.

II. THE CONCEPT OF STRESS

The word stress is used in several ways. In some cases, stress implies a state of the individual, one characterized by negative emotions such as anger and anxiety, as well as physiological arousal. These response-based definitions of stress view it as an internal event or process. In contrast, stimulus-based definitions view stress as an aspect of the environment. In this manner, people refer to stress in describing threatening or demanding life circumstances. To avoid such confusion, researchers have generally come to use the term stressors to describe the events or situations that cause the set of emotional and physiological responses called stress.

Recent conceptions of stress recognize that it is the result of a specific relationship between the individual and the environment. Stress occurs when important environmental threats or demands (i.e., stressors) are perceived as approaching or exceeding one's ability to meet them (3). Stress does not occur unless the threats or demands are construed as important, or unless the individual views them as difficult to avoid, escape, or otherwise manage. This model emphasizes the importance of not only the objective environmental circumstances in producing stress but also cognitive appraisals, perceptions, or judgments about the significance of events and one's ability to cope. Thus, external circumstances and the subjective processes surrounding such judgments are seen as important in understanding the role of stress in illness, as well as in the design of intervention programs.

The basic physiological correlates of stress have been known for many years. Selye (4) labeled the initial physiological stress response the "alarm reaction," while Cannon (5) described it as the "fight or flight response." This set of rapid physiological changes reflects the body's preparation for demanding physical action and the suppression of physiological processes not necessary in such emergencies (e.g., digestion). These changes are produced by two physiological axes: the sympathetic adrenomedullary axis and the pituitary hypothalamic adrenocortical axis.

Many of the physiological aspects of the stress response have been hypothesized to contribute to the progression of CAD and the precipitation of acute coronary events (6). For example, heightened hemodynamic force at artery bifurcations may promote endothelial injury, thereby increasing vulnerability to later development of atherosclerotic lesions. Increases in heart rate and blood pressure during stress also increase myocardial oxygen demand, potentially contributing to ischemic manifestations among individuals with underlying CAD. In animal and human studies, heightened stress-induced increases in heart rate and blood pressure have been found to be related to CAD and CHD (7–9).

Hormonal stress responses have also been implicated in CHD. The characteristic increases in circulating catecholamines, for example, may contribute to endothelial injury, as well as increasing platelet aggregation and the resulting possibility of thrombosis (6). Catecholamines also increase myocardial oxygen demand through their effects on heart rate and contractile force, again possibly facilitating ischemic episodes in persons with CAD. Stress-induced increases in circulating catecholamines may also contribute to myocardial irritability, thereby increasing vulnerability to ventricular arrhythmia (10). Furthermore, high levels of cortisol have been found to promote CAD in monkeys (11) and to be correlated with more severe CAD in humans undergoing coronary angiography (12).

Finally, a variety of animal and human studies indicate that stress promotes increases in plasma cholesterol levels (13). As a result, chronic stress may contribute to the progression of CAD through lipid mechanisms as well.

Thus, a variety of physiological stress responses are plausibly related to the development of CAD and CHD events. These mechanisms not only provide potential explanation for the many observations linking stressful environmental and personal characteristics with CAD and CHD in the research described below but also identify an additional target for interventions. Dampening the "alarm" or "fight or flight" response is likely to be useful in intervention efforts.

III. EVIDENCE LINKING STRESS AND CHD

Several plausible psychosomatic mechanisms exist by which stress may contribute to CHD, and, as will be discussed below, a variety of stress-related psychosocial risk factors have been identified in epidemiologic and clinical studies of humans. However, in most of these studies stress and similar variables are measured rather than experimentally manipulated, rendering conclusions about a causal association between stress and CHD tentative at best. Therefore, experimental studies using animal models of stress and CHD are important tests of possible psychosomatic contributions to CHD.

A. Animal Research

One of the best-developed animal models of stress and CAD involves cynomolgus monkeys. The relevance of this model of CAD for an understanding of human coronary disease is supported by the fact that the anatomy of CAD lesions and the risk factors (e.g., a high-fat diet) are similar in this species and humans. The specific experimental manipulation of stressful environmental circumstances in these studies focuses on the usual social behavior of these animals. In the wild and in captivity, these monkeys form stable hierarchic social groups. In these studies, Kaplan and his colleagues (14–16) randomly assigned animals fed an atherogenic diet to either high or low levels of social stress. In the high-stress condition, animals were frequently reorganized into new groups, thereby creating chronically unstable hierarchies with frequent dominance contests and aggressive behavior. In contrast, animals in the low-stress condition remained in stable social groups for the 2 year duration of the experiment.

As expected, animals subjected to the stress of chronically unstable social conditions developed more severe CAD than did animals in the stable, low-stress condition, as assessed through measures of intimal area on autopsy (15). An interesting finding was that the effects of social stress on atherogenesis occurred primarily among dominant male animals. As can be seen in Table 1, subordinate males were not vulnerable to the effects of stress (14). Among females, subordinate rather than dominant animals are more prone to develop CAD (17), perhaps because of different behavioral and hormonal correlates of the dominance–submission dimension in males and females. Thus, although individual vulnerabilities differed across the sexes, chronic stress clearly promoted the development of CAD.

A subsequent study by these investigators suggested that sympathetic mechanisms may underlie these results. Male animals were all subjected to the chronic social instability stressor, but one half of the animals received the beta-blocker propranolol. As can be seen in Table 2, among unmedicated animals, the dominant males again displayed significantly more severe CAD at the conclusion of the experiment than subordinate males. In contrast, neither the dominant nor subordinate animals receiving propranolol developed significant CAD. The protective

Table 1 Mean Coronary Artery Intimal Area Measurements (mm^2, ± SEM) for Dominant and Subordinate Animals in Stable and Unstable Social Conditions

	Social Status	
Social Condition	Dominant	Subordinate
Stable	0.32 (± 0.13)	0.45 (± 0.12)
Unstable	0.74 (± 0.12)	0.38 (± 0.10)

Source: Adapted from Ref. 14.

Table 2 Mean Coronary Artery Intimal Area Measurements (mm^2, $\pm$ SEM) for Dominant and Subordinate Animals Housed in Unstable Social Conditions With and Without Propranolol Treatment

Propranolol	Social Status	
	Dominant	Subordinate
Treated	0.23 ($\pm$ 0.10)	0.43 ($\pm$ 0.11)
Untreated	0.71 ($\pm$ 0.15)	0.30 ($\pm$ 0.14)

Source: Adapted from Ref. 16.

effects of the beta blocker were independent of any influence on serum lipids, blood pressure, or resting heart rate. It is likely that beta-adrenergic blockade retarded stress-induced progression of CAD by dampening the large increases in heart rate exhibited by dominant males during social encounters under unstable conditions (18). Thus, exposure to chronic environmental stressors apparently can contribute to the development of CAD, most likely through sympathetic mechanisms.

Animal research has also suggested that stress can precipitate acute coronary events in the presence of underlying coronary artery obstructions. Lown and colleagues have developed a canine model of this psychosomatic process (19). To simulate CAD, a balloon-tipped catheter was partially inflated in one of the dog's coronary arteries. In a classical conditioning procedure, the dogs were pretreated with mild but clearly stressful electrical shocks while restrained in a sling. The outcome assessed in these studies was the threshold for repetitive ventricular ectopy during electrical stimulation of the myocardium, which was a marker for vulnerability to ventricular fibrillation. Compared to animals tested in "safe" environments where they had not previously received painful shocks, animals evaluated while restrained in the sling where they had been shocked previously displayed a markedly reduced threshold for repetitive arrhythmias. These results suggest that stress can increase the vulnerability to serious ventricular arrhythmias among individuals with significant coronary artery occlusions. By implication, stress may also contribute to ventricular fibrillation and sudden cardiac death.

A similar study by the same authors underscores the potential importance of anger as a specific stress-related contribution to CHD (20). The dogs were again instrumented with balloon-tipped catheters in the coronary arteries, and measures of coronary blood flow and coronary vascular resistance were obtained. The experimental procedure involved presenting the dog with food, allowing it to eat momentarily, and then moving the dish of food away and allowing a second dog to approach and begin eating from the dish. Although the dogs were never allowed to come into contact, the procedure produced the characteristic growling and baring of teeth among the experimental animals.

In the absence of coronary occlusion, the stressor produced marked increases in heart rate, blood pressure, and coronary blood flow, which returned to baseline levels shortly after the stressful conditions were terminated (i.e, the second dog was withdrawn). When CAD was simulated through partial inflation of the balloon catheter, the stressor had similar initial effects. However, within 2–4 min after the bout of anger, dogs with the partial occlusions exhibited a drop in coronary arterial flow of 35% below baseline levels, an increase in coronary vascular resistance of over 500%, and ischemic changes in the electrocardiogram. No such changes were observed after the stressor in nonoccluded animals. Thus, a pronounced angerlike state apparently can produce significant myocardial ischemia. This finding suggests that anger and perhaps related stressful states can precipitate coronary events among individuals with underlying CAD. The results are strikingly reminiscent of the fate of John Hunter, described above.

The results from these animal models and others indicate that stress may indeed contribute to the development of CAD and the occurrence of symptoms of CHD. Although generalization to humans must be made cautiously, the elegant experimental control characteristic of these studies provides compelling evidence for stress as a potential coronary risk factor.

B. Studies of Stress in Humans

Many different stressful social processes have been examined as potential contributors to CHD. Most of these processes can be viewed as sources of stress, or as social factors that could provide some protection against the otherwise negative effects of stress. For example, changes in one's place of residence, occupation, or social class have been found to confer an increased risk of CHD (21,22,23). In the months after the death of a spouse, widows and widowers are at greater risk of CHD and coronary death than persons who have not experienced such a stressful loss. Stressful work environments have been found to be associated with increased risk of CHD, hypertension, and left-ventricular hypertrophy: a complication of hypertension that increases coronary risk (24–26). Although women working outside the home do not appear to be at increased risk of CHD compared to women working in the home, working women with the added stress of children or unsupportive bosses have been found to be more likely to develop CHD (27). Individuals who have low levels of relaxation away from work have also been found to be at greater risk for subsequent CHD (28). Thus, a great variety of potentially stressful events, roles, and circumstances appear to increase one's risk of CHD.

Similar psychosocial processes have been found to be risk factors for recurrent coronary events. For example, among survivors of initial myocardial infarction, the combination of high levels of stressful life events and low levels of social support has been found to be associated with increased risk of cardiac recurrence (29). High levels of emotional distress have been found to predict subsequent cardiac arrhythmias and even cardiac death among patients with CHD (30,31).

Recent laboratory and ambulatory studies have documented an association between emotional stress and ischemic events among individuals with CHD. Rozanski and his colleagues (32) assessed ischemia-related ventricular wall motion abnormalities in patients with CAD through the use of radionuclide ventriculography. Ischemic changes were assessed during a physical stressor (i.e., bicycle ergometer testing) and an emotional stressor. The emotional stressor entailed the patient discussing his or her personal faults with two laboratory staff members. During the discussion task, 36% of the CAD patients displayed clinically significant transient decreases in left ventricle ejection fraction, and 59% displayed ventricular wall motion abnormalities. The physical stressor had similar effects on the patients with CAD. Only 10% of healthy control patients displayed any abnormal responses to the tasks. Among the patients with CAD who did display wall motion abnormalities, the location of the changes corresponded closely to the results of coronary angiography and thallium scans. Similar effects of mental stress on transient ventricular ischemia have been demonstrated through other laboratory tests of ventricular performance (33).

Emotional or mental stress has also been found to be associated with ischemic changes observed during ambulatory electrocardiographic (ECG) monitoring. In a sample of patients with documented CAD, episodes of ischemia measured with Holter monitoring were correlated with concurrent levels of physical activity and mental stress assessed through patients' diary recordings. As can be seen in Table 3, increasing levels of physical activity were associated with increasing occurrences of ischemic ST segment depression. A more important finding was that increasing levels of mental stress were independently related to the occurrence of

Table 3 Duration of ST-Segment Depression on Ambulatory Monitoring as a Percentage of the Time Spent in Various Stressful Activities

Physical Stress	%	Mental Stress	%
Sleep	9	Sleep	9
Inactive	8	Relaxation	3
Eating/driving	15	Reading/TV	9
Usual	14	Usual	12
Light exercise	19	Stress	23
Heavy exercise	32		

Source: Adapted from Ref. 34.

ischemic episodes (34). These and other findings suggest a robust association between the experience of stress and myocardial ischemia in patients with CHD.

C. Type A Behavior

One of the most widely studied and debated psychosocial risk factors for CHD is the type A behavior pattern. This pattern is characterized by hard-driving competitiveness, impatience, easily provoked hostility, achievement striving, and a loud, rapid, emphatic vocal style (36). Compared to their more relaxed, friendly, and easy-going type B counterparts, type As are hypothesized to be at increased risk of CHD.

In the 20 years following the initial description of the type A pattern by Friedman and Rosenman, a predominantly confirmatory body of research findings had accumulated. These supportive results prompted a panel of experts convened by the American Heart Association to conclude in 1981 that type A individuals were about twice as likely to develop CHD as their type B counterparts (37). However, in the last 10 years, several notable failures to replicate the association between type A behavior and CHD have appeared in the literature (38–40). When the results of all available prospective studies, confirming and disconfirming, are combined through the quantitative procedure of meta-analysis, the type A behavior pattern is shown to be a significant risk factor for the initial development of CHD (41). However, this is true only when type A behavior is assessed through interviewer ratings rather than through the use of self-report questionnaires. Thus, although scientific support for the type A pattern as an independent CHD risk factor continues, its acceptance is somewhat less widespread and more tentative than in the past.

One important result of the controversy surrounding the type A pattern has been more fine-gained analyses of this multifaceted risk factor. When the individual elements of the type A pattern are assessed separately, it appears that hostility is the strongest predictor of subsequent CHD (42,43). Thus, chronic anger, interpersonal antagonism, and a cynical and mistrusting view of others may be the aspects of type A behavior most important to our understanding of personality as a CHD risk factor. This suggests further that other type A characteristics, such as achievement-striving and competitiveness, may not be related to coronary risk. Thus, the evolving view of coronary-prone behavior is less concerned with the original conception of the broad type A pattern and more focused on anger and hostility.

Both type A behavior in general, and hostility in particular, are believed to contribute to coronary disease by way of the physiological correlates of stress discussed above. Type As and hostile individuals are hypothesized to display more frequent, severe, and enduring episodes of physiological reactivity (6,44). This physiological arousal, in turn, is believed to facilitate the progression of CAD and contribute to the precipitation of acute coronary events. The available research is consistent with the hypothesis that type A behavior and hostility are associated with greater degrees of physiological responsiveness to stressors (45,46).

D. Stress as a Risk Factor

The converging lines of animal and human laboratory studies and epidemiologic research indicate that stress can contribute to CHD. Although the strength of the evidence may not equal the similar evidence surrounding traditional risk factors such as smoking, cholesterol, and hypertension, even skeptics must grant that long-held clinical observations have been supported by a wide array of findings. Characteristics of persons or their environments that represent an increased frequency, magnitude, or duration of episodes of stress and its physiological correlates can apparently contribute to the development of CHD.

IV. RESEARCH ON STRESS MANAGEMENT AND CARDIOVASCULAR HEALTH

A logical implication of the research on stress as a risk factor is that stress management may be a useful intervention to reduce coronary risk. Scientific study of this proposition has been underway for a number of years, and important findings are beginning to emerge. The relevant research has focused on stress management procedures to modify one important CHD risk factor, essential hypertension, as well as Type A behavior and anger. A small number of clinical outcome studies have examined the impact of these procedures on CHD events in patient populations. Related stress-management interventions may also have additional benefits for other aspects of patient care.

A. Stress Management and Hypertension

The traditional nonpharmacologic treatments for essential hypertension include weight loss, dietary salt restriction, and exercise. Recent evidence suggests that stress management procedures may be a useful addition to this regimen.

Stress management and relaxation therapies take several forms. Meditation-type approaches involve the repetition of a word or phrase while the patient sits quietly for 10–30 min at a time. Progressive relaxation techniques attempt to teach muscular relaxation through a procedure of voluntary tensing and relaxing of muscle groups. Some programs add cognitive therapies intended to reduce stress-inducing thoughts and beliefs, and also involve supervised practice in applying learned techniques to stressful events. Blood pressure biofeedback entails the continuous monitoring of blood pressure and the provision of a signal to the patient. Over time, the patient is expected to become aware of fluctuations in blood pressure and to learn to exert control.

Most currently employed interventions are multicomponent approaches, using one or more relaxation technique with training in application to daily stressors. The results of controlled studies indicate that these treatments produce clinically significant reductions in systolic and diastolic blood pressure of 5–10 mmHg, beyond any effects due to placebo effects (47). Although useful, it is also clear that stress management interventions for hypertension alone are not as effective as pharmacologic treatments, although they typically produce additional reductions beyond that obtained with medication. Thus, stress management procedures should be considered as adjuncts to traditional pharmacologic and nonpharmacologic treatments.

As noted above, work stress is associated with increased risk of hypertension and its complications, such as left ventricular hypertrophy (25,48). The results of several studies indicate that stress management procedures are useful in reducing blood pressure levels at work among hypertensives (49,50).

B. Type A Behavior, Anger, and Hostility

Stress management procedures form the core of many treatments intended to promote health through reductions in type A behavior, anger, and hostility. As in the case of hypertension treatments, the primary procedures involve relaxation therapies alone or in combination with cognitive procedures intended to modify maladaptive thoughts and beliefs.

Several dozen studies have examined the effectiveness of interventions for healthy type As. Overall, these studies have indicated that relatively brief stress management procedures can significantly reduce type A behavior (51,52). Although reductions in self-reported and interview-rated type A characteristics have been documented, the benefits of these interventions for subsequent cardiovascular health are unknown. While one might assume that reductions in type A behavior would lessen the risk of CHD, there is no evidence for such beneficial effects for healthy type As at this time.

A variety of intervention techniques have been found useful in reducing anger and hostility (53). Progressive relaxation training, cognitive approaches to modifying hostile thoughts and attitudes, and social skills training to replace aggressive behavior with assertiveness and effective interpersonal problem solving have all been found to be effective (54–56). Some evidence suggests that these procedures may be useful in reducing blood pressure as well (55,57). However, as in the case of interventions for type A behavior, the long-term health benefits of treatments for anger and hostility have not been evaluated.

C. Clinical Outcome Studies of Patients with CHD

While the research discussed above indicates that stress management techniques can be used successfully to alter risk factors for CHD, such as hypertension and type A behavior, the most compelling evidence for the use of stress management comes from studies evaluating the impact on CHD endpoints. Two major projects that have studied the impact of stress management techniques on disease outcome are the Recurrent Coronary Prevention Project (58) and the Ischemic Heart Disease Life Stress Monitoring Program (59).

The Recurrent Coronary Prevention Project (RCPP) was initiated in 1977 with a large (N = 862) sample of patients who had experienced myocardial infarction. Subjects were randomly assigned to either a control group (general cardiologic counseling) or an experimental group (cardiac counseling plus group type A counseling) that both met over a 3 year period. The type A group counseling focused on relaxation, behavioral and belief system alteration, making environmental changes, and cognitive–affective learning of type B responses. At the end of treatment, almost half (43.8%) of the experimental group showed a significant reduction in type A behavior, significantly greater than the control group (58). The cardiac recurrence rate for the experimental group was significantly less (7.2%) than that for the control group (13%). Furthermore, the reduction in cardiac recurrence was related to reduction in type A behavior: decreased recurrence was seen only in those patients who showed a significant drop in their type A scores (58).

A follow-up of the RCPP patients at the end of 4.5 years after the initiation of the project indicated continued effects of treatment (60). At that time, 35.1% of the experimental group showed a decrease in type A behavior pattern (TABP) compared to 9.8% of the control group. The experimental group continued to show a lower cardiac recurrence rate (12.9%) than the control group (21.1%). At the end of the first year of treatment and for the remainder of the 4.5 years, there was a significant difference between the experimental and control groups in the number of cardiac deaths (60). As presented in Table 4, when these data are examined for mild vs. severe prior acute myocardial infarction (AMI), the intervention apparently facilitated survival for those with mild prior AMI (61). These data suggest

Table 4 Percentage of Cardiac Deaths in Type A Treatment and Control Groups as a Function of Prior Myocardial Infarction Severity

Group	Severity of Prior M.I. (%)	
	Mild	Severe
Type A treatment + cardiac counseling	2.9	9.0
Cardiac counseling	6.5	10.4
	p < 0.05	ns

Source: Adapted from Ref. 61.

that interventions targeted to reducing TABP offer the greatest protection against coronary death for those individuals with less severe CHD.

The Ischemic Heart Disease (IHD) Life Stress Monitoring Program (59) was undertaken in 1977 to examine the impact of a stress reduction intervention on subsequent heart disease in patients who had experienced MI. Patients (N = 461) were randomly assigned to either a treatment or control group. The treatment group had their stress levels monitored monthly by phone over 1 year. When their stress level was assessed to be above a critical level (more than five symptoms on a stress inventory), the patient received a home visit from a nurse. The home visits were individually tailored stress management interventions. Results of this study indicated that the treatment group showed a decrease in stress scores over the year compared to the control group, providing evidence that the interventions were successful. In terms of health outcome, there was a significant treatment-related decrease in mortality during the intervention year and for 4 months after intervention: cardiac deaths among the treatment patients were reduced by almost 50%. The treatment had no effect, however, on readmission rates to the coronary care unit. The authors suggest that the decreased mortality rate in the treatment group was due to a decrease in out-of-hospital deaths, most often caused by circumstances other than MI, such as ventricular fibrillation. Thus, a stress management intervention helped to reduce the number of sudden deaths, which are more likely to be influenced by stress (59).

The IHD Life Stress Monitoring Program patients were evaluated for 7 years after intervention. Results of the follow-up indicated that the treated patients had significantly fewer recurrences of MI (62). However, the impact on mortality took place primarily during the time of active involvement in the program. Differences in mortality between the treatment and control group were significant between intake to the end of the second year, but not beyond that point. While the results of this project show promise for the use of stress management interventions with heart disease patients, the data should be viewed with caution due to some methodologic limitations of the study (63).

Other, smaller controlled clinical studies also support the utility of stress management interventions for coronary patients. Psychoeducational approaches to stress management have been found to produce decreased rates of CHD recurrence and death among patients (64). The combination of relaxation training and health education has been shown to reduce blood pressure and reported angina in CHD patients over a 4-year follow-up (65). Recently, Ornish and his colleagues have demonstrated that a combination of stress management, exercise, and a very low fat diet produced improvements in frequency of angina and angiographically documented severity of CAD (66,67). Thus, although few in number, these clinical studies provide provocative evidence of the potential utility of stress management procedures for the reduction of cardiac recurrence among patients with CHD.

D. Other Benefits of Stress Management

Stress management procedures have been found to be useful additions to other aspects of the typical care of the patient with CHD. For example, in a controlled randomized study, Gruen (68) found that brief supportive psychotherapy for patients hospitalized in the coronary care unit resulted in fewer days spent in the hospital and fewer arrhythmias. Treated patients showed an increased ability to return to normal activity after discharge. Stress management procedures have been found to facilitate patients' adjustment to cardiac catheterization (69), and to reduce the frequency of hypertension, delirium, and tachycardia following coronary bypass graft surgery (70–72).

Thus, stress management has multiple beneficial impacts in the possible reduction of coronary risk and management of the patient with CHD. As a result, stress management appears to be a useful addition to the tradition approaches to preventing and treating CHD.

V. STRESS MANAGEMENT IN CLINICAL PRACTICE

This endorsement of stress management must be placed in context. First, stress management must be considered as one possible intervention chosen from many possible beneficial risk reduction procedures. Choices among the alternatives must be made on the basis of risk factor profiles. Second, stress is experienced uniquely by each individual. As a result, stress management interventions must follow from a careful consideration of the sources and symptoms of stress in each patient individually. Third, the specifics of any stress management procedure must be embedded in an overall service delivery system. To ensure the maximum benefit of this intervention, it must be tailored to fit within existing systems.

To address the first issue, practitioners must recognize that as compelling as the arguments outlined above may be, other coronary risk factors must be carefully considered when assigning priorities to risk reduction interventions. For example, stress management may be a poor first choice intervention for a patient who has had an MI who smokes, has a total plasma cholesterol level greater than 300 mg/dl, blood pressure of 190/105 mmHg, and an inactive lifestyle. It is perhaps obvious that adding an increasing number of interventions requiring active patient participation will, after a point, decrease the effectiveness of any single intervention. Heavy demands on the patient are often a source of noncompliance and poor response. Thus, the decision to recommend and pursue stress management must be made in the context of a comprehensive evaluation of the individual's risk profile and the assignment of priorities to the treatment alternatives. On the other hand, stress management training may facilitate efforts to modify traditional risk factors such as smoking.

To identify patients who might profit from stress management, a variety of psychological screening procedures might be useful. Standardized inventories such as the Minnesota Multiphasic Personality Inventory (MMPI) and the Symptom Checklist-90 (SCL-90) are widely used, and can identify patients with significant levels of emotional distress typically indicative of problems with stress, such as anxiety, depression, and anger. For healthy patients, these inventories are useful supplements to a sensitive clinical interview exploring recent stressful events (e.g., change in employment or residence, illness in the family, etc.) and continuing sources of stress (e.g., marital and family relations, work, commuting, finances, etc.). In addition, interview-based assessments or questionnaires focusing on type A behavior and hostility are useful in identifying patients likely to profit from stress management. For patients with established CHD, the MMPI or SCL-90 and measures of type A behavior should be part of a more comprehensive psychological assessment, including additional evaluation of neuropsychological functioning, health-related behaviors such as activity levels, and social and work adjustment (73). Given the reciprocal relationship between psychosocial factors and the clinical status of patients with CHD, careful and thorough evaluation of these patients is likely to lead to improved care and management.

Once stress management is identified as a priority, it might seem that a standardized procedure can be applied to all patients. Although such approaches may be of some value, their effectiveness will likely be limited by the failure to consider unique features of the individual patient. Stress assessment requires a thorough and careful consideration of the likely domains of stress, including vocational, family, financial, and social factors, as well as the stress of any existing illness and its treatment. As noted above, major stressful events (e.g., relocation, loss of a job) as well as recurring, minor stressors should be identified. Characteristic emotional and physiological symptoms should be identified, as should the individual's resources in coping with stress. For example, individuals with a high level of aerobic fitness and persons with satisfactory social networks appear to be more resistant to the negative effects of stress than unfit or isolated persons. Finally, typical adaptive (e.g., exercise) and maladaptive (e.g., drinking) coping responses should be considered.

Given the variety of characteristics to be assessed, it is clear that the resulting stress management interventions are likely to vary considerably among individuals. A wide range of techniques may be relevant in individual cases, from anger management to assertiveness training to parenting skill training. Thus, a flexible approach is likely to be necessary for comprehensive care.

It is also true, however, that most individually tailored stress management programs will include some basic, core elements. Progressive muscle relaxation is a "workhorse" in many stress management interventions. This technique and its variations are not difficult to administer, and useful relaxation inductions can be delivered through commercially available audio tapes for home practice. The same is true for meditation-based procedures. Patients with severe or complex stress-related problems, or a poor initial response to simple interventions, may require treatment from a qualified mental health professional. Thus, the availability of an appropriate consultation and referral network is an important aspect of the comprehensive prevention and management of CHD.

Even the most creative, individualized program will be ineffective if it is not a coordinated part of overall patient care. There will be multiple demands on patients' time and energy, made by several different professionals involved in their care. One way to facilitate the delivery of stress management interventions in the care system of patients with CHD is to integrate it with early hospital-based procedures. As noted above, stress management procedures have multiple benefits for patients with acute MI, as well as patients undergoing catheterization or bypass surgery. If initial assessments indicate that stress management will be an important and useful component of subsequent risk reduction efforts for the patient, the therapeutic experiences and relationships established with professionals during hospitalization will provide a good foundation for the further development of stress management skills. Thus, the integration of stress management aspects of acute care and later risk reduction efforts may maximize the effectiveness of these interventions.

VI. CONTROVERSIES AND CONCLUSIONS

One potential impediment to the success of stress reduction in the prevention and management of CHD is the acceptance of stress as a risk factor. Although the public is generally open to this notion, the traditional medical community is less so. Additional, carefully controlled research would certainly be useful in encouraging openness to the role of stress. Thus, the future of stress management in preventive and clinical cardiology will be determined in large part by continued evolution of a compelling empirical foundation. The traditional biomedical or mechanistic model of CHD may need to be modified under the weight of compelling data. This is discussed in more detail in Chapter 1.

Even if stress becomes more clearly established as a risk factor for CHD and additional controlled intervention studies document the potential health benefits of stress management, the place of stress management may not be secure in the future of the prevention and treatment of CHD. Professionals supporting the use of this class of strategies must be careful to avoid promising more than can be delivered. As many authors have argued (74), the associations between behavior and health are often weak and the effectiveness of interventions intended to change behavior are often limited. The resulting effects of behavioral interventions on health outcomes, as a result, are smaller still. Stress management may be a useful addition to comprehensive approaches to CHD, but it is not a major solution to the problems posed by the CHD epidemic.

One important approach to the prevention of CHD is the prevention rather than reduction of risk factors. It may be easier and more effective to prevent hypercholesterolemia, hypertension, obesity, smoking, and inactivity than to modify these risk factors once they have developed. The question arises as to whether the same primary prevention approach is applicable to the role of stress in CHD. Certainly, stress seems to be an inescapable fact of life. Thus, this risk factor may not be preventable in the sense that smoking or obesity is preventable. What, then, would be the analogous strategy for the prevention of risk in the case of stress? The future of stress management in the primary prevention of CHD is likely to entail early intervention programs intended to equip children and adolescents with emotional and social skills to increase their abilities to resist the negative effects of stressors they will confront across the lifespan. Stressful life circumstances may not be preventable, but their effects on health may be moderated by increasing the resilience of individuals who face them. Such prevention programs have long been advocated by mental health professionals. Thus, many existing programs to enhance the emotional health of our population may ultimately reduce the scope of the major threat to its physical health as well.

REFERENCES

1. Debakey M, Gotta A. The living heart. New York: Charter Books, 1977.
2. Osler W. Lectures on angina pectoris and allied states. New York: Appleton, 1892.
3. Lazarus RS, Folkman S. Stress, appraisal, and coping. New York: Springer, 1984.
4. Selye H. The stress of life. New York: McGraw-Hill, 1956.
5. Cannon WB. The wisdom of the body. New York: Norton, 1932.
6. Williams RB Jr. Biological mechanisms mediating the relationship between behavior and coronary heart disease. In: Siegman AW, Dembroski TM, eds. In search of coronary-prone behavior. New York: Erlbaum, 1989.
7. Manuck SB, Kaplan JR, Clarkson TB. Behaviorally induced heart rate reactivity and atherosclerosis in cynomolgus monkeys. Psychosom Med 1983; 45:95–108.
8. Beere PA, Glagov S, Zarins CK. Retarding effect of lowered heart rate on coronary atherosclerosis. Science 1984; 226:180–2.
9. Keys A, Taylor HL, Blackburn H, Brozek J, Anderson JT, Somonson E. Mortality and coronary heart disease among men studied for 23 years. Arch Intern Med 1971; 128: 201–14.
10. Lown B. Mental stress, arrhythmias and sudden death. Am J Med 1982; 72:177–80.
11. Sprague EA, Troxler RG, Peterson DF, Schmidt RE, Young JT. Effect of cortisol on the development of atherosclerosis in cynomolgus monkeys. In: Kalter SS, ed. The use of nonhuman primates in cardiovascular diseases. Austin, TX: University of Texas Press, 1980.
12. Troxler RG, Sprague EA, Albanese RA, Thompson AJ. The association of elevated plasma cortisol and early atherosclerosis as demonstrated by coronary angiography. Atherosclerosis 1977; 26:151–62.
13. Dimsdale JE, Herd JA. Variability of plasma lipids in response to emotional arousal. Psychosom Med 1982; 44:413–30.

14. Kaplan JR, Manuck SB, Clarkson TB, Lusso FM, Taub DM. Social status, environment, and atherosclerosis in cynomolgus monkeys. Arteriosclerosis 1982; 2:359–68.
15. Kaplan JR, Manuck SB, Clarkson TB, Lusso FM, Taub DM, Miller EW. Social stress and atherosclerosis in normocholesterolemic monkeys. Science 1983; 220:733–5.
16. Kaplan JR, Manuck SB, Adams MR, Weingard KW, Clarkson TB. Inhibition of coronary atherosclerosis by propranolol in behaviorally predisposed monkeys fed an atherogenic diet. Circulation 1987; 76:1364–72.
17. Kaplan JR, Adams MR, Clarkson TB, Koritnik DR. Psychosocial influences on female "protection" among cynomolgus macaques. Atherosclerosis 1984; 53: 283–95.
18. Manuck SB, Kaplan JR, Clarkson TB. Atherosclerosis, social dominance, and cardiovascular reactivity. In: Schmidt TH, Dembroski TM, Blumchen G, eds. Psychological factors in cardiovascular disease. New York: Springer-Verlag, 1986.
19. Verrier RL, DeSilva RA, Lown B. Psychological factors in cardiac arrhythmias and sudden death. In: Krantz DS, Baum A, Singer JE, eds. Handbook of psychology and health, vol. 3. New York: Erlbaum, 1983:125–54.
20. Verrier RL, Hagestad EL, Lown B. Delayed myocardial ischemia induced by anger. Circulation 1986; 75:249–54.
21. Syme SL. Coronary artery disease: a sociocultural perspective. Circulation 1987; 76: 1112–6.
22. Kaplan GA, Salonen JT, Cohen RD, Brand RJ, Sume SL, Puska P. Social connections and mortality from all causes and from cardiovascular disease: prospective evidence from Eastern Finland. Am J Epidemiol 1988; 128:370–80.
23. House JS, Landis KR, Umberson D. Social relationships and health. Science 1988; 241:540–5.
24. Karasek RA, Theorell TG, Schwartz J, Pieper C, AlPredsson L. Job, psychological factors, and coronary heart disease. Adv Cardiol 1982; 29:62–7.
25. Schnall PL, Pieper C, Schwartz JE, Karasek RA, Schlussel Y, Devereux RB, Ganau A, Alderman M, Warren K, Pickering TG. The relationship between job strain, workplace diastolic blood pressure, and left ventricular mass index: results of a case-control study. JAMA 1990; 263:1929–35.
26. La Croix AZ, Haynes SG. Gender differences in the stressfulness of workplace roles: a focus on work and health. In: Barnett R, Baruch G, Biener L, eds. Gender and stress. New York: Free Press, 1987: 96–121.
27. Haynes SG, Feinleib M. Women, work, and coronary heart disease: Prospective findings from the Framingham heart study. Am J Public Health 1980; 70:133–41.
28. Wielgosz AT, Earp J. Perceived vulnerability to serious heart disease and persistent pain in patients with minimal or no coronary disease. Psychosom Med 1986; 48:118–24.
29. Ruberman W, Weinblatt E, Goldberg JD, Chaudhary BS. Psychosocial influences on mortality after myocardial infarction. N Engl J Med 1984; 311:552–9.
30. Follick MJ, Gorkin L, Capone RJ, Smith TW, Ahern DK, Stablein D, Niaura R, Visco J. Psychological distress as a predictor of ventricular arrythmias in a post-myocardial infarction population. Am Heart J 1988; 116:32–6.
31. Carney RM, Rich MW, Freedland KE. Major depressive disorder predicts cardiac events in patients with coronary-artery disease. Psychosom Med 1988; 50:627–33.

32. Rozanski A, Bairey CN, Krantz DS, Friedman J, Resser KJ, Morell M, Hilton-Chalfen S, Hestrin L, Bietendorf J, Berman DS. Mental stress and the induction of silent myocardial ischemia in patients with coronary artery disease. N Engl J Med 1988; 318:1005–12.

33. Laveau, PJ, Rozanski A, Krantz DS, Cornell CE, Cattanach L, Zaret BL, Wackers FJT. Transient left-ventricular dysfunction during provocative mental stress in patients with coronary artery disease. Am Heart J 1989; 118:1–8.

34. Barry J, Selwyn AP, Nabel EG, Rocco MB, Mead K, Campbell S, Rebecca G. Frequency of ST-depression produced by mental stress in stable angina pectoris from coronary artery disease. Am J Cardiol 1988; 61:989–93.

35. Krantz DS, Helmers KF, Nebel LE, Gottdiener JS, Rozanski A. Mental stress and myocardial ischemia in patients with coronary disease: current status and future directions. In: Shapiro AP, Baum A, eds. Perspectives in behavioral medicine: cardiovascular disorders. Hillsdale, NJ: Erlbaum, 1991.

36. Friedman M, Rosenman RH. Association of a specific overt behavior pattern with blood and cardiovascular findings. JAMA 1959; 169:1286–96.

37. Cooper T, Detre T, Weiss SM. Coronary-prone behavior and coronary heart disease: a critical review. Circulation 1981; 63:119–25.

38. Case RB, Heller SS, Case NB, Moss AJ. Type A behavior and survival after acute myocardial infarction. N Engl J Med 1985; 312:737–41.

39. Ragland DR, Brand RJ. Type A behavior and mortality from coronary heart disease. N Engl J Med 1988; 318:65–9.

40. Shekelle RB, Billings JH, Borhani NO. The MRFIT behavior pattern study II. Type A behavior and incidence of coronary heart disease. Am J Epidemiol 1985; 122:559–70.

41. Matthews KA. CHD and Type A behaviors: update on and alternative to the Booth-Kewley and Friedman quantitative review. Psychol Bull 1988; 373–80.

42. Hecker MHL, Chesney MA, Black GW, Frautchi N. Coronary-prone behaviors in the Western Collaborative Group Study. Psychosom Med 1988; 50:153–64.

43. Dembroski TM, MacDougall JM, Costa PT, Grandits GA. Components of hostility as predictors of sudden death and myocardial infarction in the Multiple Risk Factor Intervention Trial. Psychosom Med 1989; 51:514–22.

44. Smith TW, Anderson NB. Models of personality and disease: An interactional approach to type A behavior and cardiovascular risk. J Person Soc Psychol 1986; 50:1166–73.

45. Harbin TJ. The relationship between type A behavior pattern and physiological responsivity: a quantitative review. Psychophysiology 1989; 26:110–9.

46. Smith TW, Pope MK. Cynical hostility as a health risk: Current status and future directions. J Soc Behav Person 1990; 5:77–88.

47. McCraffrey RJ, Blanchard EB. Stress management approaches to the treatment of essential hypertension. Ann Behav Med 1985; 7:5–12.

48. Devereaux RB, Pickering TG, Harshfield GA, Kleinert HD, Denby L, Clard L, Pregibon D, Jason M, Kleiner B, Borer JS, Laragh JH. Left ventricular hypertrophy in patients with hypertension: importance of blood pressure response to regularly recurring stress. Circulation 1983; 68:470–6.

49. Agras WS, Taylor CB, Draemer HC, Southan MA, Schneider JA. Relaxation training

for essential hypertension at the worksite: II. The poorly controlled hypertensive. Psychosom Med 1987; 49:264–73.

50. Charlesworth EA, Williams BJ, Baer PE. Stress management at the worksite for hypertension: compliance, cost-benefit, health care, and hypertension-related variables. Psychosom Med 1984; 46:387–97.

51. Haaga DA. Treatment for the type A behavior pattern. Clin Psychol Rev 1987; 7: 557–74.

52. Nunes EV, Frank KA, Kornfeld DS. Psychologic treatment for the type A behavior pattern and for coronary heart disease: A meta-analysis of the literature. Psychosom Med 1987; 48:159–73.

53. Biaggo MK. Therapeutic management of anger. Clin Psychol Rev 1987; 7:663–75.

54. Hazaleus SL, Deffenbacher JL. Relaxation and cognitive treatments of anger. J Consult Clin Psychol 1986; 54:222–6.

55. Moon JR, Eisler RM. Anger control: an experimental comparison of three behavioral treatments. Behav Ther 1983; 14:493–505.

56. Novaco R. Anger control: the development and evaluation of an experimental treatment. Lexington, MA: DC Heath, 1975.

57. Zurawski RM, Smith TW, Houston BK. Stress management for essential hypertension: comparison with a minimally effective treatment, predictors of response to treatment, and effects on reactivity. J Psychosom Res 1987; 31:453–62.

58. Friedman M, Thoresen CE, Gill JJ, Powell LH, Ulmer D, Thompson L, Price VA, Rabin DD, Breall WS, Dixon T, Sevy R, Bourg E. Alteration of type A behavior and reduction in cardiac recurrences in postmyocardial infarction patients. Am Heart J 1984; 108:237–48.

59. Frasure-Smith N, Prince R. The Ischemic Heart Disease Life Stress Monitoring Program: impact on mortality. Psychosom Med 1985; 47:431–44.

60. Friedman M, Thoresen CE, Gill JJ, Ulmer D, Powell LH, Price VA, Brown B, Thompson L, Rabin DD, Breall WS, Bourg E, Levy R, Dixon T. Alteration of type A behavior and its effects on cardiac recurrences in post myocardial infarction patients: summary results of the recurrent coronary prevention project. Am Heart J 1986; 112: 653–65.

61. Powell LH, Thoresen CE. Effects of type A behavioral counseling and severity of prior acute myocardial infarction on survival. Am J Cardiol 1988; 62:1159–63.

62. Frasure-Smith N, Prince R. Long-term follow-up of the Ischemic Heart Disease Life Stress Monitoring Program. Psychosom Med 1989; 51:485–513.

63. Powell RH. Unanswered questions in the Ischemic Heart Disease Life Stress Monitoring Program. Psychosom Med 1989; 51:479–84.

64. Rahe RH, Ward HW, Hayes V. Brief group therapy in myocardial infarction rehabilitation: three- to four-year follow-up of a controlled trial. Psychosom Med 1979; 41:229–42.

65. Patel D, Marmot MG, Terry DJ, Carruthers M, Hunt B, Patel M. Trial of relaxation in reducing coronary risk: Four year follow up. Br Med J 1985; 290:1103–6.

66. Ornish D, Scherwitz LW, Doody RS, Desten D, McLanahan SM, Brown SE, DePuey EG, Sonnemaker R, Haynes C, Lester J, McAllister GK, Hall RJ, Burdine JA, Gotto AM. Effects of stress management training and dietary changes in treating ischemic heart disease. JAMA 1983; 249:54–9.

67. Ornish D, Brown SE, Scherwitz LW, Billings JH, Armstrong WT, Ports TA, Melanahan SM, Kirkeeide RL, Brand RJ, Gould KL: Can lifestyle changes reverse coronary heart disease? Lancet 1990; 336:129–33.

68. Gruen W. Effects of brief psychotherapy during the hospitalization period on the recovery process in heart attacks. J Consult Clin Psychol 1975; 42:223–32.

69. Kendall PC, Williams L, Pechacek TF, Graham LE, Shisslak C, Herzoll N. Cognitive-behavioral and patient education interventions in cardiac catheter catheterization procedures: the Palo Alto Medical Psychology Project. J Consult Clin Psychol 1979; 47:49–58.

70. Anderson EA. Preoperative preparation for cardiac surgery facilitates recovery, reduces psychological distress, and reduces the incidence of acute postoperative hypertension. J Consult Clin Psychol 1987; 55:513–20.

71. Leserman J, Stuart EM, Mamish ME, Benson H. The efficacy of the relaxation response in preparing for cardiac surgery. Behav Med 1989; 2:111–7.

72. Smith LW, Dimsdale JE. Postcardiotomy delirium: Conclusions after 25 years? Am J Psychiatry 1989; 146:452–8.

73. Blumenthal JA, Bradley W, Dimsdale JE, Kasl SV, Powell LH, Taylor CB. Assessment of psychological status in patients with ischemic heart disease. J Am Coll Cardiol 1989; 14:1034–40.

74. Kaplan RM. The connection between clinical health promotion and health status: a critical overview. Am Psychol 1984; 38:755–65.

15

Epilogue: A "Systems" View Toward the 21st Century

FRANK G. YANOWITZ

The Fitness Institute
LDS Hospital
and University of Utah School of Medicine
Salt Lake City, Utah

I. INTRODUCTION

As the 20th century draws to a close a number of major strategies for the prevention of coronary heart disease (CHD) and its complications have been identified. This book has provided numerous clinical guidelines and recommendations to assist practicing physicians in their efforts to prevent CHD. Issues related to management of the major coronary risk factors have been thoroughly discussed. The comprehensive therapeutic guidelines presented in the preceding chapters are based on today's knowledge of the origins and processes of atherosclerosis. Undoubtedly many of these recommendations will be fine-tuned or changed in the years to come as new contributions to our understanding of this complex disease are made. Some will be completely eliminated, only to be replaced by alternative therapies that will come into existence since the publication of this book. The science of medicine is always evolving, and concepts that make sense today will seem simplistic or even erroneous as new knowledge becomes available.

One general concept pertaining to CHD prevention that is unlikely to change in the years to come, however, is the need to focus on behavior change and lifestyle modification as the foundation for any comprehensive treatment regimen. The fundamental objective in CHD prevention, whether primary, secondary, or tertiary prevention, is to achieve long-term behavior and lifestyle changes in areas of diet, exercise, smoking cessation, stress management, and compliance with taking medications. Although the specific details of these prevention strategies may evolve with the discovery of new knowledge, the basic need to change patients' behaviors and lifestyles will always be with us. Furthermore, the pivotal role of primary care physicians in facilitating these changes will continue to be important, since the public considers physicians to be their most reliable and believable sources of health information (1,2).

Frequently, in medical practice, recommendations regarding changes in behavior and modifications of lifestyle are given to patients without taking into consideration environmental or psychosocial variables in patients' lives. The general expectation among health professionals is that health information, when provided by a credible source (e.g., a personal physician) and in an appropriate setting (e.g., a physician's office), will result in the acquisition of knowledge that, in turn, should lead to the desired changes in attitudes and behaviors (3). Likewise, the design of many group health education programs dealing with smoking cessation, weight control, exercise, and other lifestyle related issues is based on the same erroneous assumption: that changes in behaviors will occur when the appropriate health information is provided and understood. This is usually not the case, as evidenced by the very low long-term cessation rates achieved in smoking cessation and weight control, whether provided one-on-one by a personal physician or in a group setting.

Today there is a great deal of frustration and pessimism in the medical profession regarding the delivery of preventive health services, especially those concerned with modifications in lifestyle or changes in health behavior. The reasons for this are many and have been alluded to in the literature and in earlier chapters of this book (1,2,4). Although time constraints and financial impediments are certainly important contributors to this unwillingness to embrace preventive programs enthusiastically, much of the reluctance among physicians to make preventive health recommendations is due to their conviction that most patients are unlikely or unable to make the necessary changes to improve their health (2).

Chapter 1 discussed the inadequacies of the fundamental mechanistic paradigm under which the science and practice of medicine are currently based. This paradigm, the biomedical model, with its reductionist and dualist assumptions regarding the nature of reality, is considered by some to be outdated and no longer compatible with many of the 20th century "postmodern" sciences (5,6). A beginning framework for a revised medical model based on living (self-organizing) systems theory and the concept of the human patient as a biopsychosocial unity was presented (5,6). This new paradigm, supported by nonreductionist and systems-based sciences, seems especially applicable to preventive medicine because it provides a scientific rationale for nonbiological (psychological, social, cultural, environmental) as well as biological issues. These extrasomatic variables, once relegated to the "art of medicine," are of critical importance in the delivery of preventive services because they often determine the success or failure of the behavior and lifestyle changes recommended for the prevention of disease.

In this concluding chapter a systems-based model of health behavior change will be presented that integrates psychological, social, environmental, and biological variables influencing behavior. This model was first conceptualized in 1985 by Kersell and Milsum (3) to assist health professionals in developing more effective health education programs. It is presented here to illustrate the complex network of variables and feedback loops that interact to determine a patient's decision to change or maintain a given set of health behaviors. As stated by the authors, the purpose of the model is to provide a framework for understanding the behavior-change process, in order to better design comprehensive intervention strategies. The model is also compatible with the new scientific paradigm being proposed for medicine because it assumes the patient to be a "biopsychosocial entity in an open systems information exchange with the environment or, for short, an information processing system" (6, p. 156).

II. THE HEALTH BEHAVIOR CHANGE MODEL

Figure 1, adapted from work by Kersell and Milsum (3), illustrates the classes of variables and their interrelationships as they progress from left (antecedents) to right (consequents) to determine the "intention formation process," the critical step in the decision to change or maintain behaviors. Four levels of processes can be identified in which lower level variables provide input to higher level processes: I. external antecedent conditions, II. internal antecedent conditions, III. sociopsychological conditions, and IV. behavioral conditions. Examples within the first three classes of variables are given in Table 1. The following description of the health behavior change model emphasizes relevant factors that might be important to health professionals working with patients interested in developing or maintaining heart-healthy behaviors.

A. External Antecedent Conditions (Level I)

The "external antecedent conditions" represent the initial set of variables that provide input into the behavior-change process. Two different processes are represented at this level: 1. parental and hereditary factors, and 2. sociocultural environmental factors. The variables at this level are primarily related to the physical and social environments that have helped to shape the patient's growth and development; included are variables pertaining to the family, community, society, culture, and other spheres of influence. Also represented are familial and genetic factors that, along with the environmental influences, provide the general framework within which a person becomes a unique biopsychosocial individual.

It is important to emphasize that both genetic (nature) and environmental (nurture) factors can affect a person's psychosocial development as well as the resistance or susceptibly to diseases such as CHD (7,8). The old adage, "coro-

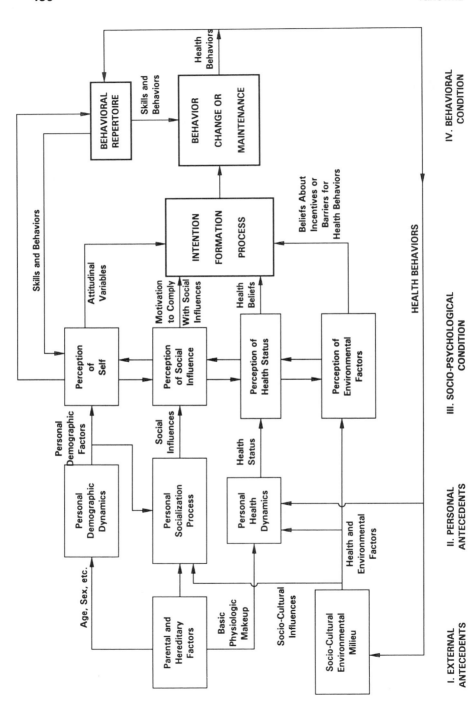

Figure 1 The health behavior change model. (Adapted from Ref. 4.)

Table 1 Variables in the Behavior Change Model

External Antecedent Conditions	Personal Antecedent Conditions	Sociopsychological Conditions
Familial/hereditary factors:	Personal demographic dynamics	Perception of self
Demographic variables	Educational achievement	Self-concept
Age	Occupation	Self-image
Sex	Income	Values and attitudes
Psychological makeup	Geographic location	Personality traits
Family structure	Sex	Locus of control: Internal vs. external
Size	Leisure time interests	Self-efficacy
Composition	Personal socialization process	Self-esteem
Type of family	Role within family	Perception of social influences
Physiological makeup	Role in community/work	Motivation to comply with social influence:
Lipoprotein phenotype	Personal health dynamics	conformity vs. rebellion or nonconformity
Blood pressure	Inherited and acquired factors	Perception of health status: Health beliefs regard-
Cardiovascular factors	related to health and disease	ing susceptibility to disease
Endocrine factors	Susceptibility or resistance to	Perception of environmental factors
Sociocultural environmental milieu	diseases and adverse lifestyles	Health care system
Health-care system	Health status variables	Work environment
Medical insurance	Blood pressure	Social environment
Access to medical care	Blood lipids	
Doctor–patient relationship	Body composition	
Behaviors and social norms of general	Cardiovascular fitness parameters	
population	(VO_2max)	
Environmental stressors		
Pollutants		
Occupational stress		

naries are made in heaven," is, therefore, not entirely correct. As illustrated in Figure 1, the various factors in Level I affect higher-level processes that characterize the patient's physical and psychosocial status (Levels II and III in the model). Factors relating to the patient's upbringing (family structure, family values, education, finances, religious affiliations, etc.) influence the conditions in Level II: educational achievement, occupation, income, leisure time interests, and various other social dynamics within and outside of the family. It is likely, for example, that the seeds of the type A personality begin to take root during this early stage in the patient's emotional development. Likewise, factors related to the patient's genetic and physiological makeup determine the "personal health dynamics," which include the blood pressure, blood lipid levels, body composition, and cardiovascular fitness parameters. Finally, the general social and environmental milieu in which the patient lives (sociocultural norms, health beliefs of the general population, and descriptors of the health care system) influences the patient's personal health dynamics, socialization processes, and perceptions of environmental factors (Level III).

B. Personal Antecedent Conditions (Level II)

Level II variables, the "personal antecedent conditions," represent demographic, social, and health dynamics that personally characterize each individual as a unique human being. Processes at this level are influenced or determined by the external antecedent conditions represented in Level I, and, in turn, they influence the thoughts and feelings that define the individual's "sociopsychological condition" in Level III. Personal demographics such as level of educational, occupation, income, and leisure time interests, for example, provide the life experiences that strongly affect the person's perception of self: self-image, self-esteem, self-efficacy, and locus of control. These cognitive variables are then the important precursors to that person's ability or willingness to eliminate unhealthy behaviors and acquire the necessary skills to develop healthy behaviors.

Variables included in the "personal socialization process" define the individual's role within the family and the broader social networks, such as work, school, friendship groups, and other community organizations. The decision to engage in a particular behavior, whether healthy or unhealthy, is often influenced by the various social dynamics that take place in the home, at work, or elsewhere in the community. The onset of smoking or the decision to stop smoking, for example, is usually influenced by peer pressures at school or in the workplace, or by parental modeling during childhood and adolescence. Health professionals need to be aware of these social influence variables in the design of effective behavior change programs. Interventions that favorably alter the environment in which the patient lives or works are often necessary adjuncts to achieving long-term success in behavior modification. It is also well known that strong social supports play an important role in the prevention and treatment of illness as well as in health maintenance (9); at the other extreme, however, the lack of social supports has been implicated in causation or progression of diseases such as CHD (10,11).

More familiar, perhaps, to the medical profession (because of the biomedical model) are the "personal healthy dynamics," which are the important mediators of an individual's overall health status and, in particular, cardiovascular health. As illustrated in Figure 1 and listed in Table 1, these biological variables are partly determined by the external antecedent conditions represented in Level I, but they are also affected (in a feedback loop) by the actual health behaviors and skills in that person's behavioral repertoire. For example, a patient's blood lipid levels at any given time are affected not only by genetic and environmental variables but also by eating behaviors that may be modified by the behavior change process itself. Cardiovascular fitness parameters such as VO_{2max} are partly determined by genetic factors that influence skeletal muscle fiber type and cardiac size, partly by sociocultural environmental factors that encourage or discourage exercise activities in the community, and partly by the actual skills acquired through participation in an exercise training program. Although intuitively obvious, the concept of improving (or worsening) biological variables as a result of feedback from a person's actual behaviors or from the external environment is much more compatible with a nonreductionist, systems view of life than with the more traditional mechanistic model (see Chap. 1).

C. Sociopsychological Conditions (Level III)

The four processes in Level III represent thoughts and feelings a person has about self, social influences, health status, and environmental conditions in his or her life. These cognitive and affective (emotional) perceptions arise as a result of the particular way one interprets the life experiences and other antecedent conditions previously discussed; they are also influenced by one another, as indicated by the many interconnections in the model, not all of which are shown in Figure 1 for the sake of simplicity. Also important at this level is the feedback from one's behavioral repertoire: previously learned skills and behaviors are able to modify a person's perceptions of self and other cognitive variables. Skills learned in cardiac rehabilitation, for example, restore not only a patient's functional capacity but also the sense of confidence and self-efficacy necessary to return to a productive life. It is at this important level that beliefs and attitudes are formed that lead to the decision to adopt, maintain, or change particular health behaviors. Health professionals interested in the delivery of preventive services, therefore, need to understand better the origins and evolution of their patients' thoughts and feelings, since these are the immediate precursors to the intention formation process and the subsequent health behaviors.

Aaron Antonovsky, a medical sociologist, has written extensively about a person's *sense of coherence*, which he defines as "a global orientation that expresses the extent to which one has a pervasive, enduring though dynamic feeling of confidence that one's internal and external environments as are predictable and that there is a high probability that things will work out as well as can reasonably be expected" (12, p. 10). Although not specifically included in the behavior change model illustrated in Figure 1, the perceptions arising in Level III, which are largely influenced by one's life experiences, are important in shaping this psychosocial variable. According to Antonovsky, the sense of coherence is the major determinant of where a person is located on the "health ease/dis-ease continuum," an objective scale that measures overall health status. A strong sense of coherence means that one has the necessary resistance resources to manage or cope effectively with the many potential endogenous and exogenous stressors encountered on a daily basis and that threaten our health. Examples of these "generalized resistance resources" (GRRs) are listed in Table 2. He further suggests that persons with a strong sense of coherence, when encountering acute or chronic stressors, are more likely to respond behaviorally with actions that include healthy lifestyle choices than those with a weak sense of coherence.

A strong sense of coherence, therefore, has certain implications about how one

Table 2   Generalized Resistance Resources (GRRs)

Physical and Biochemical GRRs
  Immunologic surveillance function
  Genetic factors
  Physical strength
Artifactual–Material GRRs: Access to money, shelter, clothing, food, etc.
Cognitive and Emotional GRRs
  Knowledge and intelligence about the world, and the necessary skills to acquire such knowledge
  Ego identity . . . "a sense of the inner person, integrated and stable, yet dynamic and flexible; related to social and cultural reality, yet with independence, so that neither narcissism nor being a template of external reality is needed" (12, p. 109)
Valuative–Attitudinal GRRs: Coping strategies (plan of action for dealing with stressors)
  Rationality: abilty to assess the extent to which stressor is a threat
  Flexibility: availability of alternative plans and strategies
  Farsightedness: thinking ahead
  Emotional affect: perceiving stressor as challenge
Interpersonal–Relational GRRs
  Social supports
  Commitment to social networks
Macrosociocultural GRRs
  Cultural stability: provides wide range of responses to stressors
  Religious beliefs

Source: Adapted from Ref. 12.

perceives the sociopsychological conditions in Level III (Table 1). Antonovsky (13, p. 16) identities three components that characterize the strength of the sense of coherence: comprehensibility, manageability, and meaningfulness. Comprehensibility is defined as "the extent to which one perceives the stimuli that confront one, deriving from the internal and external environments, as making cognitive sense, as information that is ordered, consistent, structured, and clear, rather than as noise—chaotic, disordered, random, accidental, inexplicable." Manageability is defined as "the extent to which one perceives that resources are at one's disposal which are adequate to meet the demands posed by the stimuli that bombard one." Meaningfulness refers to "the extent to which one feels that life makes sense emotionally, that at least some of the problems and demands posed by living are worth investing energy in, are worthy of commitment and engagement, are challenges that are 'welcome' rather than burdens that one would much rather do without." Individuals "high" on these three components (i.e., who have a strong sense of coherence) are most likely to have the attitudes, beliefs, motivation, and knowledge to choose behaviors and lifestyles conducive to good health. These are the output variables from Level III in the health behavior change model that influence the "intention formation process" (Fig. 1). Antonovsky has tested the validated a questionnaire that can be used by health professionals to measure the strength of the sense of coherence (13).

D. Behavioral Condition (Level IV)

The fourth and final level in the behavior change model includes the intention formation process, the skills and behaviors available in the behavioral repertoire, and the particular health behavior being considered for adoption, change, or elimination. As previously discussed, a person's attitudes and beliefs about health-related issues are formed in Level III on the basis of various perceptions he or she has about self, social influences, health status, and environmental factors. These perceptions, in turn, have resulted from a pattern of life experiences an individual has over a lifespan, shaped, in part, by genetic and familial influences and, in part, by the physical and social environments within which the person has lived. As seen in Figure 1, the behaviors themselves and any change or modification of behaviors provide feedback to influence, in a positive or negative way, the various processes that have participated in their formation. The important implication for health professionals is that the acquisition of health-enhancing skills and behaviors is likely to be self-sustaining because of the positive effects they have on the person's overall health dynamics, the sociocultural environmental milieu, and, most importantly, the person's sense of coherence.

Also important in the behavior change process is the repertoire of actual skills and behaviors acquired during a person's lifetime. These can have either negative or positive effects on the ability to change or eliminate behaviors. For example, the chronic smoker is also a "skilled" smoker, and will therefore have much more difficulty quitting even though there is the intention to stop smoking. On the other hand, someone who has just started smoking, a less skillful smoker, should have an easier time quitting once the intention to stop has been formulated, as long as that person has the knowledge and ability to recognize and resist social pressures to smoke.

Behavioral skills can also be taught to patients by health professionals to assist them in making health behavior changes. In addition to helping patients develop the appropriate attitudes and beliefs necessary to formulate the intention to make changes in one's lifestyle, health professionals should provide the educational tools needed to make those changes. It is important for primary care physicians to acquire the knowledge and abilities needed to educate their patients about exercise training, making dietary changes, stress management, smoking cessation, and so on. The recommended behaviors and lifestyles are covered in considerable detail in the preceding chapters of this book. The acquisition of practice behaviors and skills needed by physicians for the prevention of CHD in clinical practice is discussed in the next section.

III. THE PHYSICIAN BEHAVIOR CHANGE MODEL

An appreciation of the many variables and their interrelationships that make up the health behavior change model is an important prerequisite to reorganizing the medical care system to facilitate more effective delivery of preventive cardiology services. Because of the many financial and conceptual barriers that presently limit disease prevention and health-promotion activities in medical practice, however, this reorganization is not likely to occur quickly. Nevertheless, an optimistic "view towards the 21st century" is a worthy challenge for the medical profession, since the prevention of CHD and other chronic diseases is clearly within our grasp, and ever increasing numbers of the general public are interested in receiving more preventive health services.

To meet this challenge, however, many physicians will need to modify their own practice behaviors to incorporate prevention-oriented strategies in their patient care activities. Traditional approaches to altering physician behavior have generally relied on published materials and oral presentations to provide up-to-date information on various aspects of preventive medicine. However, written guidelines and lectures are unlikely to be successful in changing physicians' behaviors because they do not usually lead to the acquisition of new skills, nor do they provide the necessary feedback to achieve the desired modifications in behaviors (2). It is clear that a different approach is needed, along with appropriate financial incentives and support from the medical profession at large.

In considering the challenge of altering physician behaviors to provide more disease prevention and health promotion services, an interesting parallel can be drawn between the health behavior change model just described (Fig. 1) and a similarly configured "physician behavior change" model illustrated in Figure 2. This latter model offers a systems analysis of the processes and variables that influence the acquisition and subsequent modification of medical practice behaviors. At issue is an understanding of those variables that might lead to the desired changes in physician practices. As with the health behavior change model just discussed, four analogous levels of processes can be identified (3): I. external antecedent conditions, II. professional antecedent conditions, III. sociopsychological conditions, and IV. behavioral conditions.

A. External Antecedent Conditions (Level I)

At this initial level in the model only one process merits consideration as an external antecedent condition influencing physician practice behaviors: the "sociocultural environmental milieu." Included in this process are the various descriptors of the medical care environment that have an impact on the belief system of physicians: medical education institutions, behaviors and practice norms of the medical community, health beliefs and sociocultural norms of the general population, community health-care resources, environmental factors affecting health, and the various government and private institutions regulating health care. As shown in Figure 2, these numerous factors provide input to all three Level II processes that characterize the physician's professional life; they also affect the physician's perception of the medical care system and the various environmental factors influencing the health of the population and their patients. The skills and practice behaviors of physicians (Level IV) also provide feedback to these external antecedents and participate in shaping the medical care environment.

At this initial level the growing public dissatisfaction with a medical care system characterized by complex technology and increased specialization is likely to have an impact on medicine's future and, in particular, the practice behaviors of physicians. Changing public attitudes about health and disease are already beginning to drive the medical care system toward more primary care and ambulatory services. John Gordon Freymann sums up this new public perception when he states: ". . . the American middle class is moving rapidly toward a new paradigm of health care. Until recently, most Americans were convinced the key to health was conquest of disease through science. Their new belief is more positive: health is a natural state and the key to it lies in lifestyle and the environment" (14). Although this appears to ignore the health care needs of our nation's poor, it is clear, as Freymann points out, that middle class beliefs determine the way in which the needs of all our citizens are met. As the 20th century draws to a close there is evidence for increasing levels of awareness among Americans regarding such issues as the environment, disease prevention, and healthy lifestyles (14). This

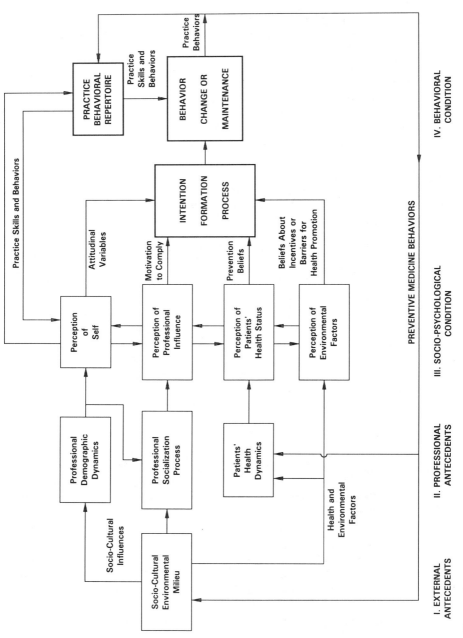

Figure 2 The physician's behavior change model. (Adapted from Ref. 4.)

awareness is linked to an increased willingness of the American people to assume more responsibility for their health and well-being (15). It is apparent that the medical profession must move towards this new societal paradigm if it is to regain public confidence.

B. Professional Antecedent Conditions (Level II)

At this level three sets of processes interact to characterize the professional life of the physician: 1. professional demographic dynamics, 2. professional socialization process, and 3. patients' health dynamics. Each of these plays a role in the practice behaviors and skills of individual physicians.

Included in the professional demographics, for example, are such characteristics as medical education and postdoctoral achievements, type of specialization, practice specifications (hospital based vs. private office, solo vs. group practice, academic vs. nonacademic, rural vs. urban, etc.), membership in professional organizations, geographic location, income, age, and sex. These variables influence the physician's perception of self (Level III) as well as the professional socialization process, to be discussed later.

One of the obvious places to start the difficult task of reorganizing medical practice to incorporate health promotion and prevention services is during physician training. Efforts to encourage more preventive cardiology practice behaviors, in fact, are beginning to take place in medical schools and in housestaff training programs as more emphasis is given to outpatient medicine, preventive medicine, and humanistic aspects of medicine. Recognizing the importance of these issues, a 1984 report from the Association of American Medical Colleges, entitled *Physicians for the Twenty-First Century*, strongly recommended that "medical students' general professional education should include an emphasis on the physician's responsibility to work with individual patients and communities to promote health and prevent disease" (16, p. 6). The federal government has also recognized the need to include more education on the prevention of cardiovascular diseases by establishing, through the National Institutes of Health, "Preventive Cardiology Curriculum Awards" in 60 medical schools during the 1980s. These 5 year stipends were for the sole purpose of developing a preventive cardiology faculty and a curriculum for educating medical students and housestaff.

In spite of these efforts, however, there is still considerable resistance and pessimism within the academic community regarding the incorporation of prevention into medical education. In a recent paper, Fried (4) pointed out that preventive medicine education does not fit in with the traditional biomedical model with its emphasis on molecular biology as providing the explanation for all diseases. He goes on to state that "biomedicine by its nature excludes prevention's world view. As long as medical education is dominated by a paradigm in which social data have no place, prevention hasn't got a chance." Fried's recommendation for successfully implementing preventive medicine into the medical education curriculum requires an expanded scientific paradigm for medicine, "a view of health and disease that specifically includes a role for psychologic and social forces—precisely those domains ignored by molecular reductionism" (4). These issues are similar to those discussed in more detail in Chapter 1.

The second process contained within the professional antecedent condition is the "professional socialization process" (Fig. 2) involving professional organizations and peer groups influencing physician behavior. Active participation of physicians in their specialty organizations is likely to have an influence on their skills and practice behaviors. Organizations such as the American Heart Association, American College of Cardiology, American College of Physicians, American Academy of Family Practice, and others regularly offer national and local symposia and distribute written guidelines that address preventive cardiology issues. Although, as stated previously, lectures and written materials, by themselves, rarely lead to long-term changes in practice behaviors, they do often lead to variables of social influence that include peer pressure and professional role-modeling influences. Physicians may be more willing and motivated to adopt preventive practice behaviors if they see such behaviors in other physicians whom they respect. Participation in the activities of state and local medical societies and health departments also increases physicians' awareness of preventive medicine issues and facilitates physician involvement in these issues.

Finally, the patients themselves are important determinants of the physician's practice behaviors. Their health dynamics are mediated in part by the sociocultural environmental milieu, in part by genetic and familial predispositions, and in part by the physician's skills and behaviors (feedback loop in the model). The particular mix of medical problems in a physician's practice influences the physician's perception (Level III) of the preventive needs of the patient population. It helps, of course, if the physician is aware of important psychosocial and lifestyle issues affecting their patients' illnesses in addition to the purely biological parameters.

C. Sociopsychological Condition (Level III)

At this level physicians' beliefs and attitudes are formed that lead to a particular style of practice behaviors and skills. As illustrated in Figure 2, these cognitive variables are directly influenced by the various antecedent conditions previously discussed in Levels I and II as well as by the feedback from the skills and behaviors themselves (Level IV). Each of the processes at this level involves perceptions formed as a result of the complex network of variables from other processes in the model. Since the purpose of the model is to aid in developing strategies for implementing preventive practice behaviors, the discussion will focus on the pertinent cognitive issues arising at this level.

The physician's perception of self includes self-efficacy, self-image, professional values, and personality factors, all of which are influenced by personal and professional demographics. Some physicians, for example, tend to view themselves as more of a figure of authority and control than an active partner in the doctor–patient relationship (15). Many patients under these circumstances actually come to fear their physicians (17). This may result in less effective delivery of preventive services because patients are more likely to perceive their roles as passive recipients of medical care rather than active participants, and physicians are less likely to give patients the necessary attention needed to modify lifestyles and behaviors. Needleman (18) addresses this issue in discussing the essence of being a physician: ". . . it is the time, be it measured in minutes or hours, that a physician is face-to-face with the person who needs his or her help. In that transaction, the one essential thing that the doctor can give the patient is attention." To cultivate and develop this "power of attention, the power to listen, to be present, to allow all the sources of perception within us to move out toward another human being," however, is no easy task. The gradual introduction of humanities and human values curricula into medical education is an important start in changing the physician's traditional perception of self. Much more needs to be done, however.

Physician's attitudes and beliefs about prevention are also strongly influenced by professional norms in their specialty and by the need to conform to these standards of care. As discussed previously, a number of specialty organizations have begun developing preventive cardiology guidelines and recommendations that define new standards of care relevant to CHD prevention. Many of these are discussed elsewhere in this book. Pertinent to the physicians' model illustrated in Figure 2, however, is that the motivation to comply with new standards is often dependent upon the physician's perception of peer influences as well as the importance given these standards by the professional organizations. This suggests, moreover, that once a critical number of physicians who believe strongly in health promotion and preventive practice behaviors is reached, the profession as a whole is likely to shift toward these views.

Finally, the physicians' perception of their patients' preventive health care needs and other health-related issues of the environment in which they live also influence their attitudes and beliefs about prevention. As patients become more educated in disease prevention issues, they ask more questions of their physicians. This is likely to motivate physicians to become more informed about these issues and more willing to offer prevention advice and services based on today's accepted standards of care.

D. Behavioral Condition

The final level in the physician's model consists of the "intention formation process" and the practice behaviors and skills in the physician's behavioral repertoire. Many physicians trained in the traditional biomedical orientation have talents that pertain mostly to the biological aspects of health and disease. These include medical history taking, physical examination, laboratory test procedures and evaluation, pharmacotherapeutics, and invasive techniques. Physicians also have, to varying degrees, humanistic skills, thought by many to present the "art of medicine" and not generally considered to be part of "scientific" medicine. If preventive cardiology is to become an integral part of the primary care physician's services, new practice skills and behaviors will be required, many of which fall outside of the boundaries of biomedicine.

The preceding discussion identified a number of antecedent conditions and processes that influence the physician's beliefs and attitudes about prevention issues. Physicians' perception of these many variables is a crucial prerequisite to the formation of the intent to practice preventive medicine. This is only the first step, however, in the behavior change process. Physicians also need the requisite skills and knowledge to develop effective prevention services, as well as the appropriate financial incentives. It is unrealistic to expect that these skills and practice behaviors will develop overnight or that remuneration for these services will be readily available. The challenge to the medical community (our institutions of medical education, professional organizations, government organizations, and industry) is to encourage the behavioral change process by focusing on the pertinent issues just discussed. The willingness to embrace an expanded scientific medical model such as discussed in Chapter 1 will facilitate this important task for medicine.

IV. CONCLUSIONS

A recurrent theme, first introduced in Chapter 1 and reiterated in this concluding chapter, is that medicine needs a more contemporary and comprehensive scientific paradigm if it is to remain coherent with today's nonreductionist, systems-based understanding of reality. The body-as-a-machine metaphor is outdated and incompatible with our current understanding of living systems. The perpetuation of the biomedical model with its primary emphasis on biological mechanisms is unlikely to eliminate the chronic diseases so devastating to our society; it is likely to continue the upward spiraling of high-technology and costly medical care, largely directed toward end-stage chronic diseases. It is indeed ironic that our current knowledge of CHD prevention, much of which was presented in this book, is more than adequate to reduce significantly a considerable proportion of the morbidity and mortality of this major disease burden. And yet, the teaching of preventive medicine and preventive cardiology, in particular, is only of minor importance in our current system of medical education. The cumulative evidence for the role of psychological, social, and environmental variables in the origins, progression, treatment, and prevention of CHD is compelling. It is time for the medical profession to include the scientific study of these nonbiological variables in their clinical, research, and educational endeavors.

To illustrate an application of these ideas, this chapter reviewed the behavior change process for both patients and physicians, to provide the reader with an appreciation of the complex network of variables that affect this process. Two parallel systems-based models, one for the patient's health behaviors and the other for the physician's practice behaviors, were presented that identified and integrated biological, psychological, social, and environmental factors influencing behavior change (3). At this time the models are more theoretical than practical, facilitating an understanding of behavior change rather than providing quantitative prediction of such changes. Nevertheless, this approach is an important first step to developing comprehensive curricula for health professionals interested in disease prevention.

In the future it is hoped that further refinements in these models might reveal the exact mathematical relationships between the important variables and permit more quantitative predictions of behavior change. This would certainly enhance the scientific practice of preventive medicine. There is reason to have cautious optimism for medicine in the 21st century.

REFERENCES

1. Dismuke SE, Miller ST. Why not share the secrets of good health? JAMA 1983; 249: 3181–3.

2. Becker MH, Janz NK. Practicing health promotion: the doctor's dilemma. Ann Intern Med 1990; 113:419–22.

3. Kersell MW, Milsum JH. A systems model of health behavior change. Behav Sci 1985; 30:119–26.

4. Fried RA. Prevention in medical education: an uncertain future. J Gen Intern Med 1990; 5(suppl):S108–11.

5. Engel GL. The need for a new medical model: a challenge for biomedicine. Science 1977; 196:129–36.

6. Foss L, Rothenberg K. The second medical revolution—from biomedicine to infomedicine. Boston: New Science Library–Shambhala, 1987.

7. Sorensen TIA, Neilsen GG, Andersen PK, Teasdale TW. Genetic and environmental influences on premature death in adult adoptees. N Engl J Med 1988; 318:727–32.

8. Williams RR. Understanding genetic and environmental risk factors in susceptible persons. West J Med 1984; 141:799–806.

9. Seeman M, Seeman T, Sayles M. Social networks and health status: a longitudinal study. Soc Psychol Q 1985; 48:237–48.

10. Blumenthal JA, Burg MM, Barefoot J, Williams RB, Haney T, Zimet G. Social support, type A behavior, and coronary artery disease. Psychosom Med 1987; 49: 331–40.

11. Cohen S, Matthews KA. Social support, type A behavior, and coronary artery disease (Editorial). Psychosom Med 1987; 49:325–30.

12. Antonovsky A. Health, stress, and coping. San Francisco: Jossey-Bass, 1981.
13. Antonovsky A. Unraveling the mystery of health. San Francisco: Jossey-Bass, 1987.
14. Freymann JG. The public's health care paradigm is shifting: medicine must swing with it. J Gen Intern Med 1989; 4:313–9.
15. Brody DS. The patient's role in clinical decision making. Ann Intern Med 1980; 93: 718–22.
16. Project Panel on the General Professional Education of the Physician and College Preparation for Medicine. Physicians for the twenty-first century. J Med Ed 1984; 59 (Part 2):1–200.
17. Levine AM. Doctors, patients, and fear. West J Med 1989; 150:723.
18. Needleman J. The essence of being a physician. West J Med 1986; 145:185–6.

Index

About the Editor

FRANK G. YANOWITZ is Associate Professor of Medicine at the University of Utah School of Medicine, and Medical Director of the Fitness Institute at LDS Hospital, Salt Lake City. The author of numerous books, book chapters, and reviews, Dr. Yanowitz is a Fellow of the American Heart Association Council on Clinical Cardiology and the American College of Cardiology, and a member of the American College of Sports Medicine, the American Federation for Clinical Research, and the American College of Physicians. Dr. Yanowitz received the B.A. degree (1961) in mathematics from Cornell University, Ithaca, New York, and the M.D. degree (1966) from the State University of New York Upstate Medical School, Syracuse.